RICK HANSON, PH.D., is a psychologist who works with couples, individual adults, and children. He has written and lectured extensively on parental stress and depletion, ways to nurture mothers and fathers, and how a couple can be both strong teammates and intimate friends while raising a family. A summa cum laude graduate of UCLA, Dr. Hanson did management consulting before earning his Ph.D. in clinical psychology from the Wright Institute. He has been president of the Board of Family Works, a nonprofit agency serving families in northern California. His personal interests include meditation, rock climbing, and having fun with his kids.

JAN HANSON, M.S., L.AC., is an acupuncturist and nutritionist whose private practice focuses on women's health and on temperament problems in children. In addition to developing protocols for preventing and reversing maternal depletion, she has written articles and presented workshops on family health and on holistic approaches to childhood illnesses. Working in the Neurochemistry Research Laboratory at the Veteran's Hospital in Sepulveda, California, when she was eighteen years old she coauthored a study that was published. She went on to receive a B.A. from UCLA and an M.S. from the Academy of Chinese Culture and Health Sciences, in addition to taking many courses in clinical nutrition, homeopathy, and laboratory assessment. She and Rick have been married for over twenty years, and they have a teenage son and preteen daughter. Jan's personal interests include her children, first and foremost, as well as playing the piano, doing arts and crafts, and going for walks with good friends.

RICKI POLLYCOVE, M.D., M.H.S., received her B.A. in zoology and immunology with honors from the University of California at Berkeley. She continued at UC Berkeley for a master's in health sciences, followed by her M.D. and residency in obstetrics and gynecology at the University of California School of Medicine, San Francisco. She became board certified by the American College of Obstetrics and Gynecology in 1984 and is on the clinical faculty at the University of California, San Francisco. Dr. Pollycove is the founding director for Education and Program Development at the California Pacific Medical Center Breast Health Center, and a past chief of the Division of Gynecology there. She is a fellow of the American College of Obstetrics and Gynecology, a member of the North American Menopause Society, American Society of Reproductive Medicine, the American Society of Breast Diseases, and past editor in chief of the *San Francisco Medical Society Magazine*. She appears regularly as a medical expert on television and radio, and is the women's health expert for MedicinePlanet.com. A mother for over eighteen years, she enjoys cooking, baking, and gardening with her daughter, Leah, with whom she also sings and plays viola.

Mother Nurture

A Mother's Guide to Health
in Body, Mind, and
Intimate Relationships

RICK HANSON, PH.D., JAN HANSON, L.AC.,
AND RICKI POLLYCOVE, M.D.

Penguin Books

PENGUIN BOOKS

Published by the Penguin Group, Penguin Putnam Inc., 375 Hudson Street, New York, New York 10014,
U.S.A.
Penguin Books Ltd, 80 Strand, London WC2R 0RL, England
Penguin Books Australia Ltd, 250 Camberwell Road, Camberwell, Victoria 3124, Australia
Penguin Books Canada Ltd, 10 Alcorn Avenue, Toronto, Ontario, Canada M4V 3B2
Penguin Books India (P) Ltd, 11 Community Centre, Panchsheel Park,
New Delhi – 110 017, India
Penguin Books (N.Z.) Ltd, Cnr Rosedale and Airborne Roads, Albany, Auckland, New Zealand
Penguin Books (South Africa) (Pty) Ltd, 24 Sturdee Avenue,
Rosebank, Johannesburg 2196, South Africa

Penguin Books Ltd, Registered Offices:
Harmondsworth, Middlesex, England

First published in Penguin Books 2002

1   3   5   7   9   10   8   6   4   2

LIBRARY OF CONGRESS CATALOGING-IN-PUBLICATION DATA
Hanson, Rick, Ph. D.
Mother nurture : a mom's guide to a healthy mind, body, and intimate relationship /
Rick Hanson, Jan Hanson, and Ricki Pollycove.
p. cm.
Includes bibliographical references and index.
ISBN 0-14-200062-0
1. Mothers—Life skills guides.   2. Mothers—Health and hygiene.   3. Self-help techniques.
4. Self-care, Health.   5. Marriage.   I. Hanson, Jan.   II. Pollycove, Ricki.   III. Title.
HQ759 .H246 2002
646.7'00852—dc21   2001058754

Every effort has been made to ensure that the information contained in this book is complete and accurate.
However, neither the publisher nor the authors are engaged in rendering professional advice or services to the
individual reader. The ideas, procedures, and suggestions contained in this book are not intended as a substitute for consulting with your physician. All matters regarding your health require medical supervision. Neither
the author nor the publisher shall be liable or responsible for any loss, injury or damage allegedly arising from
any information or suggestion in this book.

Printed in the United States of America
Set in AGaramond
Designed by M. Paul

To our parents—

    Helen and William Hanson

    Dorothy and Ray Emge

    Rosalyn and Myron Pollycove

And to our children—

    Laurel and Forrest Hanson, and Leah Harmuth

Acknowledgments

MUCH AS IT TAKES A VILLAGE to raise a child, it takes another sort of village to write a book.

First and foremost, we must express our gratitude to the many mothers who have been our patients over the years, whose insights, stories, and voices echo throughout this book. We've also learned much from the questions and examples offered by the mothers and fathers who have attended our talks. And we very much appreciate the mothers—Jennifer Abbe, Anne Marie Buckland, Lisa Demarias, Deborah Johansen, Carole Kammen, Janet Lipsey, and Pennie Sempell, J.D.—who participated in the discussions we held on the topic of community.

Numerous people took the time and trouble to read drafts of the manuscript and offer suggestions, including Scott Anderson, M.D., Debra Bell, M.D., Shoshana Bennett, Ph.D., Karla Clark, Ph.D., Caren Cole, D.C., Jenifer Cortwright, M.F.T., Vicki Darrow, M.D., Sarah Ferguson, M.D., Nancy Frease, M.F.T., Linda Gaudiani, M.D., Elson Haas, M.D., Pam Handelman, R.N., Ann Hathaway, M.D., Ifeoma Ikenze, M.D., Kristin Jokel, Evelyn Kade, L.Ac., Risa Kaparo, Ph.D., Rick Martinez, M.D., Jim McQuade, M.D., Jennifer Bean Parks, Cindy Shearer, D.A., Cherie Trombly, M.S., Bob Truog, M.D., and Shellie Wilkinson. In particular, Deb Moskowitz, N.D., of Transitions for Health, painstakingly reviewed the chapters on nurturing your body and made important suggestions.

Many other colleagues gave encouragement and constructive criticism, notably Adrienne Amundsen, Ph.D., Chris Berman, M.P.H., Michelle Borgault, M.D., Nancy Boughey, L.C.S.W., Wanda Bronson, Ph.D., Carolyn Pape Cowan, Ph.D., Philip Cowan, Ph.D., Mary Croughan-Minehane, Ph.D., Charles Dohlbaum, M.D., Ph.D., June Engle, M.D., Leah Fisher, L.C.S.W., Tina Gabby, M.D., Rachelle Halpern, M.D., Leslie Horn, Ph.D., John Kells, Ph.D., Eric Kelly, M.F.T., Phyllis Klaus, M.F.T., Jonathan Kopp, Ph.D., Judy Lane, N. Prac., Stephen A. Levine, Ph. D., Alicia Lieberman, Ph.D., Judy Loring, C.N.C., Melody Lowman, Ph.D., Kerista Luminiere-Rosen, Ph.D., Dennis Malone, Kristen Skenfield Marchi, M.P.H., Sally McGuire, Ph.D., Rick Mendius, M.D., Dayton Misfeldt, M.D., Jon Pangborn, Ph.D., Joan Patterson, Ph.D., Mary Piel, M.D., Jane Rowe, M.D., Stephen Seligman, D.M.H., Richard Shames, M.D., Mary Jane deWolf-Smith, R.N., M.F.T., Lane Tanner, M.D., and Barbara Williamson, Certified Nurse-Midwife. Although there are too many to name, we'd like to thank all of the doctors and staff at California Pacific Medical Center who generously shared their expertise and resources while we were preparing this book.

Of course, our friends and family have been a vital source of practical help and moral support. They include Nan Bakamjian, Melba Beals, Judy Bell, David Boulton, Tom Bowlin, Lynne and Jim Bramlett, Rosalie and Jim Clark, Roberta and Jim Cummesky, Daniel Ellenberg, Keith Hanson, Raven Jones, Dan and Joy Millman, Leslie Patten, Terry Patten, Michelle Rivers, and Mike and B. J. van Horn.

More broadly, we are indebted to the work of thousands of researchers and clinicians in the fields of clinical and developmental psychology, nutrition, obstetrics and gynecology, Chinese medicine, and alternative and complementary medicine. Further, as parents and professionals, we have benefited from the feminist scholars and advocates who have greatly improved the health and well-being of women and mothers.

Finally, we appreciate Alan Rinzler and Amanita Rosenbush, who offered editorial assistance for earlier versions of related books. For this book, our research assistants, Pamela Geisler and Ariel King, diligently tracked down references for complex subjects. Leslie Crawford skillfully edited several chapters and the proposal, as well as offered helpful insights from her own experiences with a young child. Amy Romanoff and Eric Kelly gave us excellent editorial and design help. While being a new mom herself, Caroline Pincus provided crucial editing and guidance, and it is impossible to imagine this book coming to fruition without her. Our agent, Amy Rennert, is the perfect balance of kindness and practical wisdom, and her editorial smarts and talents as a writer helped us make both a better proposal and a better book. At Penguin, Jennifer Ehmann and Jane von Mehren have been top-notch editors, ably assisted by Jessica Kipp, as well as warm and humane voices on the other end of the phone who clearly felt a personal commitment to the welfare of mothers and families.

Contents

Introduction

by Jan Hanson, L.Ac.

MOTHERHOOD IS A VERY PERSONAL EXPERIENCE, yet you've probably had many people who don't know you tell you how to do some part of it, from strangers on the street to professionals in print—like us. So I felt you ought to know where we're coming from, and why we wrote this book.

Being a mother has been the most wonderful, extraordinary experience of my life, and I wouldn't trade it for anything! But by the time our son was three and his baby sister was a few months old, I had been working hard and living with stress for so long with so little replenishment that it all caught up with me. I kept going every day, but I had become very drained, both physically and emotionally.

I saw variations on the same theme with my friends who were mothers. Some, like me, had hit bottom. Others felt their health and well-being were deteriorating, though some reserves remained inside. Many were still sailing along, yet even they were frazzled and tired.

But every mom I knew was surprised by the impact of becoming a parent and wished she knew more about coping with it. Many of us felt let down by our partners, who weren't helping enough at home or couldn't seem to understand what we were going through. And a number of women, including myself, had developed nagging problems that began soon after we had children—like intensified hormonal ups and downs, depressed mood, or a general sense of disturbance in the digestive tract—and these seemed impossible to get rid of while we were so busy and stressed. We told each other this was not how motherhood was supposed to be, but we didn't know what to do about it.

Neither, it seemed, did anyone else. During our pregnancies and for a few months postpartum, we received excellent care, but by our babies' first birthdays, we dropped off the radar of the health care system—as if raising a family had no real effect on a woman's well-being.

Of course, that was far from the truth. Over time, Rick and I began to realize that every mother needed to lower her stresses, replenish her body, and create a

1

strong relationship with her partner—or else she was likely to become physically *depleted,* which was exactly what had happened to me.

In retrospect, it seemed obvious: moms give so much nurturance to others that they have to receive it as well. In order to find out what mothers needed, Rick and I studied the pertinent research, talked to leading clinicians, and asked moms what had worked for them. I drew on my background in nutrition, Chinese medicine, and holistic health to develop with Rick a model of maternal depletion and recovery. We applied what we learned to the women in our practices and saw how they benefited.

Along the way, we looked for a book that could guide us, but there wasn't much available past the first year postpartum—and the deepest extent of depletion seemed to hit most mothers two or more years after their baby was born. So we resolved to create a book ourselves. Rick wrote most of it, drawing on his experience as a clinical psychologist, husband, and father; I am very glad to have a mate who's really tried to understand what women go through when we bear and rear our children. We've also had the good fortune to work with Dr. Ricki Pollycove, an obstetrician/gynecologist—and someone who was herself worn down by the demands of motherhood—whose sound medical judgment and warmhearted understanding of families are woven throughout these pages.

More than anything, we wrote the book Ricki and I wish we'd had when we became mothers! Our focus is on those years before your children are all in grade school, because that's usually when the demands on you are the greatest; and since there are already many excellent books on the postpartum months, we emphasize what you can do while you're raising a toddler or preschooler. We address your mind, body, and relationships because each of these aspects of your life is affected by motherhood. We offer a spectrum of approaches to improve your health and well-being, from mild to intensive, and conventional to alternative, since individual mothers need and want different things.

Chapter 1 gives an overview of how bearing and rearing children wear on women, and it tells how three mothers successfully used the basic Mother Nurture prescription: lower the demands on you, increase your resources, and build up your resilience. Chapters 2 and 3 present ways to cope with stress and manage the thornier emotions that often intensify with parenthood, including sadness, anxiety, shame, and anger. Chapters 4 and 5 explain how to keep your body well in the first place, and what to do if it's getting depleted. Chapters 6 through 8 focus on building teamwork and intimacy with your partner. Chapter 9 tackles the practical issue that's a big stressor for many women today, how to juggle motherhood and work. Several appendices cover topics such as how to get the most out of working with your health care providers. And if you are interested in the scientific studies we've relied on, the reference notes are posted on our Web site, www. nurturemom.com (where you will also find new information about taking care of yourself and your family, opportunities to communicate with other mothers, and sources for vitamins and other nutrients). In general, feel free to jump ahead to topics that are pressing and come back later to earlier sections of the book.

Throughout, you'll find many suggestions for boosting your health and well-being. Some are specific to mothers, while others are general methods that we've adapted to women raising children. We don't expect you to try them all, just the ones that suit you—and feel free to adapt those to your own situation. Please know that our general statements will not apply to everyone, and that this book is no substitute for professional care. *If you have an acute condition of any kind, we urge you to consult immediately with the appropriate licensed professional.*

Before we dive in, though, I'd like to create a context, since motherhood can be an emotionally charged, even controversial subject these days:

- Nurturing a mom doesn't mean doing less for her kids. When mothers improve their health and well-being, they are more able to be highly loving and skillful parents. We've tried to answer the question that gripped us soon after our children were born: *What does a mother need in order to keep giving her children the very best they deserve, year after year after year?*

- We believe that it clearly supports a mother to build teamwork and intimacy, if possible, with the father of her children. If her partner is someone other than the father, teamwork and intimate friendship in that relationship will still benefit the mother, her partner, and her children. If a mother has no partner, she could still use chapters 6 and 7 for her relationship with her children's father. (Some mothers are raising their children with another woman, but for simplicity, the masculine pronoun is used to refer to a mother's partner. We also use the terms *marriage* and *partnership,* and *husband, spouse, mate,* and *partner,* interchangeably.)

- Many of the factors that wear on mothers originate in our culture, our legal and health care systems, our economy, or in sexism or racism. Changes in these would benefit mothers greatly (please see the Afterword, p. 333), but that's a larger subject than our focus in this book.

- Mother Nurture is not just an issue for biological parents. Women who adopt children are as affected by overwork, stress, and poor replenishment as any other mother.

- Research on how motherhood affects a woman's health and well-being has been very limited. Plus, there are large individual differences among mothers, fathers, children, and families. So when we use words like *mothers* or *fathers,* we mean the mid range of a group seen with less than perfect clarity. This is not academic hairsplitting, but concern for the unique truth of each particular person.

- Many mothers are young, poor, or belong to an ethnic minority. We are middle aged, middle class, and Caucasian. Most of the mothers we know come from similar backgrounds, and our suggestions may not apply to those who do not. We hope that others will be able to build on our beginning to help all women raising children.

So much of what we have learned has come from other mothers and fathers. Parents are all in this together. Our warmest hope is that you can create a wonderful home for yourself and your family. We wish you the best!

PART ONE
Understanding the Challenges of Motherhood

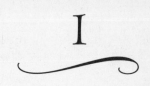

Refilling Your Cupboard

A baby is an inestimable blessing and a bother.

—MARK TWAIN

NOTHING CHANGES YOUR LIFE LIKE A CHILD, and there's really no way to prepare for it. Suddenly you're working all the time, hitting the red line on stress, and you look around and wonder, where's the support? In our practices, we see mothers every day who feel frayed around the edges, let down by their partners, and worn out—or worse. Some have developed serious physical or marital problems since becoming mothers. Many women feel that it's their fault or that they must be the only one who can't handle the strain. They figure that feeling thoroughly overwhelmed just comes with the territory.

Well, we're here to tell you that you're not to blame and you're not alone. What's more, there are plenty of practical things you can do that will help you feel better and bring more teamwork and closeness into your relationship with your partner.

In this chapter, you'll read about three women who came to us for treatment and exactly what they did to improve their health and well-being. Just as we hope to do for you over the course of this book, we helped each one of these mothers to

1. Lower the demands on her
2. Increase her resources
3. Build up her resilience

That's *mother nurture.*

And you are entitled to it. With what you give to your children and others each day, you more than earn the right to take good care of yourself. This time with your little one (or two or more) is very special, never to be repeated, and you should be able to enjoy it fully.

Further, taking care of yourself is not selfish at all. It's what you need to do in order to be at your best with your kids and still have some energy left over for your relationship with your partner. Just like in an airplane, you have to put on your own oxygen mask before you can help anyone else.

Again and again, we see a minor miracle when a woman makes some simple changes in such things as what she eats, the way she thinks about stress, or how she talks with her partner. It's not complicated or esoteric. In the chapters that follow, we'll show you easy ways that work together and add up over time to nurture your body, mind, and marriage.

How Your Cupboard Can Become Bare

The first step is to understand exactly how raising a family has affected you personally. That will give a foundation for using the tools provided in the rest of the book.

Growing Demands upon You

As demanding as parenthood has been for your mate, it has likely had even more impact on you. For starters, if you gave birth, you had the extraordinary task of building the most complex organ the body ever grows, using up to 80,000 extra calories to make your baby. If any nutrients were missing in the foods you ate, they were extracted from you and given to your child. When your baby was born, your placenta—which was a huge hormone factory during pregnancy—was dropped into the doctor's bucket, and within days after childbirth, your estrogen and progesterone dropped to a tiny fraction of their previous levels, gyrating the hormones that regulate everything from your mood when you wake up to how well you sleep at night.

If you breast-feed (about half of all mothers do—and we generally recommend it for its benefits to both you and your child), each day you use about 750 to 1000 extra calories: like running seven to ten miles day after day. Breast milk is rich in nutrients such as essential fatty acids, which are essential for your baby, but you need these, too, for a healthy body and positive mood. If you are not getting enough of these nutrients in your regular diet—and few moms with infants seem to have the time—your bodily reserves are drained every time you nurse.

Plus, as one mother put it, *Real labor begins after birth*. Each day, for twenty-plus years, you do several hundred specific child-rearing or housework tasks, from reading *Winnie the Pooh* to doing the dishes, and you probably go to bed wishing that somehow you could have done more. The more committed you are to being sensitive and responsive to your child, the more work there is. One mother told Rick: ***The biggest change was my sense that I had to always be present for and attentive to someone else, that I could never let down. I feel I am on call all the time.***

Besides being time-consuming, the work of mothers is uniquely stressful; the comedian Martin Mull once joked, ***Having a family is like having a bowling alley installed in your brain.*** Your body has been on a roller coaster, from the first changes of pregnancy to the impact of childbirth and its new shape after you've become a mother. Breast-feeding rarely proceeds without one troublesome hitch or another, especially in the beginning. You're constantly interrupted and pulled in a dozen different directions, you feel responsible for everything, things keep changing, worries gnaw at your mind, and something upsetting happens several times each day. Any wobble with your children wears on you further. You are probably the one, not your partner, who stumbles down the hall at night to tend to a baby with an ear infection, deals with child care hassles, settles most squabbles between siblings, or worries about how to handle a preschooler's tantrums. As a result, mothers consistently report more stress than fathers, or women not raising children—especially if a child has any special needs, like colic, an illness, a disability, or a challenging temperament. And, of course, the more kids, the more work and stress.

Adding to the demands upon you, there's a good chance that you've got to juggle home and work. Over half of all mothers today will return to work before their baby's first birthday—yet doing so while raising an infant increases their risk for health problems, especially if they're already stretched, such as by being a single parent.

A Thin Soup of Resources

If the demands on a person grow, her resources should grow as well. We're sure that one sort of resource has increased since you had children: the emotional fulfillment of being a mother. But otherwise, have your resources grown since your baby was born? Probably not. We're not talking about money here, but things like a good night's sleep and healthful foods and strong support from your partner. For instance, the typical mother of a young child gets about six and one-half hours of sleep a day rather than the eight or more hours most adults need—losing over five hundred hours of sleep *per year*—plus she rarely gets a chance to sleep as deeply as she needs to. This diminishes the neurotransmitters her brain needs to regulate her mood and other physiological functions.

You're probably not eating all that well, either; according to studies, less than half of the mothers of young children get three solid meals each day. It's hard to find time to exercise with little ones around. And whether you're going off to the workplace or staying home, when you've got a young family, pleasures fall away, old friends drop out of your life, and you never seem to have any real time for yourself. Even if you're ill, you usually get little chance to rest. One mother told Jan this story: *I was reading a nursery rhyme to Julie, the one about Mother Hubbard, and I had to sigh because that's how I was starting to feel: my "cupboard" was constantly being emptied and not enough was getting put back on the shelves.*

Has your partner jumped in to fill this vacuum? Maybe. Some dads are great: committed to parenthood and skillful with the kids, they do their fair share around the house and are sympathetic and supportive. But let's face it: many are not. Numerous studies have shown that the average mom works about twenty hours more per week, altogether, than does her partner, regardless of whether she's drawing a paycheck—and a mother's stress jumps and her mood drops when teamwork with her partner breaks down. You probably also handle more of the high-stress tasks, like dressing a resistant two-year-old, and carry more of the "executive responsibility" for the family by being the one who worries, plans, and problem solves. And if you're raising your children essentially alone, as does one in five mothers, you're getting little to no help from a partner at all.

Even if your partner is a strong teammate, much research has shown that the arrival of children commonly leads to a dramatic decrease in positive interactions and marital satisfaction—especially for mothers. There is so little time or energy for conversation, fun, or affection that there's a good chance your relationship no longer recharges your batteries or offers a safe haven. As one mother commented to Rick: *My husband and I work together well in terms of taking care of the kids and the house. But I don't know where he and I are when we're without them. I feel lonely inside my own marriage.* It's no wonder that couples with children report less satisfaction with their relationship than couples without kids.

Children are meant to be raised within a strong community, but compared to the times in which most of us grew up, relatives live farther away, neighbors are less neighborly, there are fewer kids nearby, and the average adult is affiliated with just one community group as compared to five in our parents' day. Compounding the problem, fathers have not entered the world of family to the extent that mothers have gone into the world of work, leaving a kind of vacuum, so there is less of the glue that once held neighborhoods together. As a result of all these factors, you're likely to have much less of the social support that could have provided practical help, lowered your stress, and buttressed your health.

In short, things have *really* changed, both in your own life once you became a parent and in the culture since you were a child yourself, and chances are you simply aren't getting the full support you need.

Vulnerable Spots in Your Armor of Resilience

In a perfect world, you could cope with all the demands upon you or with scarce resources by being Supermom. Yet that's not real. Each of us has some vulnerabilities that lower our resilience, the way a wound on a finger creates an opening for bacteria. Like a small cut that makes little difference until you do the dishes, a vulnerability may not matter much before children arrive. But then it begins to exacerbate the effects of the demands upon you; for instance, an immune system weakened by chronic stress is less able to defend you against the germs brought home from preschool. And any vulnerabilities lower your ability to handle shortages in the resources you receive; for instance, if you are even a little anemic when you enter motherhood—as ninety percent of women are—your nutritional reserves will be even further eroded by the typical low-iron diet of a mother.

Please see if any of these vulnerabilities, common among mothers, apply to you:

- *Having children at an older age.* In the last two decades, the birthrate of women over thirty has increased by about one-third, and the rate of first births for women over thirty-five has nearly doubled. Older mothers are less able to weather a pregnancy, are more prone to fatigue and illness once children arrive, and have less time to restore a hormonal equilibrium before menopause.

- *Nutritional deficiencies.* About nine mothers in ten have not consumed the U.S. government recommended amounts of minerals and vitamins before conceiving their first child. Nutritional deficiencies are cumulative, and since about 40 percent of all pregnancies are unplanned, there's often little time to remedy them before the demands of bearing and raising a child gather a full head of steam. And even if you start taking supplements, it often takes months or years to restore healthy levels of nutrients in your body.

- *Genetic predisposition.* Your relatives may have had illnesses of the endocrine system, obstetric complications, or other conditions that raise your risk for similar problems.

- *Prior health problems.* Women are more likely than men to enter parenthood with preexisting gastrointestinal, hormonal, or autoimmune conditions.

- *Postpartum depression (PPD).* At least one mother in ten will have an episode of PPD, which can increase her risk for hormonal or mood-related problems a year or two later. If you did suffer from postpartum depression after your first baby, your chance triples of having PPD again with another child.

- *General history of depressed mood.* Some women have a tendency toward depression, and this can be intensified by the hormonal fluctuations of motherhood.

- *Temperament.* Raising kids is likely to be more stressful if a mother has a high need for control or orderliness, or if she tends to be anxious or irritable.

Some unique blend of vulnerabilities affects every mother. In the chapters that follow, we'll be covering how to build up your own resilience so you are better prepared to cope with all the increased demands upon you.

Swimming Upstream

Let's step back for a minute and look at how we got here. During more than 99 percent of the time that humans (or our close ancestors) have lived on this planet, mothers raised families in small groups of hunter-gatherers. If you had been among them, your life would have moved at the speed of a walk while you provided for your needs and fulfilled your ambitions with a child on your hip or nearby. You would have eaten fresh and organic foods saturated in micronutrients and breathed air and drunk water free of artificial chemicals. Most important of all, you would have spent much of your day with other mothers, surrounded by a supportive community of relatives, friends, and neighbors. These are the conditions to which your body and mind are adapted for raising children.

Unfortunately, while the essential activities of mothering—pregnancy, childbirth, breast-feeding, worrying and planning and loving with all your heart—have not altered one bit, our world has changed profoundly, and evolution hasn't had time to catch up. We are genetically identical to the first modern humans of 200,000 years ago, and nearly identical to our earliest tool-using ancestors, who lived over two million years ago. Nonetheless, at odds with this basic genetic blueprint, most mothers today must rush about stressfully, constantly juggling and multitasking. Few modern jobs can be done with young children around, so working means spending much of the day separated from your kids—and the stresses of the unnatural schedule and pace they must then handle affect them in ways that naturally spill over onto you. Compared to our ancestors, most of us eat much fewer vegetables and whole foods, and much more white flour, sugar, and artificial chemicals, and we can't help absorbing some of the billions of pounds of toxins released into the environment each year, which even leave traces in breast milk. The so-called village it takes to raise a child usually looks more like a ghost town, so you have to rely more on your mate than did mothers in times past—but he, too, is strained by the unprecedented busyness and intensity of modern life.

If you feel like you're swimming upstream, it's because raising children was not meant to be this way. Many of the problems that seem purely personal or marital actually start on the other side of your front door.

Of course, the world is not going to change back to the time of the hunter-gatherers (and we'd miss refrigerators and telephones too much if it did!). And those times certainly had their own difficulties, such as famine and disease. But, like every mother, you can't help but feel the impact of the whirlwind we're all living in. Just how you're affected is as individual as a baby's footprint. Some mothers are fortunate to have low demands, substantial resources, and low vulnerabilities (see Figure 1). All too often, however, the demands are high, resources are low, and resilience gets worn down: a mother's "cupboard" gets emptied out and shaken and it's an uphill struggle to get anything back in. No wonder that, over time, some signs of wear begin to show (see Figure 2).

Let's take a look now at how having kids affected the body, mind, or marriage of three different mothers—plus what they did to make things better.

Compared to 1969, American parents on average have twenty-two fewer hours per week to spend with their families.

—President's Council of Economic Advisors, 1999

The Effects on a Mother's Body

A year after Judy's* second child was born, she returned to Ricki's office for a routine follow-up visit. Judy was forty-three, dark-haired, slender and edgy, with a no-nonsense gaze, and she worked full-time as a bookkeeper for a large trucking company. Her husband had moved out midway through her pregnancy, saying that he did not want another child, but she had decided to keep the baby. Ricki wondered if her ex-husband was giving her any help. Judy frowned: *Him? He takes Amanda to the park. When he feels like it.* But she smiled proudly when she added that Amanda and Matt were doing fine, and the tough mask that got her through each day dropped away for a moment, revealing a tender warmheartedness.

Ricki asked what she was eating these days, and Judy snorted. *Who has time to cook? I've got friends without kids, and they tell me they're* so *busy. I just laugh because they have no idea what "busy" really is. I usually grab a bagel for breakfast,*

---

*Identifying details have been altered in the examples given, which are sometimes composites of several mothers.

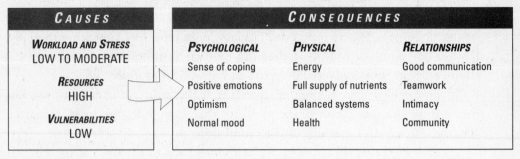

figure 1. Motherhood As It Should Be

CAUSES	CONSEQUENCES		
	PSYCHOLOGICAL	**PHYSICAL**	**RELATIONSHIPS**
WORKLOAD AND STRESS LOW TO MODERATE	Sense of coping	Energy	Good communication
RESOURCES HIGH	Positive emotions	Full supply of nutrients	Teamwork
	Optimism	Balanced systems	Intimacy
VULNERABILITIES LOW	Normal mood	Health	Community

figure 2. Motherhood As It Often Is

CAUSES	CONSEQUENCES		
	PSYCHOLOGICAL	**PHYSICAL**	**RELATIONSHIPS**
WORKLOAD AND STRESS HIGH	Feeling overwhelmed	Fatigue	Poor communication
RESOURCES LOW	Negative emotions	Drained nutrients	Tension, conflict
	Pessimism	Disturbed systems	Coldness, divorce
VULNERABILITIES HIGH	Depressed mood	Illness	Isolation

try to have a salad for lunch, and pick up some pizza or Chinese takeout for dinner. She smiled. *Besides, it keeps the pounds off.*

When Ricki began going through a checklist of physical symptoms, Judy waved her hand: *Don't bother, I'm just on edge. I wake up in the middle of the night and can't get back to sleep. Little things piss me off like never before, and I'm forgetting things I should know.* She paused and straightened her shoulders. *I'm only tired. I feel like I'm running on fumes.*

But Ricki was concerned that there was more to Judy's case than simple fatigue. In addition to the high workload and stresses of being a single mom raising two young children, Judy had several vulnerabilities: her second child was born when she was forty-two, she had had gestational diabetes, and she had a family history of thyroid problems.

Therefore, Ricki ran several tests, and they revealed that Judy's blood sugars were elevated, while her thyroid levels were at the bottom of the normal range. Judy also reported some of the symptoms of insufficient thyroid, including cold hands and feet, fatigue, and hair loss. Meanwhile, Ricki had referred Judy to Jan for a nutritional evaluation. Just from hearing about her food habits, Jan could tell that Judy was not getting enough protein. Additionally, laboratory testing revealed that Judy had insufficient vitamin B_6, which is critical for hormone balance and the production of serotonin, a neurotransmitter that helps regulate mood and digestion. Also, Judy was low on magnesium, which is essential for sleep, and taurine, an amino acid that helps a person feel both energized and relaxed.

Working together, Jan and Ricki helped Judy to:

- Lower her blood sugar levels through a low-sugar, low-carbohydrate diet.

- Restore balance to her hormones by taking a low dose of a natural thyroid medication.

- Increase her intake of protein, vitamins, minerals, and amino acids by eating in a healthier way. Jan gave Judy some tips on how to prepare quick yet nutritious meals (see chapter 4). In particular, Judy made sure to eat a lot of green leafy vegetables, which are full of B vitamins. She also started eating more seeds and beans for magnesium, and more meats for protein and taurine.

- Improve her nutrition further by taking a general-purpose vitamin/mineral supplement—as well as specific supplements for vitamin B_6, magnesium, and taurine—since it is difficult to remedy nutritional deficiencies rapidly through diet alone.

It made Judy feel immediately better to realize that her low energy, poor memory, and irritability had been due in large part to physical causes, so they no longer seemed like a personal failing. And within a few weeks, her interventions dramatically improved her sleep and energy level, and helped her feel less tense and prickly at work and with her kids. In her final appointment, Judy smiled when she told Jan, *Now when I push my gas pedal, there's something in the tank.*

Recognizing Depletion

As with many mothers who seem to have purely psychological concerns—such as irritability, poor memory, or a blue mood—there was, in fact, something awry with Judy's *body*. If there's one lesson that we've learned from working with several thousand mothers, it's the degree to which motherhood affects women physically. For example, the body of a woman generally reacts more intensely to stress than a man's does, and, like most mothers, you are probably living with more ongoing stress than anyone's body is meant to handle. It's important to realize that chronic stress is more than an unpleasant experience. It relentlessly disturbs:

- Your *gastrointestinal* system, by causing your mouth to produce less saliva, your stomach to secrete fewer digestive acids, and your small intestine to slow its contractions, which impairs nutrient absorption and can lead to irritable bowel syndrome and other digestive dysfunctions.

- Your *nervous* system, by releasing certain neurotransmitters and hormones while suppressing others, resulting in depressed mood and poorer concentration and memory.

- Your *endocrine* system, by increasing such hormones (or related substances) as adrenaline and cortisol, and by lowering estrogen, progesterone, DHEA, and the effectiveness of insulin—raising the risk for adult-onset diabetes, a poor response to stress, and other hormonal conditions.

- Your *immune* system, by both weakening it and making it overreactive, leading to an increase in viral infections and autoimmune diseases.

It all adds up over time. You're pouring out more and handling more stresses, but taking less in. It's no wonder if you feel used up, emptied out—in a word, *depleted.* Besides being a psychological experience, your body could be becoming depleted as well, which means that its vital nutrients are becoming drained and its key systems are getting dysregulated. (Researchers have found signs of depletion in mothers from both middle-class American populations and in Third World countries. Nonetheless, since the research on women's health has lagged far behind that of men, the long-term health effects of motherhood have not been well studied. Our analysis of depletion is a working hypothesis based on existing data, clinical experience, and logical inference.) Depletion is bad enough in its own right, but its effects today can also become causes of depletion tomorrow. For instance, as your mood sinks, it becomes harder to take steps to replenish yourself, like getting out of the house for some exercise. That's why it's important to take steps early on to prevent depletion in the first place: *The absolute foundation of Mother Nurture is nurturing your body.*

The demands on you may be greatest during your baby's first year, but it usually takes a couple of years for the deepest reserves within your body to run dry. Therefore, we usually see the worst slump of depletion two or three years after the first child is born, or sometimes a year or so after a second child comes along. In general, things tend to get better by the time children are in grade school. Nonetheless, some mothers—typically those who are most stressed and least supported—continue to be depleted.

Of course, depletion is not the only health problem a mother might face: you could have a medical condition unrelated to raising children, or one linked to motherhood—such as an injury suffered during childbirth—but not due to depletion. Nonetheless, any health issues become stresses that foster depletion, and depletion can worsen other bodily problems.

It should come as no surprise, then, that raising a family is associated with generally poorer health in a woman, especially as the number of her pregnancies increases. More specifically, studies have found that motherhood raises a woman's risk for:

- Fatigue
- Nutritional deficits
- Diabetes
- Gallbladder disease
- Cardiovascular disease
- Hormonal problems
- Kidney disease
- Some kinds of cancer
- A higher overall mortality rate

The good news is that these are risks, not realities. You can lower them tremendously by preventing depletion in the first place—or by replenishing yourself if you've become depleted—by using the strategies in the chapters that follow.

Depleted Mother Syndrome

Many mothers feel unnecessarily guilty about being worn out or blue, and many fathers do not really understand the full impact of motherhood on their partners. Some people might think that a mother "just has to snap out of it."

Well, if her body is seriously depleted, she can't just snap out of it! There is something physically wrong. We think she has a clinical condition that we term the Depleted Mother Syndrome (DMS). Like other syndromes such as chronic fatigue or premenstrual syndrome, DMS can:

- Appear in a variety of forms
- Be caused by different combinations of factors, depending on the person
- Take a course over time that varies from mother to mother
- Have symptoms that are ailments in their own right, such as depression
- Respond to more than one kind of treatment

How do you know if you have DMS? The gold standard, described in appendix A, is medical lab testing of your nutrient levels, plus consideration by a doctor of any signs of disturbed systems. Meanwhile, you can use the checklists at the end of this chapter to get a sense of your risk of being depleted; the greater your risk, the more vital it is to try to lower the demands upon you and increase your resources.

If you are indeed depleted, you are far from alone. Based on our clinical experience, we estimate that at least one mother in ten will go through a period of measurable depletion. If you belong to a group of women with higher risks—such as childbirth past age thirty, prior health problems, single parenthood, or poverty—your chance of developing DMS would be higher.

Motherhood is not a medical issue, but depletion is. Every year, it impacts millions of American women and their family members, and it probably leads to billions of dollars in health care expenses and lost productivity. Since the physical, psychological, and interpersonal problems of mothers often originate in one place—depletion—understanding them as a syndrome enables diagnosis, prevention, and care to be directed at their root cause.

The Effects on a Mother's Mind

Ann was twenty-seven, dark-haired, with a sturdy, large-boned figure. She came to see Rick for ideas about her strong-willed, highly active eighteen-month-old daughter. Ann had taken time off from her job managing a travel agency to stay home with Katie. Her husband, Peter, worked long days and traveled frequently as a supervisor in a commercial construction company. At night, Katie still woke up several times and would cry for hours until someone picked her up. Peter said he needed to leave early in the morning to get to work, so Ann had to get up, over and over.

Ann was embarrassed by Katie's intensity and frequent tantrums, and thought it had to be her fault that her daughter was acting that way, so she avoided getting together with other moms. Child care was expensive, plus Ann felt "lazy" using it. As a result, she spent most of the day alone with her demanding daughter. She rarely had a moment for herself, and she was constantly anxious about what Katie was going to get into next. Peter was helpful with Katie, but he was gone most of the time. When he was around, Ann felt uncomfortable saying outright how close to the edge she occasionally got, and he did not pick up on her hints.

She tried so hard to be loving and patient with Katie. But sometimes she felt overwhelmed with anger when her daughter was really defiant, *like a switch flips and I become another person,* and it was all she could do not to hit her. Then she felt ashamed of her reactions and was full of self-recrimination.

Ann had not slept well for over a year, either just waiting for Katie to wake up or restless with guilt and worry. She told Rick that she felt constantly worn out, sad, or irritable. You could see that she had once been very pretty, but now her face was lined and weary. Then she added that Katie had been adopted.

Once all this had been laid out on the table, Rick made the point that she wasn't alone, that many other mothers had similar feelings. They discussed the harsh logic of Ann's situation: even without the biological demands of pregnancy or nursing, sleep deprivation plus high stress had combined with low support to make her feel irritable and angry, anxious, guilty and inadequate, and depressed. Just hearing that her reactions were not abnormal, and that there were reasons for them, felt calming and hopeful to Ann.

Storms of Anger

Ann felt most concerned about the "amazing anger" that came over her. Rick pointed out that many parts of raising a child would irritate anyone but a saint, such as trying to change a stinky diaper while your toddler kicks and thrashes. Because they feel bad about getting mad at their kids, mothers tend to push these angry feelings down. Then they fester and grow, sometimes erupting. It's a rare parent who has never lost his or her temper with a child. The fact that Ann was worried about raging at Katie showed that she knew she mustn't hit her daughter in anger.

Rick asked how she had been brought up, since every parent is affected by experiences from his or her childhood—like "ghosts in the nursery," in the memorable phrase of the psychotherapist Selma Fraiberg. Ann had grown up in a strict and emotionally cool home. She had become very self-critical, and each struggle with Katie seemed like more proof that she was not a good person. Additionally, her younger brother was a charming goof-off who got most of their parents' attention even though Ann was well behaved and an excellent student. Katie's demands triggered resentful feelings from the past about having to be the responsible one while other people got to indulge themselves.

Fears and Worries

Ann was like many mothers who develop increased feelings of anxiety after having children. Not just the reasonable concerns everyone has—*Why is he crying? What's that crash?*—but a nagging sense of apprehension, worry, or fear. This generalized, chronic anxiety was as far is it went for Ann, but some mothers experience one or more acute conditions:

- The stresses of mothering can lead to panic attacks, which are sudden, overwhelming states of fear and physical discomfort.

- Because many aspects of parenting are beyond anyone's control—such as a child's temperament—a mother may become obsessed with irrational worries or compulsive about things she *can* control, like laying out clothes or washing her hands.

- If her child has major health problems or is seriously injured, she could suffer the symptoms of acute stress disorder at the time—such as feeling numbed, things seeming unreal, intrusive thoughts or images, or heightened reactivity—or posttraumatic stress disorder at a later point.

Feeling Guilty or Inadequate

Evidence is accumulating that being a mother may be the most important source of stress in women's lives.

—Rosalind C. Barnett, Ph.D., and Grace K. Baruch, Ph.D.

Ann and Rick also talked about how motherhood was a strange combination of feeling wonderful and worthless. You're the most important person in the world to your children and half of the all-American equation of "motherhood and apple pie." On the other hand, you feel terrible that you can't figure out why the baby is crying or like an idiot trying to get a toddler to eat cooked carrots. Others—including strangers in the supermarket—point out how you could do a better job. During the time you're home with children, you lose a source of pride and status through accomplishments at work.

The way you think about all this makes a big difference in how you feel. In Ann's mind, any little error was highlighted. Yet the many good things she did each day with her daughter were brushed aside. No wonder that, like many women, her sense of worth had declined since having kids.

Disturbed Mood

These knocks against self-esteem are just one of the many conditions faced by mothers known to cause depression. The rest include sleep deprivation, overwork, stress, changes in physical appearance, ongoing issues with children (such as problems with child care, an illness, or a challenging temperament), health concerns, marital conflict, and social isolation—most of which applied to Ann, so it wasn't surprising that she had gotten depressed

While raising children, you've got about a fifty-fifty chance of going through a period of depressed mood—lasting at least several weeks, and potentially a year or more—when you feel sad, discouraged, or emotionally numb much of the time. You may experience less interest or pleasure in activities that used to be enjoyable, and even the joys of raising a child can feel blanketed by a dark cloud. Relatively small things could seem like big problems, and it's much easier to get irritated or frustrated. You may have a loss of appetite, increase in fatigue, or disturbance in sleep. Besides being a waking nightmare for you, depression wears more on a marriage than any other health problem.

Getting the Weight off Your Mind

Ann decided to work with Rick for a few months. During that time, she took steps that we'll describe in detail in the next three chapters; they included:

- She started using cognitive techniques to argue back against overly self-critical thinking, such as listing several accurate and positive thoughts to refute a distorted and negative one. And by reflecting on her childhood, she was able to sort out sensible reactions to here-and-now situations from unreasonable responses that were amplified by the past. Because she started feeling less like a "bad mom" for needing respites from Katie, she enrolled her in a co-op nursery school a few mornings each week.

- With her extra time, she began exercising again. In particular, she returned to activities that had once given her great pleasure, like long bike rides.

- She now took little moments that she would have previously ignored to get some stress relief, such as taking a bath instead of her usual quick shower.

- Feeling greater self-respect helped her to ask Peter more firmly to get up with Katie some of the time. She also read up on methods for handling a spirited youngster and getting a child to sleep through the night. To her pleasant surprise, many of them actually worked.

These actions began showing results within the first weeks. Katie responded to Ann's change in parenting style and became more cooperative. She was still packed with punch, but now her squabbles stayed mainly within bounds. Ann's nervous anticipation of the next disaster faded, and she began feeling better about herself as a mother—and person.

Within a few months, Ann reported less sadness and more vitality. Her growing connections with other moms improved her self-confidence as a mother, as studies have shown with other women. Also, they probably increased the effectiveness of her immune system, another research finding, which helped cut down on her colds.

She began looking like her original vibrant and athletic self. She had the normal ups and downs of anyone, but she wasn't depressed anymore. She and Rick wrapped up their work together, and he asked her to keep in touch. About a year later he was delighted to receive a card from her: on the cover was a lovely picture of the baby boy that she and her husband had just adopted. Rick called to see how she was doing. They were "nuts," she admitted, but there was a bounce and sense of confidence in her voice that said she and Peter and their two children were going to be fine. All the little steps she had taken for her well-being had paid off—just like your own will, too.

The Effects on a Mother's Marriage

Couples are affected in different ways by the arrival of children: some weather the stresses and changes very well, while others are seriously strained—sometimes to the breaking point. The good news is that when there have been breakdowns in teamwork or intimacy, they can usually be repaired if one or both partners makes a real effort to work on them, and chapters 6, 7, and 8 will show you how.

For example, Maria and Alex began working with Rick when their two boys, Josh and Sam, were three and one-half and one year old. Maria was thirty-three and had worked as an operating room nurse before staying home with their sons. Her dark brown eyes were warm, and like many nurses, she had a meticulous, conscientious manner. Alex was a good deal older, forty-six. He had curly dark hair shot with gray, a complexion mottled from teenage acne, weary grey-blue eyes, and a measured, scholarly style of speaking. They had met at the hospital, where he continued to work as an orthopedic surgeon.

In their first session, Maria said that Alex never got home when he said he would. He was OK with the boys but so strict that she felt she often had to intervene. He wouldn't think for himself about what they needed, so she had to keep telling him what to do, and it seemed that whenever she turned around, he had disappeared into the study to catch up on his paperwork or messages.

On top of that, he gave her no emotional support with the issues of raising a preschooler and a toddler. She was continually weighing "a million details" about the boys. Naturally, she wanted to talk things over with him. But when she finally got him to sit down, he usually interrupted her with some superficial quick fix or rolled his eyes like she was an idiot. Her concerns were well considered, and she was flabbergasted, hurt, and increasingly angry about him treating her like an incompetent orderly.

Alex's eyes were troubled when Maria finished, and he kept shaking his head. He finally said that she needed to "quit obsessing" about the kids. He put a high value on self-reliance and felt Maria was too indecisive and needy. ***She was the best*** *nurse I ever had, so I do not understand why she cannot simply solve these child-management problems on her own.* He thought she needed to exercise better self-control and not use him as a lightning rod when it was the boys she was actually upset with. Besides, when he wanted to talk about something from work, *You can tell she's thinking about something else.*

Then he spoke even more stiffly, but the embarrassment and hurt leaked through: *Maria nurses Sam to sleep in the boys' bedroom and usually falls asleep there herself. I think our personal relationship would be improved if we arranged to end up in the same bed. I must tell you that we have not had intimate relations in a year.*

Feeling Let Down

When Alex finished, the air was heavy with disappointment. Like many parents, each of them had reasons to feel let down by the other. Maria wanted a partnership of the heart in the greatest undertaking of her life. Instead, she felt fended off, patronized, and turned into a "management problem."

Alex, however, felt he was holding up his end of the conventional bargain without a fuss—Dad makes a living and Mom runs the household—so why couldn't Maria? From his own experience as a parent, Rick explained that a new father has to change the way he looks at things: kids mean that your partner is unavoidably dependent on you (which is often uncomfortable and scary for her!), you are no longer a free agent, and you have to be aware of how your actions affect her. Second, like every father, Alex needed to recognize that he bore some responsibility for his wife's fatigue and concerns, since she was raising *his* children, and therefore he needed to give her some help with them.

Additionally, the typical disturbance in a couple's erotic relationship after children had affected Maria and Alex. There was little of the foundation of positive feelings, conversation, and nonsexual touch that most women need in order to feel comfortable making love. Even if there had been, the deep fatigue, hormonal disruption of libido, feeling pulled on all day, and logistical difficulties encountered by all new parents would still have complicated their sex life.

If you are nodding your head in recognition, you might be thinking that your partner should be willing to set aside some of his personal needs for a year or two, just like you have. But the crux for a man usually isn't the lack of sex per se, but the fact that he does not seem to matter enough to his partner to be cared about as a lover. Like many fathers, Alex felt there was as little room for him in Maria's heart as there was in her bed.

Eight Times as Many Arguments

Alex and Maria saw Rick off and on for about a year. A few weeks after their first session, in response to Alex's ongoing complaints about the lack of sex, Maria shot back: *If I can't trust you to get home on time, if I can't trust you not to be too hard on the boys, and if I can't trust you to listen to me when I'm upset, why would I trust you in bed?*

Alex hemmed and hawed. Rick asked him how he'd feel about a member of his operating team who was as unreliable about his work commitments as Alex was at home. After a pained silence, Alex said gruffly, *I can see the point.*

Kids bring an intense need for teamwork, but a mother and father often disagree about parenting practices or how to share the load fairly. As a result, researchers have found that the average couple has eight times as many arguments after children arrive—a major reason why two couples in three report a sharp drop in satisfaction with their relationship once they become parents. Struggles with your partner over child rearing are intensely distressing and can lead to psychological problems. And besides feeling awful, those quarrels wear on your health, in part by increasing your blood pressure and weakening your immune system.

Issues related to parenting last as long as kids do. If they are not resolved, the same arguments flare again and again, and they become increasingly charged. Over time, positions harden, and each person typically gets more defensive. Since each partner is more defended, the other one figures he or she had better bring the heavy artillery—which leads to even more defensiveness. Mistrust grows in vicious cycles. The fights get even worse. You once walked down the aisle thinking you could place your life in this man's hands. Now you could find yourself eyeing him as an unreliable character who must be cajoled or corralled into reasonable and helpful behavior. And it's possible that he might be thinking about you in a similar way.

A Chilly Distance

Each time either spouse feels misunderstood, let down, or angry cuts thread by thread at the emotional cords binding them together. A few months into the therapy, Maria described an episode that had occurred when Josh was just two months old. At that time she felt deeply fatigued and quite vulnerable. Alex thought it would be good for their relationship if they went out, and he insisted they leave their son with a sitter and attend an outdoor concert with people from work. She protested but felt too worn out to put up much resistance. They ended up going, despite the fact that it was a cold and windy day. She worried about her baby the whole time, and she felt chilled to the bone. She was stunned, saddened, and outraged that her husband was so out of touch with how she was feeling. As she put it nearly four years later, *I took a big step back from him that night, and I haven't come fully forward since.*

Some couples manage to mend these tears in the fabric of their marriage and preserve a strong and loving friendship. But in many cases, a chill fills the air at a time when it could have been so sweet to raise a child together. Their relationship shrinks to the size that feels safe: a bland, formal, emotionally cool partnership for raising children and little else. For example, one mother said to Rick: *My husband tried to be helpful. But I wasn't giving him much attention, I was irritable all the time, and after a while he just gave up and withdrew. I was so devoted to my children that it seemed selfish to me that he would want me to take time away from them. Eventually, once I stopped nursing and started getting more sleep, I began to feel like my old self again. But by then, my husband had been withdrawn for so long it had become a kind of permanent state. Our marriage has never been the same.*

For Maria and Alex, things hit bottom about three months into the therapy. Maria said, *I don't think he loves me anymore. When you love somebody, when you really like them, you act a certain way. He doesn't act that way and I think the reason is simple.* She paused and asked him point blank: *Do you still love me?* Alex stared at his feet and chose his words carefully: *I think you are a terrific mother and we have many interests and values in common.* He went on like this until she interrupted him, her voice rising: *But do you love me?* There was a long pause before he looked her in the eye and said, *I hope so. But I'm not sure anymore.* Maria just stared at him. He finally spoke up, getting visibly upset for the first time in their sessions: *Well, what about you? Are you interested in me—as a person, beyond the fact that I'm the father of your sons?* She answered, *There was a long time when I was actively* not *interested in you, basically paying you back for how you treated me. That's gotten better since coming here. I'm up to neutral. But I'm not yet up to real positive.*

A family therapist hears many loud and angry things. But the worst one of all is the quiet admission between two parents, said one way or another: *I don't love you anymore.* You're aware of their children, and what's at stake. His chair and hers are only a few feet apart. But they peer at each other as if across a great divide, trying to see the person once loved, or a love for oneself that used to flow so generously.

Maria and Alex looked over the edge of the abyss and did not like what they

F or many couples, the cascade toward divorce begins with the first decline in the wife's marital satisfaction after the arrival of the first baby.

—Alyson Fearnley
Shapiro, Ph.D.,
John M. Gottman,
Ph.D., and Sybil
Carrere, Ph.D.

saw: separate households, the impact on their boys, less time with their sons, financial upheaval, trying to find a new partner. They realized that the real stakes when they fought were not the overt issues on the table—whatever those happened to be that day—but the future of their marriage. They understood that they had better repair their relationship faster than they were tearing it up.

Reknitting a Marriage

Over the course of a year, Maria and Alex used many of the tools and skills that you'll find in chapters 6, 7, and 8. They each made a unilateral commitment for several months to doing what they could *personally* to have their relationship go better, independent of what the other person did. They did their best to live by the "80-20" rule: put 80 percent of your attention on the corrections you can make and 20 percent on what your partner can do better.

With this commitment as a foundation, they established basic ground rules for civility, such as not fighting in front of the children, no name-calling, and no dragging the kids into their arguments. Alex tried to "lead with empathy" when Maria was worried or upset, rather than attempt to solve her problem, and Maria paid closer attention to Alex's stories about work. As a result, they began to understand each other better. Alex saw that Maria's focus on their sons was normal and not a personal rejection, and she realized that he had lost a wife in some ways while not gaining the moment-to-moment fulfillment she had with the children.

They worked on translating their complaints about the past into specific requests for the future. They learned how to negotiate about parenting, schedules, and the way they spoke to each other. For instance, Alex started controlling his temper with the boys and Maria stopped micromanaging him. Alex agreed to come home by six on Thursday nights and take care of their sons the rest of the evening. Besides giving Maria a night off, he became immediately more understanding about what it was like to spend many hours alone with young children.

It was uncomfortable at first, but they started touching each other again with little pats and hugs. Rather than being passively resentful, Alex began gently rousing Maria after she put Sam to sleep. They started sleeping in the same bed. After several months, they broke the ice and made love again. They realized that sex wasn't going to be as spontaneous as it used to be, and they came to an understanding that they would try to make love once a week or so.

Maria asked Alex if he could please make an effort to be less stuffy. Bit by bit, he started talking with her more openly, awkwardly at first but growing increasingly at ease with it. Just the fact that he was trying warmed Maria's heart to him, and her greater friendliness in turn evoked in him more caring for her. Over time, the chill between them thawed, and the caring feelings that had drawn them together in the first place started to return. Six months after they began seriously working on their relationship, lying in bed together on a Saturday morning, Maria said three simple words to Alex that she had last spoken two years ago: *I love you.* He was startled and became quiet. Then, when he spoke, his voice was firm: *I love you, too.*

Your Path Toward Well-being, Health, and Support

Raising children is deeply fulfilling. Yet it's also intensely demanding. Compared to women who haven't had children, mothers are generally more stressed, more unhappy in their marriages, and more prone to illness. But if we've learned one thing in our personal lives and professional practices, it's that *none* of that distress or depletion is necessary! There really is an alternative path, and it's direct and straightforward: decrease the "bad"—the demands upon you—and increase the "good"—your resources and resilience. The actions you take will work together. For example, research shows that getting more support from your partner can boost your own physical and psychological health.

We know it's hard to take care of yourself when you've got a little one (or ones) on your hands. We've each been there and we see it all the time in our practices. But nurturing yourself *is* altogether possible, even with kids to manage and a household to run. In the chapters to come, you'll see how to get the stress relief, nutrition, health care, teamwork, and intimacy you need. That will prevent depletion and build up your well-being so that this wonderful time in your life is as good as it can possibly be. That's what Mother Nurture is all about.

Key Risk Factors for Depletion

In order to see where your risks for depletion lie—and therefore where to focus your efforts—please check the boxes that apply to you. Wherever possible, chapters are indicated in which you will find help for that issue. And to get a sense of your overall risk for depletion, add up the number of boxes you marked. Five or fewer factors suggest low risk, six to fifteen factors suggest moderate risk, and sixteen or more factors suggest high risk.

HIGH DEMANDS UPON YOU

Physical

[   ]   Have had two or more children

[   ]   Less than eighteen months' spacing between any two children

[×]   Breast-fed one or more children over eighteen months

[   ]   Breast-fed during pregnancy, or two children during the same period

[   ]   Became pregnant and carried to term less than three months after weaning

[×]   Disturbed sleep over past three months, or averaged less than seven hours per day during that period (*chapter 4*)

Child-related

[×]   Currently caring for a child under three years of age

[×]   Care for a child eight or more hours a day

[   ]   Have a child with a challenging temperament—e.g., spirited, stubborn, aggressive, fearful

[   ]   Have a child with chronic physical or psychological problems

Associated factors

[   ]   Unreliable or mediocre child care (*chapter 9*)

[   ]   Care for others besides children—e.g., ill spouse or parent

[   ]   Returned to work twenty-plus hours per week before baby was one year old (*chapter 9*)

[   ]   Currently working for pay thirty-plus hours per week or full-time student (*chapter 9*)

LOW RESOURCES COMING TO YOU

Physical (*chapter 4*)

[   ]   During pregnancy(ies), ate fewer than three meals per day, or few fresh vegetables, or little protein

[   ]   Since birth of first child, nutrition has been mediocre or poor

[   ]   Little use of vitamin/mineral supplements

[×]   Little or no exercise

Psychological (*chapter 2*)

- [×] Little time for breaks
- [×] Little use of stress relief techniques: progressive relaxation or meditation
- [ ] Do few personal enjoyments or pleasures
- [×] Little or no spiritual or religious orientation

Interpersonal

- [ ] Single parent
- [ ] Partner travels frequently (*chapters 6 and 7*)
- [ ] Low sense of teamwork or cooperation with partner (*chapters 6 and 7*)
- [ ] Partner does little child rearing or housework during evenings or weekends (*chapters 6 and 7*)
- [ ] Low sense of emotional intimacy with a partner (*chapter 8*)
- [×] Little affection or sexuality with a partner (*chapter 8*)
- [ ] Little tangible support from relatives
- [×] Little sense of connection with other mothers
- [×] Little sense of connection with community institutions supportive of families (e.g., a mothers club)

PERSONAL VULNERABILITIES

Prior to pregnancy with first child

- [ ] Extensive dieting or eating disorder (*chapter 4*)
- [ ] Generally mediocre or poor nutrition (*chapter 4*)
- [×] Little use of vitamin/mineral supplements (*chapter 4*)
- [ ] Significant exposure to toxic chemicals (*chapter 4*)
- [×] Hormone problems—e.g., thyroid disorder, diabetes, or severe PMS (*chapter 5*)
- [ ] Gastrointestinal problems—e.g., irritable bowel syndrome, ulcer, digestive parasites (*chapter 5*)
- [ ] Immune system problems—e.g., severe allergies, asthma, arthritis, lupus (*chapter 5*)
- [ ] Significant depression or anxiety (*chapters 3 and 5*)

[ ]   Family history of hormone, gastrointestinal, immune, or reproductive problems (*chapter 5*)

[ ]   Family history of psychological problems (*chapters 2 and 3*)

[X]   Highly sensitive, anxious, or rigid temperament (*chapters 2 and 3*)

During any pregnancy carried to term

[ ]   Complications such as preeclampsia or toxemia

[ ]   Serious obstetric complications

Since children

[X]   One or more children born when mother was thirty-plus years old

[?]   One or more episodes of postpartum depression (*chapters 3 and 5*)

[ ]   Regular use of tobacco (*chapter 4*)

[ ]   Alcohol abuse—e.g., needing to drink daily to cope, averaging over fifteen drinks per week (*chapter 4*)

[ ]   Regular use of illegal drugs (*chapter 4*)

[ ]   Significantly overweight (*chapter 4*)

PART TWO
Nurturing Your Mind

Whether it's middle-of-the-night feedings, daily battles with your toddler over wearing shoes, or a call from kindergarten to say that your daughter's taken a bad fall off the jungle gym, as a whole, raising children will probably be the most stressful experience of your life. And it can stir up some of the most painful feelings you've ever experienced, including intense sadness, anxiety, shame, and anger.

Chapter 2 covers strategies for coping with parental stress. The idea is first to get immediate relief, and then—over the long term—build up your psychological resilience: the capacity to cope with and recover quickly from stresses.

Next, chapter 3 focuses on the normal but difficult emotions that typically increase in the first years of parenthood, like sadness at the loss of a part of your old life before children, or anger at your husband's casual assumption that you'll watch the kids Sunday while he watches football. You'll see how to release these feelings and replace them with more positive ones.

Of course, addressing your inner experience—be it a general sense of stress or a specific emotion—will not itself change challenging circumstances such as a colicky baby or problems with child care. But it can help you deal with them more effectively, or at least endure them with grace. Similarly, a psychological intervention may not improve a health problem that's dragging you down, but the mind and body are interconnected, and upgrading your "software" can often improve your "hardware" as well; you'll find specific help for health starting on page 95. And in part 4, we'll explore a key source of stress relief: a supportive relationship with your partner.

Reducing Your Stress

Nobody likes being stressed, but mothers often seem to have a hard time doing anything about it. First, it might look like nothing can help. After all, you're kind of stuck for now with having to grocery shop with a fussy toddler in tow or juggle home and work. But while it's true you no longer have the kind of control over your life you once had, it's important to remember that no matter how bad it gets, there is always *something* you can do to soothe your nerves and boost your spirits. Right now, for instance, try shifting in your seat, loosening tight clothing, or taking a full breath. Do you feel even a little better? It's a small thing, but it shows you *can* affect your own stress level.

Second, you may be experiencing some resistance to taking time to be good to yourself, either from within you or from the people around you. Well, you're certainly not alone there. Many women were raised to put everyone else's needs first, and they can have a hard time asserting their own. And for mothers it just gets worse. Your commitment to your children's welfare is so primal that it's hard to pay attention to yourself—how can you even *think* about taking a bath or a nap when your kids need you?—plus other people can make you feel guilty for daring to try. A client of Rick's with a two-year-old plus a newborn was talking with her own mom about how tired she was. Her mother interrupted impatiently, *That is just mothering, you may as well get used to it,* and then changed the subject, as if she were passing down some unwritten rule of motherhood: *I suffered, and so must you.*

To us, this view is crazy. Nurturing yourself is what enables you to be at your best for your children. One mother told us: *The times I have really blown it with my kids have all come when I was at the end of my rope. I remember moms with older kids telling me to take care of myself. I thought, "yeah, sure," and kept on going full tilt. But they were right, and I wish I had accepted that earlier.* Further,

---

You Matter

Please consider these questions:

When you were growing up, how did your parents or others treat your needs and wants? How has that affected you?

Currently, how do you treat your own needs and wants? Deep down, how much do you feel they matter? Take a few minutes to imagine going through your day as if your needs and wants really mattered; how would that change your day?

In the "pie" of your typical day, how big is the slice that is lived just for you? When you feel like you really matter as a person, what seems like a wise and appropriate size for that slice?

---

mothering is not a hobby you picked up for fun. You work hard for the sake of your children and family, and that entitles you to respect, care—and stress relief.

Short-term Stress Relief

HELMER: First and foremost, you are a wife and mother.

NORA: That I don't believe any more. I believe that first and foremost I am an individual, just as much as you are.

—Henrik Ibsen,
A Doll's House

Even in the middle of the most insane day, there are lots of things you can do that will immediately lower your stress level and help you both feel better, and create a small space in which you can begin to figure out how to lower your stresses over the long term. Additionally, getting the needle on your personal stress meter out of the red zone stops the current wear and tear on your body, and it helps prevent your brain and hormones from getting so sensitized to stress that they overreact to it in the future.

That's why we recommend that you try to *feel good* as often as you can, at least several times each day. These experiences are more than enjoyable: they help protect your body against future stresses, improve problem solving, and stop downward spirals. The occasional getaway for a weekend is great, but regular, daily, positive experiences will make much more difference for you over the long run.

Below, we've listed lots of ways to get your stress meter into the green. Many of them will take only a minute or so, and you can do the ones that take longer while nursing, tending to children, doing housework, or driving. And we heartily encourage you to use whatever stress-reducing techniques you have discovered on your own as well.

ONE-MINUTE SOOTHERS

- Take four long, slow breaths, and as you exhale, imagine that a gray cloud of stress, worries, or troubles is leaving your life, and as you inhale, imagine that peace and love and wisdom are filling you up.

- Take your shoes off, rub the bottoms of your feet with your knuckles, and massage the joints and tips of your toes.

- Smell something nice, like an orange or your child's hair, or put on a dab of perfume.

- Roll your head around to loosen your neck.

- Splash water on your face.

- While standing, bend over to touch the floor, shake your arms loosely, and straighten up slowly as you take in a big breath.

- Look at something pretty.

- Knead your neck and shoulders.

- Nibble something good.

- Rub your eyes and the bones around them gently.

- Hug your child or partner for one whole minute.

- Stretch your mouth open as wide as you can, like a lion roaring, and then let your face relax.

- Remember a good joke.

- Repeat a favorite saying or prayer to yourself.

FIVE-MINUTE SOOTHERS

- Make yourself a cup of tea.

- Lie down, close your eyes, and imagine a warm, golden balm settling over you, softening the edges of your feelings, and gently carrying away any distress.

- Listen to your favorite music, from Bach to the B-52s.

- Ask someone for a sincere compliment.

- Step outside and watch the play of sunlight dancing on leaves, or the moon and the stars.

- Do a few minutes of stretching or yoga.

FIFTEEN-MINUTE SOOTHERS

- Take a long shower.
- Read a magazine.
- Go for a short walk and look for beauty.
- Arrange flowers in a vase.
- Cuddle up with your children or your partner.
- Call a friend for a quick chat.
- Be especially loving with someone.
- Lie down for a brief nap.
- Meditate for fifteen minutes.
- Exercise, dance, stretch, or do yoga.

THIRTY-MINUTE SOOTHERS

- Read a good book.
- Take a bath—maybe with bubbles.
- Watch a TV show.
- Go for a walk.
- Treat yourself to a good nap.
- Trade a neck rub or foot massage with your partner.
- Do some art or a craft.
- Play a musical instrument.
- Put some flowers in every room in the house.
- Call a friend and really talk.
- Make love with your partner.

When you are a mother, you are never really alone in your thoughts. A mother always has to think twice, once for herself and once for her child.

—Sophia Loren

ONE-HOUR SOOTHERS

- Go for a run, swim, or bike ride, even if you have to arrange special child care to get an hour to yourself.
- Get a manicure.
- Go out to lunch with your partner, a friend, or a good book.
- Visit your church or temple.
- Browse through a bookstore.

- Provide a simple charitable service to someone in more need than you.
- Go for a walk in a park.
- Prepare a really nice meal just for you or treat yourself to a special lunch.

Long-term Stress Relief

Immediate stress relief feels great, but it's also important to build up your psychological resilience for the long term. The essential method is simple: first, *let go of the "bad,"* like tension, sadness, or troubling thoughts. Then, when you have released these burdens on your mind, you will have created a space in yourself in which to *take in the "good,"* such as positive experiences of happiness and self-worth. You can prevent or reduce depletion by the regular practice of these fundamental stress-reduction techniques. And over time, that practice will make a lasting difference in your own psychology, leading to improved mood and greater insight into yourself and other people.

You can let go of stress in each part of your inner world, including your body sensations, mental images, emotions, desires, and thoughts. Let's begin with the body.

Relaxing Your Body

There are many ways to relax your body even in the middle of a busy day. You've already seen some in the section above (e.g., stretching), and here are additional ideas:

- A few times each day, sweep your attention through your body, noticing the places that are tight or uncomfortable, and consciously relaxing them. Key places to look for tension include your eyes, jaws and tongue, diaphragm (located just below the rib cage), and pelvic floor.
- After going to bed but before falling asleep, you can systematically relax the parts of your body. Just bring your awareness to each part—left foot, right foot, left ankle, etc., all the way up to your scalp—and let it relax.
- Breathing techniques are great ways to relax. The easiest one of all is to just take a big breath and let it out slowly. Or inhale deeply and hold it for a few seconds before exhaling gradually, and then try not inhaling for a few seconds after you exhale. Perhaps imagine that your breath is going in and

out of some tense part of your body; for example, you could get a sense that you are breathing into a tight neck or nervous stomach.

Occasionally try to breathe from your diaphragm by placing your hand on your stomach just below the arch of your rib cage and having each inhalation push your hand away from your backbone. This is an especially good technique for letting go of anxiety.

You could experiment with techniques from yoga, such as: inhaling through the nose and exhaling through the mouth; inhaling through your left nostril (closing the right one gently) and exhaling through the right nostril (closing the one on the left); taking several breaths by following a rhythmic count: inhale for five, hold for twenty, exhale for ten, and hold the exhalation for ten (adjust the pace of the count for your own comfort); or breathing rapidly and forcefully in and out of your nose for half a minute or more.

- When lying down, imagine being very heavy, so weighty that you are sinking down into the earth.

- Imagine that your hands are getting very warm, as if you had a cup of cocoa between them or were holding them before a cheery fire; this is particularly helpful for going to sleep.

- Tense your arms or legs for a few seconds and then relax.

Resources for Letting Go

The Relaxation Response by Herbert Benson

Focusing by Eugene Gendlin

Being Peace by Thich Nhat Hanh

The Relaxation and Stress Reduction Workbook by Martha Davis, Mathew McKay, and Elizabeth Eshelman

Using Mental Imagery to Release Stress

We are mainly aware of our verbal thoughts, but actually, most of the brain is dedicated to nonverbal processes. That realm is a vital part of who you are, and by becoming more able to enter the fertile, wise world of images, daydreaming, and fantasy, you'll gain both stress relief and self-knowledge. Whenever you get tired of the yammering voice in the back of your head—the one that just said, "What voice?"—you can try one of these suggestions:

The quickest way for a parent to get a child's attention is to sit down and look comfortable.

—Lane Olinghouse

- Recall or imagine a relaxing experience. Maybe you're on a tropical beach, feeling the warm sun and a gentle breeze playing on your skin, with the soft murmuring of happy people—perhaps your children—nearby. Or you could be walking across a mountain meadow, surrounded by wildflowers and the sound of babbling brooks, with the crisp smell of distant snow in the air. Try picking images of situations that are the opposite of the ones that are causing you stress. For example, if you feel like you're unable to solve a problem with your child, you might imagine successfully skiing down a challenging slope, or if you feel unable to break out of a sticky situation at work, imagine sailing freely under gorgeous skies.

- Visualize little faucets at the tips of your fingers and toes, and your body filled with colored liquid. Open the taps and let the liquid drain out, taking with it all of the tension within you. Notice any remaining liquid, indicating stress that is not yet released, and encourage every bit of it to drain away.

- Imagine stresses or upsetting experiences flowing out of you each time you exhale, like a smoggy cloud exiting whenever you blow out a breath. Or get a sense that you are standing in a warm and beautiful river, and that the water is cleansing you of stresses, carrying them away and out to sea.

- If you've had an upsetting experience that you'd like to let go of, imagine putting it on a rocket and sending it to burn up in the sun, or on a big red balloon that disappears into the sky, or on a raft that floats down a river to the sea. If it's meaningful to you, you could imagine releasing the experience to God.

- If an ongoing situation is stressing you out—let's say one of your in-laws is passing judgment on how you are raising your child—imagine using a pair of glowing magic scissors to cut apart the connection between you and the situation.

Letting Go of Feelings

One of the challenges of motherhood is finding good ways to express your feelings. After all, you can hardly tell a child that you feel depressed or that his whining makes you want to scream. And sometimes it's not the right time or place to lay out all your feelings about your partner.

The problem, though, is that emotion is like a river. When it's allowed to flow, it stays clean and clear; but when it's dammed up, it grows dank and dark. Fortunately, there are two ways to let your feelings flow without the consequences that sometimes come from communicating directly: expressing them within your own mind, and expressing them symbolically. (We'll discuss direct communication with your partner in chapters 6, 7, and 8.)

Expressing emotion within your own mind. The safest way to express emotion is to yourself, which doesn't reveal how you feel to anyone else. As a start, and as best you can, try to name your feelings to yourself. (Please see the box on self-observation.) Normal emotions include joy, surprise, curiosity, lust, love, peacefulness, sense of worth, triumph, religious exaltation, fear, sadness, anger, and shame. Also acknowledge the intensity of the feeling. For example, the spectrum of anger includes mild annoyance, exasperation, irritation, resentment, hostility, and rage.

Further, can you notice more than one emotion present at a time, especially the softer, more vulnerable feelings beneath any angry ones? In order to identify your deeper feelings, relax and let your awareness sink down into the younger layers of your personality; see what might be similar there to your current situation, perhaps intensifying your reactions to present-day events. For example, feeling let down by your partner could be amplified by experiences in which important people were not understanding or supportive when you were a child. If those early experiences stir up feelings of embarrassment or shame, remember that much as every child is innocent and good, you are innocent and good yourself at your roots. Try to bring an attitude of compassion for yourself to all that you see. Sometimes there will be a memory or image of some episode, but often there will simply be a feeling that has a young quality to it.

Paradoxically, feeling your emotions fully helps to let them go. Try to own them, even the most difficult ones, inside your mind: *This is my anger, my sadness, my frustration. I'm out of my mind with worry about the baby. I really do feel let down by my partner. I feel embarrassed, trying to pump milk at work.* In essence, you let yourself feel bad for a moment in order to feel good for a long time. (For an extended experience of expressing emotions within your mind, try the "safe room" exercise in appendix C.)

Of course, it's hard to claim your feelings as your own if you can't accept them in the first place. As one mother put it: *The worst part of it is I get mad at myself for how I'm feeling. This is supposed to be a happy time, so I think I must be doing something wrong if I'm grouchy or sad.* Often our reactions to our experience are more stressful than the experience itself, like feeling ashamed of being needy or angry at getting irritated once again. We suffer *that* we suffer, frustrated with our experience or guilty about it. For example, one mother said: *I feel mad at Tyler for making me mad. I just want to feel happy with him, not irritated. I'm upset about*

Self-Observation

At any moment, you can separate from your experience and observe it like a neutral witness, as if a part of you had stepped out of the movie of your life and now sat ten rows back, watching the drama on the screen: ***OK, I'm getting really irritated here with Jesse's whining, I'm thinking it's hopeless, I really wish he would hush up, a part of me would like to swat him, I feel bad about that, I'm getting into that whole thing about how I'm a crappy parent, it makes me really tense.*** Rather than BEING your experience, HAVE it. When you detach from it, it's immediately less stressful.

Try to observe your experience in little snapshots while you're on the go or by taking a break for a few minutes to tune into yourself. Notice the details in your inner world, especially the body sensations, emotions, and desires—not just the chatter of verbal thoughts. Notice the layering in your experience, with softer, younger, more fundamental material underneath more angry, adult, or superficial preoccupations.

Notice how your experience continually changes. Most of it is not that significant, but a largely automatic cascade of one thing triggering another. If anything disturbing comes along, you can remain detached, watching as it inevitably, happily becomes something else.

being upset so much! Instead, see if you can have compassion for your feelings. They occur for real reasons, triggered by hard situations today or by the painful residue of difficult experiences you had as a child, and they are not your fault. Imagine being as kind to your inner self as you'd be to someone else who's upset, like your child or a dear friend. You can be a dear friend yourself to the distressed parts within you.

There is nothing shameful about a feeling itself, and accepting it is not at all the same as acting on it. When a person resists her feelings through suppression, denial, or minimization, they keep sticking around, like a preschooler pounding on a closed door. But when you accept them and express them to yourself, the door opens, the pounding stops, and the feelings move on.

Expressing emotion symbolically. In this mode, you do express your feelings outwardly, yet still not directly to the person they concern. The most obvious way is to write them down without editing or censoring yourself, remembering that no one will see these words but you. If you like, you could write in large letters with crayons to bring out the younger feelings below the surface, or use your nondominant hand (the left one for most people). In a more structured way, you can draft multiple letters to a person (*not* to send) in which you focus on different feelings such as hurt or anger. You could then release your writings through physical action, such as by throwing them away, cutting them into pieces and flushing them down a toilet, or burning them and scattering the ashes. As you do this, you may want to speak some words of release, in your mind or out loud, such as: *I am letting go of these feelings. As this paper burns, my anger is turning into smoke. I am cleansed inside. Good-bye, feelings!*

Or you might draw pictures—which is about exploring and expressing your inner world, not trying to make good art. Take a moment to get a sense of what you are feeling, and then let it flow through you and onto the page. Don't be concerned if there seems to be no logic to it. Let your hand movements be big and free. If it helps, you could speak out loud or make sounds while drawing. You can be completely abstract, or you can do loosely representational drawings, such as you in relation to another person. You can also combine pictures and words, such as a cartoon of a typical argument with your spouse, with balloons over the heads that show what each person is thinking or feeling.

Venting out loud is another form of symbolic expression. Please do this only when no one can hear you (especially your kids)! The shower might be a good place, the top of a hill, or inside your car (as long as you can continue to drive safely). If you feel you are losing control or getting lost in a negative emotion, stop venting and do what you need to do to calm down. You can also vent through physical action, not words. You could tear paper, smash your pillow against your bed over and over, hit something soft, or jump up and down. Again, do this only while no one can see or hear you, and be sure not to hurt yourself.

Finally, you could express your feelings to someone else. Pick a person with whom you feel safe, tell him or her your purpose in talking, and ask for whatever would make you feel comfortable, such as a promise to keep things confidential. You are not looking for advice, but for someone to hear you out so you can move on; nor do you want to fan the flames of your feelings, since your purpose is release. As you speak, try to sense that the emotions are leaving you, that your listener is drawing them out of you. You can ask him or her to help you let go by saying things like *I got it, I hear you, yes, OK.*

Riding the Wave of Desire

Many times a day, there is probably a collision between the normal desires you have as a person and the realities of life with children. In addition to being lovable, fascinating, delightful, etc., kids are sometimes unavoidably frustrating. You desperately want them to just eat their supper, and all they want to do is smear it in their hair. You want them to come here but they crawl away, or to hug Grandpa but they hide behind your legs. Children grab hold of your life and oblige you to do one thing after another that is a million miles away from your personal preference at the moment. Meanwhile, long-term plans for your career or a remodel or a long vacation get postponed. Each one of your wants is like a wave that starts small in the mind, builds to a crest of action, and then subsides when it is fulfilled or you decide to let it go. When wants are frustrated, especially on a regular basis, it creates stress. Relief comes from knowing how to ride them lightly, and how to let go when it's time to move on.

There is nothing wrong with wanting itself, whether it's our most fleeting wishes or deepest values. At bottom, every one of our wants is positive, even if some might be expressed in a problematic way. For example, Rick had a client who was troubled by her overprotective need to have her five-year-old in sight at all times. Her compulsion was founded on a healthy desire to keep her child safe, and eventually she learned more reasonable ways to feel secure about his safety. At its core, her want was always positive.

But trouble comes when a parent clings too tightly to her wants. Children bring one surprise after another, disrupting order, cleanliness, schedules, and plans. They also make you more dependent on others who have needs and agendas of their own, such as your partner or nursery school teachers. As a mother, you probably have less control over your life than you've ever had, and accepting this fact helps prevent stress right from the start. As a mother of four-year-old twins told Rick: *I'm not obsessive, but I like things tidy and I like knowing what's going to happen. The clutter and constant changes drove me crazy for a long time. Finally I realized I had to give up. Now I insist on my bedroom being neat and just do what I can with the rest of the house. I try to remember that the big picture is going fine with the boys and not get too caught up in the little details. And I use work as a refuge: at least there, things happen on time!*

Pursuing healthy wants provides a positive model for children. On the other hand, many wants are unattainable or inappropriate, and we need to release them and shift to a different plan. Here's how:

Step back. You can observe a want just like you can observe a feeling. That bit of distance alone can lower the dial on your stress meter. You'll probably notice many desires, some nested within others, some pulling in opposite directions. Every aspect of this bubbling stew is normal, including the wilder or darker wants all of us have. In particular, you'll see how wants that are rooted in early life experiences can be transferred into the present; for example, you may find yourself yearning for things from your partner that you missed getting from your father.

Clinging is the root of all suffering.

—Second Noble Truth of Buddhism

This process of transference occurs for everyone, but it is intensified when you have kids because you are drawn into the kind of situations you experienced as a child. The problem is that wants that are normal for a child—like being the center of someone's universe—just aren't going to be fulfilled to the same degree in adult relationships. Through self-observation, you can separate the unattainable wants of a child from the adult wants that have a chance at being satisfied.

Try to be kind to yourself about any of your wants, but especially those that come from childhood. The stronger these young desires are, the more likely it is that they were not treated with sensitivity when you were little. They really should have been; every child deserves that kind of care. If you take an attitude toward them that is dismissive, cold, or shaming, you are doing to yourself what should *not* have been done to you in the first place. Instead, try to be like a good mom to the young parts within you, sympathetic and understanding, while gently making it clear that it's just not possible to fulfill those wants today.

Relax. Usually, the more important the want, the more it is felt in the flesh. When you relax your body, your wants become less insistent.

Release feelings about not fulfilling the want. Notice any frustration or disappointment about not getting what you want. You can let go of these much like you would any other unpleasant emotion, using the techniques described in the previous section.

Release the want itself. You could remind yourself of the reasons why it is not possible or wise to pursue it, perhaps even writing a note to yourself. You can say good-bye to it in your mind, out loud, to another person, or in a letter to yourself. You could imagine that it is draining out of you like water into sand. Fundamentally, you can just surrender to never having it fulfilled.

Move on to a new plan. This might be a small matter—like taking a break from trying to shovel peas into your toddler—or a fundamental shift in your deepest values. You can make the new plan feel solid by saying it to yourself, writing it down, or telling someone else. Focus on its benefits and imagine it going well.

Liberating Insight

Untrue, illogical, or overly negative thoughts just increase your stress—and insight into them is like waking up from a bad dream, usually to good news, as one mother found out: *I got a message at work that the day care staff had phoned me. I called them and called them, but their line was always busy, so I left and drove over. It's true, I usually assume the worst. I was sure Jasmine had gotten hurt, and I worried about all the horrible possibilities the whole way. When I got there, they said she was fine, they'd had some trouble with their phones, and they just wanted to ask me about my payment last week. I felt a little silly about getting so worked up.*

Seeing stresses as opportunities. Let's say your fifteen-month-old squirms and fusses when you try to put him in his car seat. It's natural to feel frustrated and annoyed. But it's also possible to regard the situation as an opportunity for learning new skills, developing greater patience, enjoying a feeling of accomplishment, deepening your sense of compassion and love, and even experiencing spiritual growth. Even though it's a cliché, it's still true: seeing both sides of the coin—the challenges *and* the opportunities—will improve your well-being and how you cope.

Talking back to the voice in your head. Just because a thought arises in your mind does not mean it's worth believing. All you have to do is catch the unrealistic thoughts that are making you stressed and replace them with true, logical, and positive ones. Many studies have found that this kind of self-talk is one of the most powerful ways to handle stresses effectively. You are sticking up for yourself inside your own mind by focusing on the objective facts, defending against unfair attacks, and giving encouragement. (See the box for some of the beliefs that can help a mother to cope well with stress.)

Most of the time, you'll stand up to stressful thoughts inwardly, within your own head. But it can also help to put it in writing: just draw a line down the center of a piece of paper, write an untrue, illogical, or negative thought on the left side, and then list two or more true, logical, or positive ones on the right side. Whether it's in your mind or on paper, try to make a strong case for yourself, arguing actively with negative thoughts, refusing to let them defeat you. With practice, you'll be talking back to them so quickly and naturally that you'll hardly notice it.

Let's try this method with some different categories of stressful thinking. When you start becoming able to recognize the *type* of thought that's raising your blood pressure, you've got a jump on letting go of it.

- *Exaggerating the problem*

NEGATIVE THOUGHT
Baby-sitters never work out.

POSITIVE ALTERNATIVES
So far, there's been a problem only one time in five.

Even when that one flaked out, all it meant was that Bob and I didn't get to go out.

Maybe an older person would be more responsible, like a college student.

Beliefs That Help Mothers Cope

The real problem here is just _____ . It's a hassle, but not life or death.

Things could have gone much worse.

It's not permanent.

Things will get better.

I have handled this in the past and I can handle it again.

I will figure something out.

I have resources all around me.

I can create more resources if I need to.

Determination will get me through this problem, just like it always has.

Even if I can't change the situation, I'll grow from it.

I am a good person.

I am doing my best.

- *Focusing on the negative*

NEGATIVE THOUGHT
   The teacher said Johnny was "rambunctious," and I feel so embarrassed.

POSITIVE ALTERNATIVES
   She also said he was sweet, smart, helpful, friendly, creative, and liked by
      everyone. Almost everything she said was positive.
   Nobody has ever complained about Johnny being aggressive, wild, or mean.
   So what if he gets rambunctious, that's normal for a three-year-old.

- *Discounting the positive*

NEGATIVE THOUGHT
   It doesn't mean anything if people like me at work because they're still mad I
      took time off for the baby.

POSITIVE ALTERNATIVES
   If people like me, it means I am likable. No one is forcing them to like me.
   Every woman at work told me she thought it's great I took the time off.

- ***Dooming the future***

NEGATIVE THOUGHT

I'm going to have to put the baby in day care forty hours a week because I'm never going to find a good part-time job.

POSITIVE ALTERNATIVES

Good part-time jobs do exist. I've seen them advertised.

I know people who have them, and they have less on the ball than I do.

I've only been looking for three weeks.

I can try changing my resume, working with a personnel agency, or doing temporary work.

- ***Overgeneralizing***

NEGATIVE THOUGHT

Men don't listen.

POSITIVE ALTERNATIVES

OK, my dad didn't listen, but that alone does not mean my husband doesn't.

All men are not alike just like all women are not alike.

I can remember times when men listened to me.

My husband listened to me when _____ , and when _____ .

I chose my husband in part because he is different from my father.

I can talk to my husband about listening, and I couldn't do that with my dad.

- ***Attributing negative intentions to others***

NEGATIVE THOUGHT

My kids are trying to manipulate me.

POSITIVE ALTERNATIVES

They just want what they want and are trying to get it.

They are not old enough to be crafty and manipulative.

It's OK that they are trying to persuade me, and it's OK for me to say no.

Mindfulness. Through becoming more aware of your thoughts in everyday situations, you'll get better at catching the ones that cause you stress—and then letting them go. We also recommend you try meditation: in addition to being wonderfully relaxing and a proven method of lowering blood pressure, it's a great way to practice observing the stream of thoughts and feelings, like an endless train passing by, without jumping on board (please see the box on meditation opposite).

Pinning down the sources of stressful thoughts. You've probably noticed that stressful thoughts bubble up from particular sources in your mind, such as the inner critic that often gets louder when a woman has children. Many of these sources lurk in the shadows, outside of your conscious awareness. Shining a light on where a thought comes from helps you judge its credibility, much like you'd be skeptical of a news bulletin about the wonderful health benefits of one brand of infant formula when you found out it comes from the manufacturer; thoughts from certain sources in your mind should be considered guilty until proven innocent! As soon as you can identify where a stressful thought comes from, you have a head start on letting it go. Sources of stressful thoughts include:

- *Beliefs about motherhood.* You could look back on the hopes and dreams for motherhood and family you had during your first pregnancy. Were any of those unrealistic and worth letting go of today? You might also list, in your mind or on paper, some of the beliefs about how a mother *should* be that give you stress, such as *A good mother never gets angry at her children* or *I should always look as put together as my mother did.*

- *Gender.* Volumes have been written on how being a woman or a man shapes the way a person thinks. For example, women often add to their stress by telling themselves that they are responsible for the feelings of others. Take a moment to reflect on the messages you got as a girl from your parents, other people, or our culture about how you were supposed to be. How have these messages affected your thinking in ways that increase your stress?

- *Temperament and mood.* If you tend to be cautious or anxious, your thoughts will overstate problems and underemphasize how well you can cope. If you are inclined to depression or sadness, your thoughts are more likely to contain themes of loss, defeat, or helplessness. If you often feel aggressive or irritable, you'll have more thoughts about how other people are challenging or threatening. When you understand these things about yourself, you can routinely put in a correction factor, like: *I know I'm in a*

Meditation

Meditation has been practiced in various forms for thousands of years. You may already have tried meditating. If not, we can suggest a simple yet fundamental method:

Find a comfortable place to sit in an upright position, perhaps on a pillow or chair. Set aside twenty minutes or more if you can; even five minutes could be helpful, though you will generally go deeper the longer you sit. Try meditating for one minute if much longer seems overwhelming.

Close your eyes and take a big breath. Roll your head around, or otherwise adjust your position to feel comfortable. Sweep your attention through your body and relax any tension.

Breathing in and out through your nose, focus on the physical sensations of the breath, your belly rising and falling, the air going in and out of your throat, the coolness of the exhalation on your upper lip. Let your focus on your breath be a kind of anchor that enables you to witness the waves of passing thoughts and feelings without getting caught up in them. You need not struggle with this stream or try to control it. You are only being with it, letting it come and go, focusing on your breath.

If you do get swept along, no matter, it happens to everyone who meditates, and just return your attention to the breath. It may help center you to count your breaths for a while, from one to ten, and then start over; if your attention wanders before you get to ten, just start the count again.

As the minutes pass, you may find your thoughts quieting and a sense of spacious peacefulness emerging, like the way sediments in a pond settle to reveal clear water. But if this doesn't happen at first, it's all right: it will with practice and time.

When the moment comes to end your meditation, you can return gently to the outer world, sitting for a moment longer with your eyes open, breathing, letting the experience linger. As you meditate more regularly, this sense of peace will stay with you during your day.

bad mood today, so of course everything looks like a huge problem. But it's really not.

- *Subpersonalities.* The mind is like a big committee—though sometimes it may seem more like a zoo! All of these "subpersonalities" are trying to help you, but some of them just increase your stress, like the one that says your home has to look perfect before anyone can come over. By understanding your subpersonalities, you'll be more able to detach from those that wear you down. You can tune into a subpersonality by imagining that part of yourself and then asking what it thinks, feels, or wants—as if it were a person in its own right. If you talk with it respectfully, its viewpoint will usually become less insistent, but if you argue with it, it will just stiffen or go underground. You can also imagine or write out a dialogue between two subpersonalities—such as the part of you that is ambitious for a career and the part of you that wants to stay home with your child—or even among several parts of yourself, such as the critic, the vulnerable child, and the nurturing parent, as you can see in the dialogue in the box opposite.

- *Beliefs from childhood.* We all formed many ideas and expectations when we were little that we still tend to apply unconsciously to ourselves and the world. For example, one of Jan's clients was the oldest of eleven children, a kind of junior mother to her siblings, and it has been hard for her not to assume that everything in her family today is her responsibility. It can feel wonderfully liberating to realize how a stressful belief from your childhood can be wrong at the present time. The thinking of a child draws conclusions from a handful of individuals and applies them to a whole world full of very different people; it presumes that the self is small and weak compared to others; it overemphasizes negative experiences (one scary time with a dog is more memorable than ninety-nine good ones); and it makes all-or-nothing rules that oversimplify the complexity of adult life. Today, you can truly afford to let go of those beliefs. You have so much more choice about who you are with, and you have so many more ways to take care of yourself. The world is safer, people are kinder and more trustworthy, and you are more capable than you've probably thought.

Taking in the Good

Now that you've seen how to let go of stressful experiences, we can explore how to replace them with positive ones. Every day has dozens of little opportunities—such as moments of pleasure, achievement, or love—to replenish yourself psycho-

Sample Dialogue with the Inner Critic, Vulnerable Child, and Nurturing Parent

CRITIC: Listen to that baby cry! You screwed up again. As usual!

VULNERABLE CHILD: I'm sorry, sorry, sorry.

CRITIC: Quit whining. You're pathetic.

NURTURING PARENT: Hold on here. She didn't make Susie cry. It's not her fault.

VULNERABLE CHILD: Yeah!

CRITIC: Yes, she did. She never feeds her right.

NURTURING PARENT: No way. The doctor said she was doing a great job.

CRITIC: It doesn't matter. It's her job to do everything right.

NURTURING PARENT: EVERYTHING???!! That's nuts. She's doing great as a new mom, so shut up.

CRITIC: I'm just trying to get her to be perfect.

NURTURING PARENT: She IS a perfectly good mother already. Every mother has to learn things, and it's only harder when she is getting yelled at by you.

CRITIC: She still shouldn't have let the baby cry.

NURTURING PARENT: She absolutely did not "let" the baby cry! All babies cry, no matter how perfect their mothers are. Susie just woke up and wants some love. See, she's settling down, Carol is really helping her. She's doing a great job. As usual! I know you're trying to help, but you're over the top. Get off her back!

logically. Each of these is an oasis where you can rest briefly and refuel yourself for the challenges ahead.

Since mothers are supposed to be self-sacrificing, it might feel wrong to savor the good moments. But letting yourself enjoy them does not take anything away from anyone else. Try to be aware of any reluctance to linger with a nice experience, such as thinking you are supposed to be on the go every second. Or resistance to accepting a compliment, as if that would be vain or, *If they really knew the*

I see women's spirits getting weaker and weaker when they don't fill their pitchers up, when they don't recharge.

—Shoshana Bennett, Ph.D., Founder, Postpartum Assistance for Mothers *truth about me they wouldn't be so nice.* Or discomfort with receiving recognition or love, as if that would make you seem needy. You can use the methods you've already learned to let go of these like you would any other negative thought or feeling.

Throughout your day, really try to pay attention to positive events. For example, notice everything you're accomplishing. Or has your child been especially cute, your partner acted supportively, or someone praised your work? Try to infuse ordinary events with positive meaning. For example, it is possible to see making a meal or folding laundry as gifts of love that can make you feel good about yourself, not merely as repetitive chores.

We're not talking about million-dollar moments, but the small change of everyday life. In a fundamental sense, the person you are is the distillation of all the experiences you've ever had. By consciously putting new, good ones in the emotional memory bank each day, you build up an increasingly positive balance.

So when a tasty dish is set before you, dive in with a big spoon! As your day unfolds, make sure that positive events register as positive *experiences.* Stay with those experiences a few seconds or minutes longer than you normally would. Let your body relax around the good feelings, be filled with them, and soak them up like a sponge. If you like, you could imagine that they are being placed in a treasure chest in your heart, and you can take them out and feel them again any time you want.

You could also set aside specific times for reflecting on the good things in your life. For example, you might like to do a brief meditation at the end of each day in which you look back for happy moments and successes, and then allow these to sink in. Or you could do this through writing in a journal (please see the box).

Out with the Old, In with the New

Going a step further, you could actively dislodge old, bad experiences from their places in emotional memory by replacing them with new, good experiences. One mother offered this example: *Growing up, people told me I wouldn't amount to much. So when Jorge's nursery school teacher told me I was a good mom, I just brushed it off. "No," she said, "I really mean it, I've watched you with him for a year and I can see that you are really good with him." We were alone in her office, she put her hand on my arm, and I started to cry. I was embarrassed, but she was so sincere I decided to believe her. Something melted inside me, and I realized that I did at least one thing in my life right, and I have felt better about myself ever since.*

All you have to do is be aware of both experiences at the same time—the

A Journal for a Mother

Many mothers have found that keeping a journal is a wonderful way to create a record of this special time. It's also a good way to carve out a specific occasion each day for reflection and renewal. Sometimes it even helps you work through an issue. You may already be experienced with keeping a journal. If not, here are some suggestions:

- Pick a blank journal to write in that feels friendly and comfortable, unless you prefer to write on a computer or typewriter. Make sure your privacy will be respected so you can express yourself freely. And try not to be judgmental about what you say or how it all comes out.

- In addition to writing about whatever comes to mind, you might like to reflect regularly on questions such as: What did I accomplish today? What was enjoyable? What's one way I was a loving, skillful mother? What did I learn or how did I grow?

- Explore different styles of self-expression, such as poetry, drawing, dialogues between parts of yourself or between you and another person, letters that you will never send to your partner, mother, or others, and so on.

- Some people like to re-read what they wrote that day, or periodically look back at entries from months or years before.

- There are many lovely books about journaling, such as *Keeping a Journal You Love* by Sheila Bender, *Leaving a Trace* by Alexander Johnson, and *The Artist's Way* by Julia Cameron.

present, positive one and the old, unpleasant one—and let the new one be a more powerful experience than the old. Then you'll have an internal sense of the good, current experience dissolving and replacing the painful, old one, of finally getting fed where you are hungry inside. You'll be giving yourself today some of what you didn't get, but should have gotten, as a child.

In particular, try experiments in which you do something out of character that challenges a negative belief, and observe the results. For example, if you normally feel nervous about being assertive, because deep down you expect to be punished for it in some way, you could try being one notch more direct, blunt, or forceful with your partner, a friend, or a coworker. If the experiment goes badly (but make sure it's a fair one!), maybe the old belief is true after all. If it goes well—which is what usually happens—then let the good news sink in. This process is probably the single most effective method of personal growth we know, and every day has opportunities to use it.

Cultivating Positive Experiences

In addition to taking in the good experiences that come your way in the natural course of life, you can create new sources of positive experiences.

A regular personal practice. The options include spiritual or inspirational reading, meditation, yoga, prayer, writing a poem, attending twelve-step meetings, knitting, art, crafts, exercise, a peaceful walk with the dog, or simply a long bath. Whatever form it takes, a personal practice creates an experience—often a profound one—that routinely nourishes you. Perhaps you had a practice that fell by the wayside once children arrived; if so, it could be time to take it up again or find something else that's doable in the life you have today. And if you've never had a personal practice, we strongly suggest you develop one that works for you.

Rather than taking on something too ambitious that fades out in a few weeks, it's better to have a modest practice that you can stick with most days. Some mothers wake up a little early in order to have a quiet time to themselves in the morning, and that might mean making sure you get to bed at a sensible hour the night before. Your partner may be willing to take care of the kids at a regular time while you do your practice; you could exchange the favor, or he might simply be happy to support you in this way with nothing wanted in return. Or you could trade with another mom to watch the children.

Once you start raising a family, you have to make your practice a priority, or it will be pushed aside. Finding other people with a similar interest—such as in a church, reading group, or art class—is a good way to help yourself stay committed, plus it enriches the whole experience. But they need to understand that you've got other commitments as well, and there may be times when you can't join them.

Reaching out to others. Studies have shown that one of the most powerful ways to reduce stress, especially for a woman, is to have the experience of feeling connected to another person. If you don't have them already, try to form friendships with people—especially moms—who you'd be comfortable talking with when your stress meter starts redlining. Perhaps you could think of someone who's called you during a hair-on-fire moment; she would probably be understanding and supportive if you gave her a ring when you're feeling frazzled. You don't even have to talk about whatever it is that's stressing you—just being able to chat will probably help you feel a whole lot better in a few minutes.

Since raising a child today is often quite isolating, especially if you're a stay-at-home mom, it can help to think systematically about how you could connect with other people. An obvious place to start is with your relatives; for example, having a baby brings many women closer to their mothers. On the other hand, relatives can also meddle and criticize. Paradoxically, knowing that you can close the door to unwanted comments or advice enables you to open up to relationships with your family and in-laws. If someone starts saying something you'd rather not hear, remember that it's *your* child, that you understand him or her better than anyone else in the world, and that it's all right for your parenting values to differ from those of the other person.

Neighbors are another good source of companionship and practical support. If you're not meeting people in the natural flow of your day, you might need to go out of your way to strike up a conversation. You could invite neighbors over for a casual meal, or see if there's a neighborhood association.

Playgroups, babysitting co-ops, and mothers' clubs are great ways to meet other parents. To connect with one of these, ask around, look in the phone book— or start one yourself! Nursery school parent associations, sports activities (e.g., soccer, T-ball, gymnastics, martial arts), or youth groups such as Tiger Cubs are similar opportunities to get to know new people.

Of course, you can meet people in situations that don't have anything to do with parenting. These include religious and civic organizations, charities, environmental groups, and so on. Fundamentally, whether you're shy or outgoing, there are many ways develop a greater sense of community with others.

Scheduling good times. If you do not make time for fun and enjoyment, the world and your children and partner will claim every second you are awake. There are lots of ways to grab a little time for yourself. For instance, a patient of Jan's told her: *After I've dropped Jason off at nursery school, I'll come home, make some eggs and toast, and then sit down and eat my breakfast alone. It's just this little ritual I perform for myself. It seems so basic, but what makes it special is doing it in peace and taking the time to really enjoy it, as opposed to gulping down breakfast cereal with the kids at the table, all the while trying to remember if I put the extra cookie in their lunch.*

You could make a deal with your partner about breaks for each other, perhaps for half an hour in the evening, or for several hours each weekend. For example, one of Ricki's patients has a monthly dinner "with the girls" in which they all get dressed up and go out to a nice restaurant.

And you could make sure there are times with your kids that are especially enjoyable for *you*. Make a mental list of what you most like doing with your children, and go out of your way to do those activities on a regular basis. Plus dream up a wish list of new things you'd *like* to do with your kids, and then do at least some of them. It doesn't have to be a big-ticket item. At a talk Rick gave, one mother laughed when she said, *My dream is to go shopping at Wal-Mart with my kids WHILE MY HUSBAND WATCHES THEM!*

Focusing on being, rather than doing. Sure there's a lot to do, but you might be running around like the Energizer Bunny much more than you need to: maybe you've got a perfectionistic streak, or you may think you need to "make it up to my child" if you feel guilty about needing to work, or you might stay busy as a way to avoid certain feelings.

The Enjoyment of Being

Consider these questions:

When you are busy doing, what do you feel like? Energized, numb, tense, driven, productive, weary?

What inside you draws you into the role of a doer? A sense of duty? Habit? A reluctance to ask others to do more? Concern about what people might think if you do less?

Try these suggestions:

Consider your worth to others in terms of who you are rather than what you do.

Try being more of a benign and loving presence, a humorous and supportive observer, and let others do more of the problem solving and task accomplishment.

Try an experiment for a week: set aside a time each day, twenty minutes or more, when you can just be with your child without trying to accomplish anything. What happens, and how does it feel?

Ask each person in your family to start doing one small thing that you've done in the past, so that you can do one thing less.

I don't think the quiet mind is very far away for anybody.

I don't think the place of stillness is very far away for anybody.

It doesn't matter whether you're chopping wood or sitting on a meditation cushion.

It doesn't matter whether you're in intensive retreat or you're living a very creative and vital life. What's important is that your home is in stillness.

—Christina Feldman

Every so often, we hope you get a chance to stop all that doing for a bit. Perhaps the In Box is empty, the baby's asleep, the bills are in the mail. The urgency of the daily round falls away and a quiet fills the air. Your thoughts slow down, no longer grabbed and jostled by tasks. You are present in *this* moment, not worried about the future. You feel freer, less bound by your burdens, less limited by your roles. The edges soften. Each breath comes like a wave on the seashore, rising and falling, the ocean abiding. There is peace, contentment, warmth, and happiness, just here, just as you are. In this state of mind, you can do tasks as well, but the pot gets stirred or the phone answered in a way that feels much less stressful.

As you relax doing, you will usually experience a growing sense of your innermost being. This core of the self is a fundamental property of the human nervous system. It may be overlooked, but it cannot be tainted or destroyed. All you can do is to uncover it, to allow it to come forward into your daily life. It is always loving, peaceful, and wise, a bottomless well of clarity and strength, detached from the daily craziness, a refuge of nourishment and quiet humor, your own true self.

Experiencing the fact that the essence of your personality is not what you might secretly fear it is provides instant stress relief. Your essence is not bad, unlovable, dreary, empty, or stupid. It is, in fact, radiant with goodness, beautiful to others, and deeply intelligent.

Essential being is an extraordinary resource for anyone, but especially for a mother. In the turbulence of the typical day, your innermost being is a place to watch the storms within you, or between you and others, swell and crash and blow over. From within your being, compassion comes naturally for family and friends, all living things—and for yourself. It lets you hold your own sorrows and pain with a tender concern, helping you remember that you are doing the best you can, that you have already come through a lot simply to stand here today.

For many people, their essential nature is also a window within to the Divine, and they feel most available to God when grounded in their deepest being. One does not need to believe this in order to reap the benefits of cultivating a depth of being. But you may be a person who feels that the spark of God is what gives your essence its light, providing the most profound form of nurturance in your life.

Whatever your spiritual orientation may be, including none at all, a child can help awaken a sense of your innermost being. Children arrive, in the words of Wordsworth, "trailing clouds of glory." The eyes of a child are radiant with a mysterious illumination, and a mother can always replenish herself by letting in that light.

There is no pleasure in having nothing to do; the fun is in having lots to do and not doing it.

—Mary Little

Key Ideas from This Chapter

- Your inner experience matters in its own right, plus nurturing yourself is the foundation of caring for your children.
- The accumulation of moments of stress makes a world of difference, so do small things throughout the day to keep your stress meter out of the "red zone."
- More fundamentally, systematically focus on letting go of stress in your body, mental images, emotions, desires, and thoughts. For example, try to let go of unrealistic expectations about the sort of mother you are "supposed" to be.
- You can be active in your own mind, ultimately in charge of it, like the skillful rider of a high-spirited horse.
- Try to accept your inner experience for what it is; there is nothing shameful about whatever arises unbidden in the mind: accepting it is not the same as acting on it.
- Reflect on how your childhood is affecting you today; bring compassion to the young parts of yourself; try to sort the intensified "young" reactions from the more moderate, here-and-now ones; try to let go of the deepest, youngest level of an upset, like making sure you get the tip of the dandelion's root to prevent it from growing back.
- Let positive experiences sink deeply into your emotional memory banks, soothing and even dislodging negative ones.
- Commit to daily practices, like meditation or journaling, that nurture you and deepen your capacity to stand apart from the inevitable, endless ups and downs of your inner and outer worlds.
- If it's meaningful for you to do so, you can nourish and draw on a spiritual awareness in the middle of raising your family.

Transforming Painful Emotions

Insanity is hereditary—
you get it from your children.

—Sam Levenson

CHANCES ARE PARENTHOOD HAS BROUGHT ON some of the most intense feelings you've ever had. Suddenly everything's different: you have awesome new responsibilities and in so many ways you aren't the person you used to be—and you will never be her again. It's easy to feel that your emotions are happening *to* you, that you've got no control over them. But in fact, a century of psychological research has discovered numerous ways that you can consciously change how you feel.

In this chapter, we'll be looking at methods for turning around feelings of sadness, anxiety, shame, and anger. Since motherhood can be both numbing and emotionally chaotic, it's sometimes hard to know *what* in the world you're actually feeling; take a look at the box on page 61 for a map to the landscape of your emotions. You can focus on the sections in this chapter that fit your emotional concerns, and within each one, we'll cover a range of difficulties, from mild to severe.

Turning Sadness into Contentment

Feelings of sadness, including depressed mood, are common among mothers. For example, at least one in eight will experience clinical depression, and some studies have found that roughly half the mothers of young children today will suffer many of the symptoms of dysthymic disorder (milder but more chronic depressive feelings). Everybody feels sad sometimes, just like some days are cloudy, and often your mood will change on its own. But when an emotional "low front" settles in and stays with you longer than it should, it's time to take a more active approach for the sake of your well-being.

Mourning Your Losses

Most women would say they're supremely grateful they had kids, that they could never have imagined how wide open their hearts would become, that their children have brought an inexpressible richness to life. But that doesn't mean there aren't always losses as well, whether it's needing to put a hold on your career, less closeness with your partner, or simply never having a free hour to yourself. Mothers often find it very hard to give way to the feelings they have about such losses, if only because they think that would be selfish or self-pitying. But those emotions can't simply be brushed over or they will drag your mood downward. Each of us needs to acknowledge losses and allow the feelings that come with them to flow and be released in a healthy way.

In the box on page 63 you'll find a six-step process for letting go of feelings of loss. You can do these steps in one sitting, or spread them out over several days or weeks. Feel free to adapt them to suit your own needs.

Unlearning Helplessness

Because there's so much about mothering that's beyond anyone's control, a mom can begin to acquire a sense of "learned helplessness," a feeling of powerlessness and pessimism that lowers her energy and mood, and makes her feel less confident about taking action to solve her problems. Many studies have found that learned helplessness is a powerful source of depression. The antidote is "learned optimism," an attitude that focuses on what you *can* do, on your successes, and on the future. With learned optimism, you believe in yourself and your ability to make good things happen either out in the world or inside your own head. It's a self-fulfilling prophecy: when you think there's a fair chance you'll succeed, you're more willing to try.

Therefore, *try to pay attention every day to the good news about:*

- *Yourself:* your positive qualities and virtues, your honest efforts, the results you did indeed produce, and the ways you've been true to your deepest values. For example, if you're feeling depressed about a hassle with your in-laws about where the children go for Christmas, you might focus on the patience you've shown, your sincere attempts to resolve the issue, the fact that you got people at least to agree that you'll spend Christmas morning at home, and that you've always been motivated by wanting the best for your children.

- *The world:* the resources available in your partner, extended family, friends and neighbors, other mothers, church or other institutions, libraries, and the natural world. For instance, if you feel stuck with a child care situation that isn't working well, you could think about the many other forms and settings of child care, including home day care, nursery schools, after-school programs, baby-sitting co-ops, swapping with other families, adjusting work schedules with your partner so there is more time to take care of your kids yourselves, or doing home day care yourself.

The Landscape of Your Emotions

Most of us experience just about every possible human emotion at least once a year, but some feelings are more of a "home base" to which we keep returning. To find out exactly where on the emotional landscape your mind tends to settle, you can use the techniques of self-observation discussed in the previous chapter. The major emotions come in many shadings and intensities, and here is a kind of map:

- **Sadness.** Wistfulness, loss, regret, hurt, the blues, moping, sorrow, grief, melancholy, depression

- **Anxiety.** Worry, obsessions, compulsions, apprehension, fear, dread, panic, terror

- **Shame.** Self-consciousness, embarrassment, guilt, sense of inadequacy, humiliation, worthlessness

- **Anger.** Frustration, irritation, annoyance, disdain, contempt, resentment, getting mad, rage, hatred

- *The future:* the positive scenarios that *could* realistically happen. Let's say that your three-year-old son is extremely stubborn and hates transitions. You might reflect on these facts: he will naturally become more flexible and easygoing over time, he will gravitate to friendships and situations that feel predictable and safe to him, and that's all right, and his strengths of thoroughness, determination, and caution will bring him success in school and adult life.

Learned optimism means redefining the game into one you can win, focusing on what is in your power to accomplish rather than what is not. Once you have goals you can succeed at, take some sort of *action,* either inside your mind or out in the world. When you're active, rather than passive, you feel better and you keep learning how to be ever more skillful at coping. For example, if you have to get up with your colicky daughter, you can use the time to fantasize about nice ways to refurnish the room when she gets older, or to come up with new funny songs to sing her. If you're tired of changing diapers but potty training your two-year-old is going nowhere, you could reframe your purpose to seeing if you can stay completely calm during a diaper change.

Talking Back to Sadness

Extensive research has shown that talking back to negative thoughts can actually lift a sad or depressed mood. We suggest that you track down your own depressive thoughts and come up with positive alternatives. Here are examples of several kinds of unrealistic thoughts to get you started.

- **Assuming there's nothing you can do**

NEGATIVE THOUGHT
I'm stuck in the house all day.

POSITIVE ALTERNATIVES
If the weather is all right, I can put Simone in the stroller and go for a walk.

If the weather is bad, we can go for a drive. Or go to a mall and window-shop.

I could invite some other moms to come over.

Even if I'm alone in the house with Simone, I can make that better by playing music, watching some TV, talking with a friend on a headset phone, or lots of other ways.

Mourning Past Losses

1. Look back at everything that has happened to you since conceiving your first child—at the changes in your body, career, friendships, finances, or marriage. Name your losses by listing them on paper or in your mind.

2. Write or think about the resources you drew on to cope with your losses. These include both external (e.g., friends, your mother, a savings account) and internal ones (e.g., patience, religious faith, self-knowledge).

3. Write or think about what you've learned or how you've grown from your losses.

4. Tell your partner or a trusted friend about your losses, how you coped, and how you've grown.

5. Imagine going into the safe room in your mind (see appendix C) and really grieving your losses. Or if you like, find a comfortable place in your home or outdoors and grieve your losses out loud. Either way, try to really let yourself go. Sense that the feelings related to your losses are flowing out of your body.

6. Imagine that the learning and growth related to your losses are sinking deeply into you, becoming a positive part of yourself.

- ***Feeling bad about things beyond your control***

NEGATIVE THOUGHT
Brenda keeps getting ear infections. I must be doing something wrong.

POSITIVE ALTERNATIVES
She's sick because of germs, not me.

I've done everything the doctor has said so far. I've taken really good care of her.

I'm very sorry she's in pain. Feeling concerned and sympathetic is natural, but getting upset is not going to help her.

- ***Assuming the future will be the same as the past***

NEGATIVE THOUGHT
My husband left me, and I'm never going to find another partner.

POSITIVE ALTERNATIVES

He's not the only man who has ever liked me; other men will like me, too.

I can put myself in situations where I'll meet good people. I don't have to sit home waiting for the phone to ring.

My next relationship will be better than the last one since I will look for a different kind of man, and I will use the things I learned from my marriage.

- ***Brooding about a loss***

NEGATIVE THOUGHT

I can't stop thinking that I'm missing important time with my son while I'm at work.

POSITIVE ALTERNATIVES

Being at work makes the time with him feel more special.

I know stay-at-home moms who get cranky with their kids because of all the time spent alone together; there are some advantages to Carlos because I work.

If I'm serious about spending more time with him, maybe I should stop obsessing about it and start figuring out how to cut back my hours.

Resources for Learned Optimism

Learned Optimism by Martin Seligman

The 7 Habits of Highly Effective People by Stephen Covey

Warriors Don't Cry by Melba Beals

The Little House on the Prairie series, by Laura Ingalls Wilder

My Left Foot by Christy Brown, or see the movie

Under the Eye of the Clock by Christopher Nolan

Star Trek II: The Wrath of Khan

Many Ways to Feel More Contented

There are many ways to break the spell of sadness on your mind. Here are some suggestions.

Enjoy your children. It's easy to get so caught up in the tasks of daily life that you can miss opportunities to enjoy your kids. But there are always at least a few occasions each day when you could take the time for an extra cuddle or linger a few seconds longer when they're being extra lovable. You can also plan activities that you particularly enjoy yourself, something besides knocking down a tower of blocks over and over.

Accommodate the changes in your life. There's a kind of wishful thinking in our society that says a woman can simply graft motherhood onto her old life with nary a change. But if you don't accommodate to the changes that children bring, it's like trying to hold back the tide. For example, you can't interact with young children with the same mind-set that propelled you forward in your career, keep your house like you used to, or (usually) get back your old figure. It's just not possible. Raising a family takes up *space* in a person's life. It has to replace some things and push others to the edges, especially during the years when your kids are little.

You can help yourself by seeing what, if any, wishful thoughts still linger in your mind about somehow returning to business as usual. Or unrealistic expectations about motherhood that you are straining to live up to. Or any ongoing underestimates of the new needs that have come with children. If you find any of these, you can use the methods you learned in the previous chapter, such as talking back to unrealistic expectations or letting in the reality of new priorities.

Laugh away the tears. Sometimes it's so awful it's funny. One mother told Rick: **I'd had a string of bad days, and this was another one. Just as I got the baby to sleep, I heard a noise in the kitchen. My boyfriend was on the phone in our bedroom, so no one was watching Tucker. I found him squirting catsup on the floor and fingerpainting with it. He looked up and smiled proudly! It was so ridiculous, I started laughing and laughing. We had to clean it up, but it was the first time I'd felt good in a week.**

You can draw on your sense of humor in lots of ways. Just taking a few big breaths while you smile gently can improve your attitude. You could try to spend more time with lighthearted friends or coworkers, watch comedies, or read a humorous book about motherhood. Perhaps imagine the weirder moments in your day as if they were scenes in a sitcom with a laugh track. None of these is a miracle cure, but over time they can help. And it's good for your kids to hear you laugh!

Shine a light. Bright light, particularly sunshine, can lift your mood, especially

P arents are often so busy with the physical rearing of children that they miss the glory of parenthood, just as the grandeur of trees is lost when raking leaves.

—Marceline Cox

"Top Ten Topics for Future Presentations
at Our Mothers' Club"

This was a tongue-in-cheek list of future topics offered to the
membership of a mother's club:

10. Breasts—Here Today, Gone Tomorrow

9. Hips—Gone Today, Here Tomorrow

8. Timesaver—How to Starch Business Suits So You Can Sleep in Them

7. Dinner in a Diaper—New Product Idea

6. 365 Meals You Can Make with One Hand

5. Sex After Kids—When, Where, How, and *Why?*

4. How to Turn Spit-up Stains into Fashion Statements

3. Styling Techniques for Unwashed Hair

2. Baby Talk—I Understand It, and It Scares Me

1. How to Stop the Crying—Yours!

if you get gloomy during dark winters. Try to spend more time outside during day-light, clean dingy windows, or pull the drapes back. Even brighter lights might help.

Get exercise. Regular aerobic exercise (i.e., three or more times a week, half an hour each time) will increase the serotonin in your brain and lift your mood, sometimes as much as an antidepressant would.

Keep good company. Few things can improve your mood like the empathy, kindness, and emotional support of other people; for suggestions on how to connect with others while raising a family, please see page 54. If you are wrestling with a loss, look into a support group; for example, most counties have groups for women who have become single mothers or who have lost a child. (Support from your partner is covered in chapters 6, 7, and 8.) And above all, really try to notice the support that's actually there for you, including all the little things; studies have found that *perceiving* support is a key to alleviating mental and physical distress.

Have some fun. A mother tells this story: *My sister came to town; Jeff watched the kids, and we went out to dinner. Afterward, on a whim, we stepped into a lo-*

cal jazz club. We had a great time, and it reminded me that a whole world exists outside of shopping for groceries or going to work.

How much fun did you have this week? If it wasn't much, make a list of activities you enjoyed before you had children, and think about how you could start doing some of them again. It's usually surprisingly easy; you just have to make a commitment to yourself, as one mom did: *I've always loved riding fast downhill on my bike . . . the feeling of the wind and the freedom are so exhilarating! But when I got pregnant, the bike went into the garage. Every so often, after Carson was born, I'd think wistfully about going for a ride, but there never seemed to be enough time. One weekend, though, I was feeling just blah, and sick and tired of being blah. I decided to get the bike out and to heck with everything else. Well, when I got going again, that old thrill came right back. I couldn't stop smiling. My whole mood changed. Since then, I try to ride every day, even if it's only down the street and back. It's a little thing, but it makes me feel so much better.*

Make a contribution. When you're depressed, putting out more energy is about the last thing you'd ever want to do. But by finding some form of community service—such as volunteering once a month to serve meals at a homeless shelter or tutoring a disadvantaged child—you'll feel good about yourself, spend time with other people, be distracted from your own pain, and even access a kind of self-nurturing source inside as you nurture others.

It will be gone before you know it. The fingerprints on the wall appear higher and higher. Then suddenly they disappear.

—Dorothy Evslin

Look on the bright side. When you appreciate what you have, rather than longing for or grumbling about what you don't, feelings of contentment naturally fill you. A mother told Rick a story about straightening up her six-year-old's bedroom one night. The usual debris was everywhere and she was grumbling to herself about him: *Why won't he pick up this stuff? Don't I remind him over and over? Why clean up at all? He'll just clutter it up again. I'm sick of housework.* Then she happened to turn over a *National Geographic* magazine whose cover showed a famine-stricken mother holding an emaciated, naked child. In an instant her perspective changed as she compared her own life to that of the woman in the photograph. She suddenly appreciated the dirty socks on the floor because they meant her children had clothes to wear at all. She thought about the other good things her family had, how they were safe and could enjoy life. Days later, when she was feeling down, she thought back on the realizations she had had that evening and became grateful again for her good fortune, which immediately helped her feel better.

Sprinkling moments of thankfulness throughout your day is like taking sips of cool water while working under a hot sun. Try to notice the little occasions of beauty, pleasure, or growth. You could say some kind of grateful blessing at a meal. You could tell another person what you appreciate about him or her, or about life in general. In the morning, you could take a moment to ask the universe or God for what you want, and then just before bed you could take another minute to appreciate what you've got. Or set aside more extended occasions to reflect on all the good things in your life (see the Mother's Meditation on Gratitude in the box).

Extremes of Mood

At one time or another, many mothers will experience forms of sadness that are so intense or chronic that they are in the clinical range. Please see if any of the descriptions below apply to you, and if one does, you should consult with a professional right away.

- *Postpartum depression (PPD):* Depressed mood continuing past the "baby blues" (three to seven days postpartum); suffered by at least one in eight mothers. Often accompanied by severe anxiety or panic, spontaneous crying, agitation, insomnia, obsessional thoughts, disinterest in the baby, or suicidal thinking. In the extreme, there may be psychotic delusions, often related to the baby. Making things worse, it is common to feel guilty about being depressed at a time when a mother is "supposed" to be happy.

  Good books and support organizations for PPD are listed in appendix B. After an episode of PPD has seemed to resolve, there may still be an underlying disturbance in the endocrine system, or unstable or low mood; these possibilities should be discussed with your doctor if you have ever had an episode of PPD.

- *Dysthymic disorder:* Chronically low mood that occurs during most of the day, more days than not, for at least two years. (But remember, you don't have to wait two years before seeking help!) Some days can feel OK, but then the dark cloud descends again. Often coexists with anxiety, feelings of guilt or inadequacy, brooding about the past, or major depressive episodes.

- *Clinical (major) depression:* Feelings of extreme sadness or despair lasting two weeks or longer, accompanied by hopelessness, fatigue, disturbed sleep or appetite, poor concentration, difficulty making decisions, feelings of worthlessness, withdrawal from family or friends, or suicidal thinking. When you add up the number of individuals who get depressed, the typical length of a depressive episode, and its impact on both functioning and experience of life, women worldwide are more burdened by depression than by any other health condition. About 8 percent of mothers are clinically depressed at any given time, and this rate jumps to 12 percent among women who

A Mother's Meditation on Gratitude

Set aside a quiet time during which you can reflect on some of the many things you could be thankful for. As a starting point, you might read the passage below to yourself or out loud, adapting it to your situation as you like.

There really is so much to be thankful for.

I am grateful for my children, for the delight and love they bring, for the sweet smell of their hair and the soft touch of their skin. For the first time they smiled at me or walked into my arms. For the meaning they bring to life. For receiving my love and lessons. For being their own persons, for giving me their own love and lessons. Having them at all is a miracle, and the rest is details.

I appreciate myself. For the love I have given my children, all the diapers changed, all the dishes done. For the long hours I've worked, the hoops I've jumped through to keep all those balls up in the air. For the efforts I've made, the many times I've stayed patient, the many times I've found more to give inside when I thought I was empty.

I appreciate my partner. For the ways he has loved me, the fun we've had together, the humor and the companionship. For the times of support, understanding, and sympathy. For sweating and suffering too.

I feel thankful for the life I've already had, for the good parts of my childhood, for everything I've learned, for good friends and beautiful sights. For the roof over my head and the bread on my table, for being able to have a life that is healthier, longer, and freer than most people have ever dreamed of. For this beautiful world, where each breath is a gift of air, each dawn a gift of light. For the plants and animals that die so I may live. For the extraordinary gifts of evolution I carry in each cell of my body, for the capabilities accumulated during three and a half billion years of life's presence on our planet. For the wonder of the universe, for all the atoms in my body—the carbon in my bones, the oxygen and iron in my blood—that were born in the heart of an exploding star billions of years ago, to drift through space, to form a sun and planets, to form the hand that holds this book and the eye that reads this word. For all that was in order for me to be. For grace, for wisdom, for the sacred, for spirit as I know it. For this moment, this breath, this sight. For every good thing that was, that is, that ever will be.

have recently given birth. Of course, the percentage of mothers who will *ever* be clinically depressed is higher than that. Also, the number of mothers who have depressed mood but do not meet the stringent criteria for clinical depression will be greater than those who are clinically depressed.

Depression is best treated through the teamwork of:

§ *You.* Sometimes the first step is the hardest: admitting to yourself that you are in fact depressed. But once you do, you can reach out to the many resources that can help you. Remember what worked the last time you were depressed; you probably found some things that helped, and there's a good chance they'll work this time, too. Stick with it, and you will almost certainly feel better.

§ *Your partner.* He can support you through understanding, extra help, affection, and encouragement. It might help him to read about depression in such books as *An Unquiet Mind* by Kay Redfield Jamison, M.D., or *Noonday Demon* by Andrew Solomon. He also needs to take extra care of himself in order to keep being supportive of you. (It's important, as well, to reach out to your friends.)

§ *A therapist.* There is more evidence that psychological factors cause depression than biochemical ones, and studies have shown that psychotherapy is as effective or better for many people than antidepressants (and without the side effects), plus generally more successful at preventing relapse. And a person can certainly take an antidepressant while going through therapy; a combination of treatment methods is sometimes more effective than either one alone.

§ *A physician.* Depression is a common complication of insomnia, chronic pain, illness, or medications (including oral contraceptives), and you should rule out these possibilities with your doctor. For the physiological treatment of depression, including antidepressants and herbs such as Saint-John's-wort, please see chapter 5. In general, depression should be addressed through a combination of social support, stress reduction, optimizing physical health, psychotherapy, and, if necessary, medication.

• *Bipolar disorder:* Fundamental instability in mood, marked by at least one manic episode. Features of a manic episode include abnormally elevated or irritable mood, decreased need for sleep, grandiosity, distractibility, racing thoughts or speech, bursts of activity or agitation, or sudden shifts in mood (e.g., from euphoria to anger).

Key Ways to Turn Sadness into Contentment

- Take time to mourn the things you've lost since becoming a mom.

- Pay attention to everything that's going well.

- Talk back to helpless, pessimistic thoughts.

- Keep your sense of humor and perspective.

- Make it a priority to get out and have some fun.

- Find support among friends.

- Take time to be grateful.

- Get professional help for depression or other mood disorders.

Bipolar disorder and major depression carry a serious risk of suicide. The death of a mother by her own hand is a devastating loss and a lasting wound for her children, and there are *always* better options. Psychotherapy and medication are highly effective, and people usually rally behind a mother when she lets them know she's really hit bottom. If you have been contemplating suicide, even abstractly (e.g., "the children would be better off if I were gone"), please immediately tell someone who cares about you as well as get professional help from a licensed therapist.

Turning Anxiety into Security

As a mother, you have a sense of total responsibility for the life and well-being of your vulnerable child. But you are unable to do much about many things that can affect him or her, such as diseases in other children, how other people drive, workplace policies, or your partner's moods. No wonder you sometimes feel anxious!

Even seemingly small matters can have large stakes, as a single mother with a five-year-old son described: *When I dropped Nick off at soccer camp, I realized I'd forgotten his shoes. The coach said he couldn't play without them, so I left Nick there and raced off to get some shoes, with his parting words ringing in my ears: "This is the worst day of my life." Instead of driving twenty minutes each way to home and back, I figured it was best to try some stores nearby. But nothing was open because it was Saturday morning. I got so nervous about all the time this was taking that I yelled at other cars, "Hurry up, move!" All the while I could see Nick standing alone on the sidelines, watching the other children, the minutes ticking by. I get so worried about letting him down: his dad has already done that big time, and I just can't stand the thought of me doing it, too.*

Feelings of anxiety can also be triggered or increased by experiences you had as a child. For example, Rick worked with a mother whose son's fiery temperament was just like her dad's. Even though she knew intellectually that Tommy was just a four-year-old, it made her body feel panicky whenever he got mad.

A heightened sense of vigilance after children is normal, Mother Nature's way of keeping your children safe from the local tiger. But anxiety that is "over the top" feels awful. It also wears on your body and mind, and it can lead you to be rigid, controlling, or overly cautious with your children. Let's explore some effective ways to feel safer and more secure.

Talking Back to Anxiety

One powerful method for feeling better fast is to spot the inaccurate, illogical, or overly negative thoughts that make you anxious and replace them with positive ones. By now, you're probably getting pretty good at this technique. Here are examples of the kinds of thoughts that tend to make mothers nervous, with some sample talk-back rebuttals. We really encourage you to try this technique with your own anxiety-provoking thoughts.

- ***Overestimating the chances of a bad outcome***

NEGATIVE THOUGHT
He drives faster than me, so the baby is not safe in the car with him.

POSITIVE ALTERNATIVES
My husband drives no faster than most other people, and he has never been in a serious accident.

He has driven many more miles than me; as a more experienced driver, he can afford to drive a little faster.

We have a good car seat, and he is always careful to hook the baby in. He has promised to drive extra carefully with the baby in the car.

- ***Assuming there's been a catastrophe***

NEGATIVE THOUGHT

They're late, they haven't called, something terrible has happened.

POSITIVE ALTERNATIVES

Maybe he was delayed getting Henry out of day care.

They've been this late before.

I know I tend to get worked up with worry, so I can't assume there is actually a real threat just because my body is panicky.

- ***Overgeneralizing***

NEGATIVE THOUGHT

Amy hangs back in kindergarten, so she won't have many friends growing up, and she'll be lonely all her life.

POSITIVE ALTERNATIVES

"Slow-to-warm" is a normal temperament. Amy is a normal five-year-old.

There are lots of slow-to-warm people in the world, and many of them have happy lives and good friendships. There is no reason it can't be the same for Amy.

Her teacher and I can probably help her find a friend in her class.

Retraining the Worry Impulse

Chronic worrying is a form of anxiety. It can become an almost automatic response, but the good news is you can retrain it. It just takes practice. Here are some of the best ways we know to change worried thoughts.

See the safety in the world. Try to make yourself pay attention to all the reasons why you *should* feel safe, secure, and confident. You could make a mental list of the resources within you (intelligence, character, determination, good-heartedness) or in your environment (strong marriage, savings, friends, etc.). Notice how things usually work out all right; remind yourself that people who have been there for you in the past are likely to be there for you in the future, too.

Be realistic. Try to think through whatever it is that you are worried about in a rational way. Ask yourself, *What's the chance of this actually happening?*

> We are, perhaps uniquely among the earth's creatures, the worrying animal. We worry away our lives, fearing the future, discontent with the present, unable to take in the idea of dying, unable to sit still.
>
> —Lewis Thomas, M.D.

Take action. Occasionally, worrying is just a disguised way to avoid acting. One mother was rueful as she admitted to Ricki: ***I think I'm obsessing about the different ways to get Jamie to sleep through the night partly because I'm afraid to just pick one.*** And sometimes we believe in a corner of the mind that worrying itself will ward off threats: ***If I relax about the baby, that's when something awful will happen.***

But it's only real action that will solve the tangible problems that are making you anxious. Perhaps talk through your concerns with your partner or a friend and make a plan for what you'll actually *do.* Being active rather than passive will probably help you feel better.

Cultivate an attitude of acceptance. The painful truth is that many of the forces that will shape our precious children's lives are out of our hands, whether it's the intellectual potential or temperament they were born with, the vulnerabilities in their bodies, or the accumulated effects of thousands of interactions with other children. There's peace in surrendering to this fact.

Don't overreact to your body. The brain draws conclusions about the world in part by reading the body's signals; in a sense, it reasons that "the world is scary because my body is nervous" rather than "my body is nervous because the world is scary." This kind of thinking helped keep our ancestors alive in the wild, but today it's like looking for road hazards by staring at the speedometer.

It's especially important for a mother to watch out for this tendency since depletion and stress make your body more reactive and "jumpy." Notice any inclination in yourself to be preoccupied with your body or hypersensitive to its sensations; if you find one, try to put in a correction factor in the other direction, such as ***I know I have a nervous stomach, so I need to remember that I should not assume that Ivy is really sick just because I feel queasy when I hear her coughing.***

Budget worry. Maybe it's reasonable to have the same thought ten times, but more than that has got to be overkill. Instead, make an appointment with yourself to worry. It could be an hour from now. If an alarming thought arises before then, tell yourself that you'll be open for business in a while, but right now the person who staffs the worry window is on her break. Or pick a specific period, say for twenty minutes each morning, when you will worry about a particular issue. Keep to that schedule and try to worry hard within it. For the rest of the time, tell your anxious thoughts that you will give them your attention only during their regular appointment.

Derail your train of (anxious) thought. Our worries often have a mechanical, repetitive quality, like a train going around a circular track. There are a number of ways to bring them to a halt, including snapping a rubber band on your wrist, thinking about something that requires concentration (like counting down from one hundred by sevens), repeatedly reciting a prayer or mantra, or shouting "Stop!" in your mind. You can do distracting activities such as making cookies with your toddler, playing a sport, or reading a novel (with a happy ending!). Simply focusing for a minute or two on some aspect of your environment, such as the grain on a wooden table or the steam coming off a cup of tea, is deeply calming. Or you could meditate (see p. 49), which has been shown to be quite effective in lowering anxiety. (If worrying keeps you awake at night, please see our suggestions about sleep in chapter 4.)

Settle your body. Breathing techniques (see p. 37), massage, or simply a hot shower can reduce anxiety and lift your overall mood. Cutting down on caffeine or eliminating it entirely could also make a big difference. Instead of coffee, try some soothing herbal teas such as chamomile or peppermint.

Talk it out. When you tell someone about your concerns, you get them out of your head and into the open where you and the other person can judge how serious they actually are. It'll make you feel better to hear that others have similar fears, and you can also find out how they handled them.

Dealing with Traumatic Stress

Lots of things with children will give your nervous system a jolt: a sudden yelp of pain from the other room, an unexpected call from the preschool director, a dog on the sidewalk lunging at your stroller, and so on. After a few minutes, the fright wears off, and everything settles back down to normal. But sometimes, the shock of an event, or series of related events, is so great as to be truly traumatic. For example, studies have found that mothers whose children have had serious illnesses or traumatic experiences often experience intrusive and intense images or memories, problems concentrating or making decisions, a heightened reactivity, or physical symptoms such as a pounding heart or headaches.

Though less dramatic than having a child in the hospital, other stressors can still have traumatic effects, as one mother described: *Mike and I got a baby-sitter for our first night out since Terrell was born. I went over all the instructions and gave her the phone number for the restaurant. When we got home, we heard the baby crying and crying. The baby-sitter said he woke up soon after we left and had been crying since, nearly two hours! Incredibly, she hadn't thought she should call us. I rushed upstairs and finally settled Terrell, but I felt terrible. Since then, I haven't been able to leave him with anyone but Mike. It makes me feel trapped in my house, but I don't care, I can't let it happen again.*

Even trauma that is not directly related to child rearing—such as experiencing abuse as a child, sexualized assault as an adult, or spousal abuse*—can cast a shadow over your life as a mother. For example, putting your child in a setting that's like the one in which you were traumatized, such as being left alone with a male caregiver, can make your heart pound. Trauma can also be vicarious, especially if you witnessed it as an impressionable child. One of Rick's clients saw years of loud, drunken fights between her parents, one of which put her mother in the hospital. She said that, *When my kids yell at each other, I feel frozen inside and far away. That's when it's really hard to just be a mom.*

If traumatic stress is affecting you, here are some ways to help yourself cope:

- *Really acknowledge the intensity and seriousness of what had happened,* rather than telling yourself that you are weak or flawed to have let it get to you.

- *Share your experience with others* who care about you. Besides helping you feel better, research has found that talking about a traumatic experience can strengthen your immune system.

- *Consider joining a support group,* such as one for adults who were abused as children, or for parents of children with serious illnesses.

- *Take extra care of yourself,* with good meals, plenty of rest, and time to relax. Try to maintain familiar routines as much as you can.

- *Seek professional help* if you feel panicky, troubled by intrusive thoughts or images, or unable to continue functioning in your job or family. Both counseling and medication have been shown to be quite successful with traumatic stress and other forms of anxiety.

Turning Shame into a Sense of Worth

It's easy to feel like you're falling short. Your kids think that *you* are the solution to every problem. There's more work to do in a day than anyone could possibly finish. Few of the people in the different parts of your life are really aware of the jug-

> Motherhood brings as much joy as ever, but it still brings boredom, exhaustion, and sorrow, too. Nothing else ever will make you as happy or as sad, as proud or as tired, for nothing is quite as hard as helping a person develop his own individuality—especially while you struggle to keep your own
>
> —Marguerite Kelly and Ella Parsons

---

*It is estimated that 7 to 38 percent of girls have been sexually molested, 25 to 50 percent of women will be the victim of attempted or completed sexual assault, and 25 to 50 percent wll be battered by an intimate partner. (These estimates vary because of the groups studied and the definitions used by researchers.)

gling you've got to do in the other ones, so it's hard for them to be understanding when you can't keep every single ball in the air. It's natural to think that your children reflect on you, as a mother related to Rick: ***We were sitting in the pediatrician's waiting room, my baby started to cry, and I couldn't settle her down. I caught looks from other mothers that made me feel I was doing everything wrong.*** And your own mother may be a tough act to follow; in a national survey, over half of the women said they were doing a worse job as a mom than their own mothers had done, compared to just eleven percent who thought they were doing better.

These seeds of shame find fertile soil in the minds of many mothers. Because girls and women are bombarded with messages that equate appearance and worth, the weight gain and shifts in your figure that are almost universal after having babies can lower your self-esteem. The demands of raising children can make it hard to spend time with your friends, diminishing the sense of worth that many women derive through social connection. One mother told Jan: ***Now I spend many hours each day with no one to talk to besides my baby. Before, there were lots of people to joke or talk with at the office, and just doing that reminded me in lots of little ways that I was making a difference.*** Trained as a female to put the wants of others first, and now putting your child's needs far ahead of your own, it is a short step from "my wants don't matter" to "my *self* doesn't matter."

Plus, each of us has personality characteristics that make a person extra vulnerable to the challenges to self-worth that come with children. Do any of these apply to you?

- You set high standards for yourself.
- You are easily mortified or humiliated by criticism.
- You depend on approval from others for a sense of worth.
- As a child, you received frequent criticism or abuse from parents, coaches, teachers, siblings, or other kids.
- You have a relentless inner critic.

Every mother feels at least occasionally embarrassed, self-critical, inadequate, guilty, or remorseful. A bit of this is inevitable in any parent with a conscience, since raising kids is such a complicated and difficult business that everyone makes some mistakes. But if you're feeling guilt or shame that's undeserved, it's no good for either you or your children. Getting unfairly critical or angry with yourself lowers your well-being, makes it harder to cope, and leaves a bruised sadness inside. Therefore, it's really important to feel as good about yourself as you truly deserve.

Talking Back to Shame

If you berate yourself for being less than a perfect mother, think about what you would do if you heard another person speaking to a friend or, heaven forbid, your child the way you speak to yourself. Surely you would stick up for your friend or your child; why not yourself? Here are a few examples.

- ***Linking your worth to your child's behavior***

NEGATIVE THOUGHT

Mark is melting down and people are staring. I'm a klutz as a mother.

POSITIVE ALTERNATIVES

Mark is out of line but I am not. I am not Mark.

Most people understand that kids from good parents sometimes misbehave.

People who know me think I'm a good parent. If strangers come to a snap judgment, that's their problem.

- ***Comparing yourself to your mother***

NEGATIVE THOUGHT

I'm just not handling things as well as my mom did.

POSITIVE ALTERNATIVES

My memories of my mother are those of a child, with little real idea of the mistakes that occurred out of my sight. I probably look pretty good to my kids, too.

She did not have to juggle home and work. She received more support from neighbors, relatives, and the community. She felt safe with us playing outside, and she didn't have to drive us everywhere. Considering what I have to deal with, I am actually doing very well.

- ***Feeling bad about being needy***

NEGATIVE THOUGHT

I need so much from my partner and my relatives. It's shameful that I can't manage on my own.

POSITIVE ALTERNATIVES

Mothers throughout history have always relied on tremendous support from others. That's the normal state of affairs, and that's what my child needs me to do.

Key Ways to Turn Fear into Security

- Replace anxious thoughts with hopeful ones.

- Retrain the worry impulse.

- Take action to change the things that concern you.

- Routinely relax your body.

- Get professional help for chronic anxiety or experiences of traumatic stress.

There's a nutty idea in our culture that everyone is supposed to be super-self-reliant. Most other societies emphasize community much more than ours does.

While I do get some help, the truth is that I handle almost everything on my own.

- ***Equating your fundamental value as a human being to your performance as a parent***

NEGATIVE THOUGHT

I blew it today when I yelled at Keith during his tantrum, and I feel like a bad person.

POSITIVE ALTERNATIVES

What I do is not who I *am*.

I blew it for about fifteen minutes. That's a tiny fraction of a life. And the part of me that came out is just a small aspect of my total personality.

I can repair what happened.

Forgiving Yourself

We all make mistakes. And the more complicated, ambiguous, and changeable the task—in other words, the more it resembles motherhood—the more mistakes we are bound to make. Most of them are little ones: forgetting to bring along snacks for a walk in the park, missing a meeting at the preschool, leaving a baby in a wet

---

Steps of Self-Forgiveness

1.   Name the thing that you feel guilty or ashamed about.

2.   Reflect on the total situation, including your part in it, and sort out in your mind what you are legitimately responsible for. Separate out the rest as beyond anyone's reasonable control, bad luck, or the responsibility of others. Regret may be warranted for those pieces of the puzzle, but not self-criticism, shame, or remorse.

3.   Take complete personal responsibility for what is appropriate. Notice any emotions that come with the sense of responsibility, such as sadness, relief, guilt, embarrassment, or shame. Let yourself truly feel them for a bit. When it seems right, let them go, using the techniques you've learned.

4.   Resolve to yourself what you will do about the parts you are responsible for. Sincerely decide how you will acknowledge your responsibility to others, make amends, or act differently in the future.

5.   Now, let in a sense of forgiveness for yourself. You've taken responsibility for your part, you've felt bad about it, you've figured out what you can do, and it's all right to move on. In your mind, you can tell yourself things like *I am forgiven for* _____ , or *You are forgiven for* _____ , or *I forgive myself for* _____ . You could imagine your children or partner forgiving you. You might imagine that a nurturing being of great integrity—perhaps a specific person such as your mother or a kind of guardian angel—understands everything that has happened and forgives you completely. Or, if this is meaningful to you, you could ask for God's forgiveness and allow that grace to fill your heart.

---

diaper for too long. But there isn't a parent alive who hasn't made at least one big mistake with a child, whether screaming and yelling, missing a safety hazard, or simply being too busy to really pay attention.

One of the hardest parts of raising children is watching ourselves make the same mistake over and over. It seems so unforgivable! But it takes time to change. There are four unavoidable stages in any kind of learning or personal growth, and we need to be easy on ourselves in the process. Let's suppose you've been snapping too harshly at your kids:

Stage 1, Unconscious Incompetence. You're not aware that there's a problem.

Stage 2, Conscious Incompetence. You realize you shouldn't be doing it, but you just can't stop yourself. This is by far the most uncomfortable stage.

Stage 3, Conscious Competence. The inclination to snap harshly still arises within your mind, but you catch it and do something different, like take a big breath and speak more calmly.

Stage 4, Unconscious Competence. The tendency doesn't even arise. Sometimes it's even hard to remember that you used to act in a different way.

The fact that change takes a while doesn't make you a bad parent. Errors come with the territory of raising a family, they are unavoidable, you are trying to correct them, and you deserve to be forgiven for them. If something is bothering you, you could talk about it with someone who knows you well as a mother, like your partner, good friend, or your own mom, and then ask that person for forgiveness. You can also forgive yourself, using the essential steps of self-forgiveness in the box on page 80.

Nurturing Your Sense of Worth

The factors that might make you feel guilty or inadequate—from frustrating struggles with a child to critical looks from other parents—are busy every day, so we think you ought to *actively* nourish your sense of worth. Here are some suggestions.

Carry a picture of yourself as a child. You take pictures of your children with you wherever you go, and one look is probably all it takes to feel a surge of love. But you were once such a little person yourself, and within you today is still a precious being that deserves to be treated with love and respect. One of the best and simplest ways we know to keep that feeling alive—of your innate worth and the need to be kind to yourself—is to find a picture when you were a baby or young child and carry it with you. You might put it in front of the driver's license in your wallet. Each time you reach for some cash or a credit card, that innocent little face will remind you that you are the same dear person, just older and more seasoned by life.

Appreciate your accomplishments. As you go along, try to pay conscious attention to the things you get done. And as a sample of a typical day, you could keep a running list one day of all the tasks you've completed, down to the details. Review it in the evening, maybe with your partner, to see the incredible number of things you take care of every day.

Meditations on Your Worth

You can do the mini-meditations below separately or in combination. Just find a place where you can be quiet for a few minutes, close your eyes, and begin.

- Think back over the last hour and recall as many things as you can that you accomplished. Think back over the past day or so and recall some ways you held your temper, had patience, were determined, or otherwise showed good character.

- Imagine how much you matter to your children. Think about the many ways they depend on you. If you went out of town for a week, what would be missing in their lives?

- Visualize one or more people who care about, like, and respect you. Take a moment to imagine each one of these persons speaking from his or her heart about your good qualities. Let it really sink in that you are seen and accepted, wanted and cherished.

- See if you can experience a sense of connection with these people or others. You could feel this in your body, or visualize lines of energy linking you together, or have an intuition of the philosophical and scientific truth that all seemingly separate things blur into and depend on each other. If you can, let that experience of connection extend from these individuals to other people, perhaps to the entire human race. Try to sense that you belong to that larger family. Finally, see if you can shift from looking outward at all these people to their perspective, in which they have a connection with *you*.

- In particular, imagine your connections with other moms, starting with those closest to you and extending ultimately to all mothers alive today. Feel how you are joined to these women by shared experiences and commitments. It is an honorable community, the wellspring of humanity, and you are a valued member.

- Let an awareness grow of your innermost being, inherently good and wise, your essential self. Nothing can taint that inner being or alter its quality. Let a sense of its worth fill you. In the deepest sense possible, who you *are* is that being, and its worth is your worth.

- You could imagine God within you and you within God. Sense that radiance as it is expressed through you, a profound source of your life's meaning and worth.

Take some credit for how well your children are doing. Unless something is terribly wrong, your children are thriving, and you have had a lot to do with that. From time to time, take a few minutes to reflect on the many ways you have nurtured and guided them.

Pay attention to positive feedback. Many times each day, your children, mate, coworkers, or friends offer you a compliment, appreciate your work, give you affection, or let you know they like you. It could be obvious—a child running to give you a hug—or implicit, like being asked to be copresident of your mothers' club. But in either case, it is sincere and real, and you deserve to take it in.

Ask for acknowledgment. This may seem a little bold, but there is no law against asking for legitimate recognition, appreciation, or praise. You could take the plunge with your partner or a friend and ask for some positive feedback about how you are doing as a mother. Or, if you're paid a compliment, say thanks and then ask if the person might be able to explain a bit why he or she sees you that way.

Reflect on your fundamental worth as a person. Take a minute or more every day as a small sanctuary in which you focus on the goodness inside you. You could also try one or more of the meditations on worth that are listed in the box.

Sticking Up for Yourself with Others

One mother of a bouncy two-year-old told Rick this story: **We were houseguests with my husband's best friend, his wife, and their three children. Their home is very nice, with lots of expensive bric-a-brac. I was a nervous wreck, keeping Lily out of trouble. The wife kept making little comments, always with this sweet smile, about how she got her own children to behave well. By the end of the weekend, I was ready to wring her neck.**

For some reason, all sorts of people—perfect strangers, nonparents, your mother-in-law, etc.—feel entitled to comment freely about how a woman could do a better job as a mother, yet they wouldn't dream of giving the same level of advice to a shopkeeper, plumber, architect—or father. There's a place for gentle suggestions if they're welcome, but unwanted advice contains the implicit message that whatever you are doing is wrong. That message comes through in other ways as well: nasty looks, criticisms from relatives, comparisons to other parents, and so on. Besides being embarrassing, these comments can prey on your mind, breeding self-doubt and a sense of inadequacy. Here are some useful strategies for dealing with them:

- Anticipate situations that are likely to generate judgments about you or your children. For instance, maybe it's wiser to leave the kids home with a sitter when you go out to dinner with your husband's parents.

- Brush off a comment with one of your own, such as *Yes, there are lots of ways to be a good parent.*

- Take pressure off yourself by postponing judgment about what was said. Later on, within your own mind or by talking with a friend, you can see if there is any wheat amidst the chaff.

- Ask your partner to stick up for you (if that's a problem, please see chapters 6, 7, and 8).

- Confront the comment directly. You can address the values that underlie it by asserting your own, as in, *Actually, John and I think it's more important for a child to feel loved than to have good manners.* You can back up your views with scientific research, such as *No, many studies have shown that going to babies when they cry helps make them more secure and confident when they're older.* If you have to, you can go right to the heart of the matter: *Mom, you did the best you could and I love you a ton. But, in some ways, I've decided to raise Sandy differently.*

- Tell the person commenting that you would rather not hear any feedback or advice unless you specifically ask for it.

- Remind yourself of several specific ways you are clearly a good mother.

Treating Yourself Well

We know many mothers who dote on their children and are loving with their partner but have a really hard time doing anything nice for themselves. For instance, Sasha, a mother of two, had worked nearly full-time throughout her kids' early years for a number of catering companies on an as-needed basis. When her youngest was still in preschool, the economy had a downturn and catering work dried up. She and her husband decided that she should not look for work for six months and be a full-time homemaker instead. She told Rick: *Even though I'm home, I still always have to be doing something. I make lists and check things off: Fold the laundry, call the dentist, get some milk. I feel totally guilty if I'm just sitting, even for a few minutes. I can't relax and read a magazine or call a friend. If I did, I'd feel like a goof-off.* Jenny laughed at herself in Jan's office while telling a similar story: *I love a sale, and I always get the kids stuff they don't really need. But I cannot bring myself to buy a new pair of loafers to replace the funky ones I've had for five years.*

Do you find it hard to do nice things for yourself? If so, we suggest you experiment with deliberately going against the grain; doing so will make a strong state-

Key Ways to Turn Shame into Self-Worth

- Understand the psychological factors within you that make you prone to feeling inadequate; try to get some distance from them, and even let them go.

- Stick up *for* yourself *to* yourself (e.g., talk back to shame).

- Actively forgive yourself for being human and imperfect, and for not changing overnight.

- Carry a picture of yourself as a child.

- Notice all the things you get done each day.

- Reflect on how well your children are doing and take some credit for that.

- Try hard to take in positive feedback.

- Stick up for yourself with others.

- Do nice things for yourself; if you act like you have worth, you'll start to believe it.

ment in your mind about your worth. For example, buy a bottle of luxury shampoo instead of your usual, more sensible brand. Tell the kids that it's your turn to listen to something besides Raffi. At lunch, occasionally splurge on some exotic appetizer. Try taking a longer but prettier way home from work, even if that means dinner will be fifteen minutes later. You don't have to eat with a video on every night simply because that's how your toddler likes it. Or get your partner to watch the kids Saturday morning while you take a long bath.

Turning Anger into a Peaceful Heart

Elaine had three children ages two, four, and seven, and she worked full-time as a computer programmer for a large brokerage company. She had been meeting weekly with Rick for several months, talking about her marriage with Dennis, before she felt comfortable enough to tell her deepest, darkest secret. Normally self-controlled and forthright, her voice was sad and hesitant: *Sometimes I get pretty mad at my kids. Like yesterday. I was making lunches for day care, and running late. I heard Leo and Nick start screaming at each other. Dennis had already taken Ariana to school, so I go into the living room and they're fighting over some stupid toy and Leo shoves his little brother and he falls and hits his head on the floor. I pick up Nick and just start yelling at Leo. He looks scared but I keep yelling any-*

way, I'm so tired of him pushing his brother around. He started crying and I stopped yelling. I got a little calmer and we talked about what had happened and how he couldn't hit or shove his brother. It was OK, but I felt upset for a long time afterward. The person I was most mad at for the rest of the day was me.

Let's be realistic: it's completely normal to get angry with your children. Or with your partner, the in-laws, the staff at preschool—or yourself. Studies have found that the more children a woman has, the more time she spends with them or doing housework, or the more hassles she has with child care or her kids, the more angry she's likely to be. There's no need to feel guilty about anger itself. The real question is, what can you do about it?

On the one hand, anger is a healthy emotion. It shines a bright light on things that should be different—like a child's incessant whining, a partner's broken agreements, or some stupid workplace policy that keeps you from your kids—and energizes you to try to change them. Bottling up anger numbs your other feelings as well, and it wears on your health. Acting like you are not mad when you really *are* is inauthentic and teaches kids to put on a false face themselves—not a good lesson.

On the other hand, anger takes you on an emotional roller coaster that stresses your body and can leave you feeling bad for hours. And no other emotion has such an impact on relationships. When Mom or Dad gets mad, that's scary and often overwhelming for kids since their parents are so big, powerful, and important. In a marriage, frequent anger is very wounding; after a while, anyone would start wanting to step back from a person who's mad a lot of the time. There's a saying that getting angry with someone is like throwing hot coals with bare hands: both people get burned.

Fortunately, there's a healthy middle path for a mom between tight-lipped self-censoring and boiling-over rage. In this section, we'll be looking at a number of ways to work with anger wisely, *inside your own mind*. (Chapters 6, 7, and 8 address anger in an intimate relationship.)

Stop Things from Building Up

We usually get mad in two stages. First there's the priming: tension, frustration, bodily discomfort, fatigue, gripes, etc., mount up like a growing pile of dynamite. Then comes the firecracker that sets it all off: *I got home from a hard day at work, the little one was getting a cold, her big brother was whiny and clingy, and the phone kept ringing. Then the garbage disposal stopped working and the sink wouldn't empty. That was the last straw. It's stupid, but I jabbed the drain over and over with the end of a wooden spoon, I was so mad!*

During the priming phase, try to defuse things *before* there's a blowup. Here are a few ideas.

Don't overgive. For example, don't agree to chair the annual fund-raiser at the preschool when you don't really want to and then resent it later. One trick is to imagine asking your future self, the one who will be stuck with the work, how she will feel and what she would like you to do. Another is to adopt the blanket policy of never agreeing to anything until you've had some time to think it over.

Blow off steam as you go along. Try not to accumulate a residue of irritation from individual interactions. Let's say you've just had the usual struggle to wash your daughters' hair. Before shifting gears into the next thing, you could rinse your face with warm water, do something loud and goofy with your child, or shake your arms and exhale vigorously.

Take a break before you get to the breaking point. Most people become quite frayed by the time they've been alone with a young child for three or four hours. Make it a serious priority to find some way, *any* way to give yourself a break before your pot boils over. Maybe you need to arrange a regular get-together with another mom, schedule some child care in the middle of the day, or use the video baby-sitter for half an hour.

Understand What's Making You Angry

When you're mad, there's typically more to the story than just anger. Let's say it's Wednesday after work, you're in the store with your three-year-old son, and all you want to do is get home, make some dinner, and relax. But he wants some candy, you say no, and he throws a major tantrum. People are staring, you feel mortified, somehow you get him out of the store and into your car, and then you really yell at him. In that moment, the intensity of your anger is at least a six or seven on a ten-point scale.

But now let's change some of the elements of the situation. Suppose it's a Saturday morning instead and you're feeling rested and relaxed. How intense do you think your anger would be in that case? Probably less: maybe one to three on the anger scale. Or suppose that you're at home, not out at the store, when he throws his tantrum; no one is watching you and you don't have to care what anyone is thinking. How angry do you think you'd be then? Again, probably less. Fatigue and embarrassment amplified your feelings by five or so points that had nothing to do with the actual seriousness of your son's misbehavior. And when you understand the "amplifiers" in your life, suddenly you're able to be a lot less mad.

Sorting out the various factors involved lets you see how much a situation is actually worth getting mad about. If it's really just a "one" or a "two," feeling any angrier than that is needless aggravation. This sorting also helps you protect your children or partner from getting blasted about things that don't have anything to do with them: it's not their fault that a coworker was a pain in the neck or you got stuck at the house waiting for a phone company guy who never showed up.

Let's see how to deal with common factors that add topspin to a mother's anger.

If you think your child is manipulating you. Manipulation involves deception, and most children below the age of seven or so have not yet developed the cognitive abilities required to be deliberately deceptive. Your child just wants what he wants, and you happen to be in the way. In the normal course of development, he needs to try different ways of getting what he wants in order to find out what works. When you hold your ground and say no, he gets a little lesson that he has to find a different want, or a better way of getting it. Of course, it could take dozens or even hundreds of repetitions before the lesson sinks in; in that case, the situation is definitely tiresome, but it's not manipulation.

If you see something in your child that you don't like in yourself. One of Rick's clients, Wanda, had grown up in a strict and traditional home, and she was always getting into trouble as a little girl for her tomboy ways. Over time, she learned to push down her more aggressive and independent parts and act like a highly "feminine" girl. Then, years later, she had a daughter herself. To her dismay, Tawny wanted to run around with the boys, yelling and building forts and sword fighting. She was blunt and outspoken with other kids, and had no interest in acting nicey-nicey just to get along. Wanda often felt deeply embarrassed by her daughter. She told Rick: *Part of me is rooting for Tawny, but another part is horrified, and it says a girl is just not supposed to act like that! In a way, I keep waiting for some big punishment to come down on her, like people yelling at her. Even though it never happens, it keeps making me nervous. So I'm always after her to be different. It's like I'm afraid of getting punished when she acts that way.*

By becoming more aware of the sources of her reactions to Tawny, Wanda was able to address Tawny's misbehavior for what it was without the added layer of being upset about her daughter's tomboyishness. She also remembered that it had upset her to have grown-ups angry with her when she was a kid, so it wasn't going to be any good for Tawny, either. When Tawny was pushy or too wild, what worked for Wanda was compassionate firmness, saturated in love for the wonderful qualities in her high-spirited daughter.

If you're prickly about any challenge to your authority. You are the ultimate authority until your child is eighteen, and he needs to know that. If you feel confident and matter-of-fact about your authority, you'll usually be able to exercise it without having to make a big deal about it. It sounds backwards, but reminding yourself deep down that you have much more power than your child, and that you have plenty of ways to make it stick, makes it less necessary for you to prove it. It's also healthy for a child to challenge his parents periodically in order to clarify the limits of his autonomy. Excess anger on a parent's part about that natural process slows down a young child's learning, and it often makes an older child or adolescent particularly oppositional.

If your partner is a lightning rod for your irritation with the kids. Some of this is inevitable, especially if you're spending long stretches alone with young children. It's just a lot easier for him to be a kind of shock absorber if you let him know that you're venting about the children, and not angry with him personally. And you can deal with your irritation with the kids directly, by doing what's possible to change things so they're less grating on you.

If your kids are a lightning rod for your irritation with your partner. Merely becoming aware of this usually makes it stop since it's about the last thing most moms would ever want to do. And it's a wake-up call to address issues forthrightly with your partner.

If issues with your job are spilling over onto your family. Please take a look at pages 325 to 332 in chapter 9.

If your childhood is getting mixed into your anger. Like getting really mad at one child picking on another because that's what happened to you. Or becoming tense and irritable at meals because your dad would usually be drunk by then. At this point, you know lots of ways to deal with childhood issues transferred into the present, so simply naming them to yourself will start you on a path of separating them from the here-and-now realities of your life and working with them in their own right.

If you're taking things too personally. Young children generally have no idea of their impact on their moms and dads. It's not realistic to expect the same empathy or consideration for yourself from your child that you would from another adult. Kids are like a force of nature; it's not *personal* when a bull knocks over dishes in a china shop.

And it's not just your kids. The intentions we attribute to others make a big difference in how we feel. An ancient Chinese parable says it well: *Imagine you are sitting on a small boat on a river in the fog. Suddenly there is a loud crash against your boat and you are tipped over into the cold water. You come up sputtering and see that another boat full of laughing people has intentionally run into you; how do you feel? Now imagine the same situation, the same crash and dunking, but this time you come up sputtering and see that a submerged log has drifted into your boat; how do you feel?*

For better or worse, the world is basically one log after another—whether it's your son's snit fit, policies at the preschool, or your boss's latest brainstorm—and none of it is about you personally. Even reactions that seem to be about you, such as a partner's criticism, were set in motion long ago, shaped by a biology, culture, and individual history that have nothing to do with you. Nobody likes getting whacked by "logs," and of course it makes sense to manage them as skillfully as possible. But if you can treat them more like impersonal facts, they won't make you as angry.

If you feel frustrated. Motherhood contains inescapable frustrations, and frustration is a major trigger for anger. For example, there's no way anyone could possibly do everything on your daily to-do list in one day; you can't pursue your career while staying home, but you can't be with your kids while you're at work; and you can't *make* your partner see it your way if he genuinely disagrees. All completely normal—and routinely maddening. One way to cope is to admit to yourself, and perhaps others, that you cannot change the situation: basically, you give up. Doing so usually brings a kind of peace. It also sends a healthy message that you can't do it all, and you shouldn't have to try. And it sometimes gets other people, such as your partner, to help out more.

Another way to cope with frustration is to lower your standards: if you're more willing for your son to wear yesterday's grass-stained jumpsuit, you'll feel less cranky about the seven interruptions that got in the way of the laundry. You could also focus your attention on what you are doing or could be doing to improve the situation rather than on the places where you're being stymied. Or think about the future when the source of frustration will have ended: most things involving children really do get better over time.

Put On the Brakes

If you've ever screamed at or spanked your child in anger, you know that sick feeling you get later, after you have calmed down and start thinking about what you've done. Reasonable people can disagree about corporal punishment (we believe there are always better options), but no reputable professional thinks it's fine for a parent to vent his or her anger through raging at or hitting a child. Besides wounding a child psychologically and sometimes physically, it makes a mother feel awful about herself. Instead, walk away from the situation, put yourself on a time-out, yell into a towel or pillow, or call your husband or a friend. If you still have trouble controlling yourself, you're not alone. Most counties have anonymous telephone hotlines running twenty-four hours a day for parents to blow off steam and get practical ideas about child rearing. These hotlines can also refer a mom to support groups or other community resources, such as low-fee child care.

In less extreme situations, you might like to consider taking up the practice, for a day or longer, of not speaking to your children in an angry way. We are definitely not suggesting that you suppress your emotions, but rather that you:

- Sense down to the more vulnerable feelings—like fear, hurt, or disappointment—that usually lie beneath anger, and focus your awareness on them.

- Express whatever might be appropriate to your children about these softer feelings by saying things like: *I feel really scared when you run ahead at the mall, like something bad might happen to you, and to me that would be the worst thing in the world.* Or: *I feel hurt and sad when you scream at me.*

- Do whatever you need to do in the way of correcting, reprimanding, or disciplining your child, but without losing your temper.

If you like, you can adapt this approach to your partner as well. No matter who you use it with, this practice will help you become more aware of the deeper feelings beneath anger, and more comfortable and skillful at expressing them. It's also easier for a child, or your partner, to let in what you have to say.

But we do not mean at all that you should turn anger toward others against yourself. Some mothers yell at themselves in their head, or even out loud. Some go further, pulling out their hair, abusing laxatives, or hitting or cutting themselves. If you ever do that sort of thing, please know that you are far from alone. Millions of other women have had similar issues, and feeling angry with yourself or ashamed for doing it just adds to the problem. As a first step, you should tell someone, such as a close friend, your partner, a parent or relative, or a counselor on a telephone hotline. But after that, please contact a therapist and get some professional help. The person in the world who least deserves your punishment is *you.*

Ask Your Heart

A client of Rick's told this story: *I was arguing with my husband about going back to work and he wanted me to stay home. I was getting madder and madder, but something else was happening, too. It was like a part of me was watching the whole thing very calmly. After a while, I ran out of steam, and for a minute there was just that calmness. Then I did something I'd never done before. In a way, I asked the calmness for what it thought. Immediately, there was the sense of an answer, that the right approach was to be strong and confident and just go forward with what I knew to be right without quarreling about it, just start looking for work with self-respect and see what I found and then make my decision based on what was real. I didn't just hear how I needed to be, I felt that way. He asked what I was thinking and I told him, while I was feeling strong and confident, kind of digni-fied. He grumbled a little but didn't blow up again, and he seemed to accept more what I was saying. I spent about a month looking around for work. Once in a while, I'd think back to the experience and feel that sense of strength and confi-dence again. I found a pretty good job and we talked about it. It felt right to me, and he got some of that feeling, too. I took it and I've been real happy that I did.*

Anger is like a storm at sea. On the surface, waves are roiling and spray is fly-ing. But deeper down, it's much calmer. At almost any moment when you're an-gry, you can look down there for wisdom and guidance. To make those depths tangible to yourself, we suggest you ask your heart what might be a better way to handle the situation that's making you angry. Just put your awareness into the area of your heart and imagine asking a specific question—*What should I say? What does she really need here? What would be best for everyone?*—or simply be open to your heart's perspective. Let both the meaning and the feeling of the answer fill you, pushing the surface froth of anger to the margins of your mind.

⌐

With the rush of changes and responsibilities in your life, it's no wonder you have some intense emotional responses. Sadness, anxiety, shame, anger: these come with the territory of deep caring for your family, but with just a bit of sus-tained effort, you can certainly keep them from overwhelming you. The truth is, there is fundamentally nothing you can't handle by reaching in for the strength that resides within you, and by reaching out for the support of others who care about you and your children.

Key Ways to Turn Anger into Peace

- Don't let things build up—don't overgive, blow off steam as you go along, etc.
- Understand the thoughts or ways you are perceiving things that are the true sources of your anger.
- Try to sense down to the softer emotions beneath anger, like hurt or fear; acknowl-edge those to yourself or express them to others.
- If you feel like you're going to blow up, walk away or call a friend.
- Get professional help if you are directing anger at yourself in harmful ways, such as cutting.
- Ask your heart for guidance.

PART THREE
Nurturing Your Body

Taking good care of your health probably feels like one more thing to add to your long, long list. It's often really hard—with everything else clamoring for your time and attention—to take the actions that would add up to long-term wellness. That's why the next two chapters have lots of options so that you can pick the ones that are the easiest to work into your life.

Chapter 4 focuses on prevention and on commonsense practices—like more sleep or better nutrition—that will keep you feeling well. Chapter 5 addresses what to do if you're already getting depleted and how to replenish and balance your nervous, gastro-intestinal, endocrine, and immune systems.

If it seems like your health has started to head downhill right in the middle of trying to raise a family, it's a horrible feeling. Your support may not be the greatest, and now your body is letting you down, too. Besides being scary, it's that much harder to push through for your children. Thankfully, there is a lot you can do to nourish and settle the very roots of your body, to prevent and to heal the drainage and dysregulation of depletion.

Staying Well

Health is a state of complete physical, mental, and social well-being and not merely the absence of disease or infirmity.

—*Platform for Action of the Fourth World Conference on Women*

ALANA, A THIRTY-THREE-YEAR-OLD REALTOR with two daughters aged six and two, came to Ricki for her annual gynecological visit. Alana showed off pictures of her children, whose red hair matched her husband's, and she laughed softly as she added, *They've got his feistiness, too.* Before doing the exam, Ricki asked how she was feeling, and she said, *Fine, I guess.* Alana paused, and Ricki could tell that she didn't want to seem like she was complaining or unable to cope, so she told Alana that raising her own young daughter had worn her out more than a hundred-hour-per-week obstetrics residency. *Yes,* Alana replied, *it's just been very physically taxing, like running myself to the ground, pushing my body to the edge of its capacity. For example, I hardly notice what I eat but I'm really careful about the girls. I stay up late to pay bills or just relax since it's the only time, but then it all starts again early the next morning. It's all making me feel more and more run down.*

Ricki nodded in understanding, having heard essentially the same story literally thousands of times before: a dedicated mom working harder than she ever has, with less time than ever to eat well or sleep or exercise, letting her own needs fall to the lowest priority. On most days, Alana was taking out more from her body's reserves than she was putting back in, so she was becoming gradually more depleted.

No one wants her experience of raising children to be shadowed by fatigue, nagging aches and pains, or emerging health problems. Not only is it a shame, it's also harder to function at a high level at home, at work, or in a marriage when you're running yourself into the ground. Many mothers have more or less resigned themselves to this condition, but the fact is that with only a few changes to your routine, you can be just as healthy after kids as you were before. The moms we know who stay energetic, avoid illness, and keep some reserves in their "health bank" do these essential things:

- Get enough sleep.
- Eat right.
- Exercise regularly.
- Keep a basic balance in their lives.
- Avoid health hazards like smoking.
- Have regular checkups.

Getting Enough Sleep

There's an old saying: *The journey of a thousand miles begins with the first step,* and the journey to health starts with sleep. Most people need at least eight hours of sleep each day; a person with a hardworking, stressful life—like a mother—usually needs even more, and it is vital to make sure you're getting enough. Insufficient sleep can lead to gastrointestinal troubles, a weakened immune system, and slow repair of strained or sore muscles acquired through routine activities like hauling children out of car seats. It also causes poor concentration and memory, lowers mood, and shortens a person's fuse.

When Your Children Are Little

If you've got a baby or toddler, these steps should help you get more sleep:

Ask Dad. There's no good reason why a father shouldn't cover a significant portion of the nighttime parenting, half if possible. Apart from breast-feeding, a father can feed, walk, or settle a baby just as well as a mother can.

Unfortunately, some dads try to make the case that they have to function at work so they should be let off the hook at night. But you also have to function during the day. If you work for pay, your job performance matters as much as his does, and if you stay home, your hours are probably more stressful than his are. Besides, the stakes in any day of parenting—the mind and heart of a precious child—are usually more significant than whatever is on the table at work. Twenty years from now, those projects and career moves will be long forgotten, but a happy and productive person will be walking the earth thanks to all the caring—

and well-rested!—attention his parents were able to give him. So, if anything, you need more sleep than your partner does.

If he doesn't understand this on his own, your best chance of getting your message across lies in feeling clear in your heart that he should pull his weight at night, and making your case in a serious and determined way. If he still won't help, that suggests larger problems, which are discussed in chapters 6 and 7.

Sleep when the baby does. If you are staying home from work, do your best to sleep when the baby does during the day. You may need someone to watch any older children. It may also mean cutting back on housework for a few months, but your sleep is more important than a tidy home!

Consider shifting the father's sleep schedule. Sometimes the solutions are a lot easier than we think; they just take a little flexibility and a willingness to try something new. For example, when their kids were little, Rick started going to bed early with Jan and them, and then got up at 4 or 5 a.m. to work or study. This helped Jan get to sleep soon enough to survive nighttime parenting, and it gave Rick and her time in bed with each other.

Ask your partner to take the baby in the early morning. You could get more sleep while Dad can spend more time with his child. Kids are often at their best first thing in the morning; even so, your husband may get some eye-opening experiences with what it's like to try to accomplish anything while tending to young children, which could help him understand better why the house isn't always picked up. After an hour or two, the baby might be ready for a nap with Mommy, letting you have a really long stretch of dozing or sleep. Again, this will take some arranging, but it's often a pretty simple change.

Tailor sleeping arrangements to the unique needs of your family. It's common to feel pressured to take the advice of experts or other parents on sleeping arrangements, but what's important is to choose a method that feels right to you and your partner. Each of the main approaches—baby in the parents' bedroom ("cosleeping") or down the hall—has its pluses and minuses. Cosleeping worked for Jan and Rick's family for years, yet Ricki found that both she and her daughter got more rest once Leah was sleeping sweetly in her own room. Let's briefly review the pros and cons of each approach (you can skip ahead if you've already made up your mind).

From the child's standpoint, cosleeping is usually the most desirable option. During our evolutionary history, youngsters who strayed at night risked being attacked by predators. Consequently, it's natural for young children to protest intensely when they are made to sleep by themselves, and for their parents to feel uneasy if they can't hear their child's breathing. Studies have found that cosleeping

There was never a child so lovely but his mother was glad to get him asleep.

—*Ralph Waldo Emerson*

is associated with children who are more likely to sleep better, be less fearful, handle stress well, behave in school, and be independent. There are also practical advantages. Parents often do not have to rouse themselves as much at night; many mothers barely wake if they roll over to nurse a baby, and their partner can sometimes keep sleeping. And one study found that the risk of Sudden Infant Death Syndrome (SIDS) in cosleeping arrangements was one-fourth as likely as down-the-hall arrangements when obvious risks were avoided (e.g., parental obesity, use of tobacco, abuse of drugs or alcohol, soft mattresses, or blankets that could be pulled over the baby's head).

On the other hand, having a child sleep in her own room may enable her to rest better if one of her parents snores. Mom and Dad will be awakened less often themselves by a child's gurgling, coughing, and snorfling. A mother and father have the need and the right to get sufficient sleep, and even if one were to focus strictly on the child, it benefits her to have well-rested parents. There is also more time for parents to talk and snuggle together alone, and more easy opportunities for lovemaking; moving the child out of the bedroom can be a kind of statement for the couple that their marriage has important parts to it besides raising kids.

The bottom line is that a particular arrangement may work for one child but not her brother, or for a parent at one time but not another. It's also important to consider the context in which sleeping occurs: other children, number of bedrooms, jobs, parental illness, and so on. You may be able to adjust one of those external factors, such as work hours, in order to have the sleeping option you'd like most, or you may realize that you have to live with a less-preferred sleeping arrangement for the sake of the greater good of your family and yourself. Your best guide is your own instinct and intuition, and don't let anyone—whether a know-it-all relative or a well-intentioned professional—talk you out of your deepest sense of what you, your child, and your family need. Nor is there any call to feel guilty: you will have thoroughly considered your options and made the best possible choice you could. Please see the boxes for tips on making either arrangement work for you.

When the Baby Is Sleeping but You're Not

Usually by the end of a child's first or second year, she's sleeping through the night (Yes! Yes! Yes!). But many mothers still have a hard time falling asleep in the first place, or toss and turn in the middle of the night, or wake up early and not be able to get back to sleep. There are plenty of effective steps you can take to sleep well again.

Making Cosleeping Work for Mom

- Try different options to find the one that brings you the maximum sleep:

  Child between mom and dad. Maximum snuggles with child, and prevents him or her from rolling off the bed. But most likely to keep parents awake and separate from each other, and may increase chance of SIDS if risk factors are present.

  On the other side of Mom. Allows parents to snuggle. Easier for Dad to sleep through nighttime feedings. But can make Mom feel she's solely responsible. If your bed is off the floor, child might roll off it.

  On the other side of Dad. Also allows parents to touch easily. Draws fathers into night-time feedings parenting. If you are bottle-feeding at night, Dad can do so as readily as Mom, and she can get some sleep. Same caution as above about child falling out of bed.

  In a crib near your bed. Creates more separation between parents and child, perhaps enabling each to sleep better. If a crib is placed next to your bed, one side can be lowered as long as the crib is firmly positioned with no chance whatsoever of the baby falling through the crack.

  On a futon or small mattress on the floor near your bed. Works even better if parents place their own mattress on the floor. Nighttime nursing is a simple matter, and babies are usually not roused by movement in their parents' bed. But make sure a family pet won't get on top of the baby.

- Your child's signals will often tell you when he'll resettle without you doing anything. In general, see if he can settle on his own. But if he needs some food or comfort, try to get it to him quickly, before he, or you, rouses fully, and then each of you can drift easily back to sleep.

- Cosleeping need not interfere with the parents' sexual relationship. Many couples are comfortable making love quietly, under the covers, while an infant sleeps in a crib or futon nearby. Or they find another location in the home. If a mother and father want to make love, they'll find a way, regardless of where the baby sleeps (please see chapter 8 for more discussion of sex after children).

- There are many ways to transition from cosleeping to down-the-hall. You can make the child's bedroom more inviting and yours less so. For example, Jan and Rick started out with their mattress on the floor next to comfy pads for each child (on either side); they ended up with getting nicer furniture for the kids' bedrooms, raising their own mattress off the floor, and the kids using thin pads. With a toddler, you can start putting her to sleep in her own room with the understanding that she can come down the hall in the middle of the night to crawl into a little bed next to your own. Bedtime routines can be elaborate and fun in the child's room, and boring in your own. You're the parent, you're the boss, and you can have it go the way you want.

Watching what you eat. Some moms feed the kids first but then eat a big meal later in the evening that can make their stomachs restless midway through the night; see if you can eat dinner at least three hours before going to bed. You might also try reducing or eliminating caffeine, especially in the latter half of the day. Alcohol may initially relax you, but it can wake you later on. Even chocolate isn't so good right before bed, since it contains caffeinelike substances. Finally, don't take stimulating supplements, such as B vitamins or ginseng, in the evening.

Then there are the foods that you *could* eat for a good night's rest: many people find that rice or warm milk helps them get to sleep.

Lowering your stress. Sleep disturbance is one sign that a person is overly stressed. For example, cortisol normally rises in the morning to prepare you for the activities of the day, but with too much stress, this hormone will kick into gear extra early, waking you at 3 or 4 a.m. The solution is to do whatever is necessary to lower stress overall (using the tools in chapters 2 and 3), and to try to settle down your adrenal hormones (see p. 187 in the next chapter). Other than a life-or-death emergency, nothing is more important for a mother than getting enough sleep.

Getting exercise. Exercise during the day or right after work can bring good sleep at night. But be careful about exercising in the later parts of the evening, since it can stimulate your body and make it harder to fall asleep.

Relaxing your body. One mother offered this suggestion: ***I find that taking a nice warm bath with my baby—and a little lavender in the water—relaxes us both. It's a signal to our bodies and minds that it's time for bed. Also, it "kills two birds with one stone."*** Once you're in bed, try one or more of the relaxation techniques on pages 37 to 38.

Using psychological techniques. These methods can help you sleep better:

- Do mentally restful activities during the hour or so before bedtime, like reading casually, watching TV, or taking a bath. Don't pay bills at night—or talk about them with your partner!

- Try to avoid arguments just before bed. You and your partner could agree that it's all right to table a discussion until the next day.

- Sit in a sleeping child's bedroom for a while, watching him or her breathe, and let your thoughts relax and wander.

- Meditate before bed, even for just a few minutes.

- Keep a pad and pen by your bedside to write down any thoughts or reminders for the next day, so you can get them out of your head.

- If nagging worries push forward in your mind when you settle down to

Making Down-the-Hall Work for Mom

- Get a baby-room sound monitor and place the speaker next to the person who is "on duty" each night, hopefully Dad some of the time.
- Decide if you want to let yourself fall asleep in the child's bed (assuming it's not a crib), either when you put the child to sleep or if you get up at night to settle her back to sleep. It's cosleeping, albeit in the child's bedroom, with the pluses and minuses of that arrangement. Some men feel abandoned or miffed if their partner falls asleep with the child, and some mothers do so to avoid dealing with their intimate relationships (though Rick has seen couples in which this pattern is reversed).
- If you are not getting in bed with the child, place a comfortable chair next to her bed. Try not to crouch or hold the child in an awkward position, since you risk throwing your back out—not uncommon among mothers whose backs have been weakened by overwork and depletion.
- Make the child's room pleasant and peaceful for you, since the two of you are going to share it some of the time. Lovely pictures and night-lights, sweet-smelling sachets, or soft pillows can help you feel nurtured at night.
- Have the time with your child be as soothing as possible for you, not just her. A rocker can feel deeply relaxing. Softly singing songs, even ones you make up on the spot, can de-jangle nerves and lift a mood. Or murmur your hopes and dreams for your child, yourself, and your family.
- Try the various methods that can help a child to sleep, from standard ones like musical mobiles to exotic techniques such as running a blow dryer on low (not pointed directly at a child).
- If you've decided to see if you can train your child to sleep through the night, (e.g., with the Ferber method), try not to get too upset by the process. If it hasn't worked in a week or so, you should try a different method, for both your peace of mind and your baby's well-being. During that time, do what you can to treat yourself and your child really, really well.

sleep, like imps slipping past weary guards, make an agreement with yourself that you will think about them the next day. Also, try the techniques for dealing with anxiety discussed in the previous chapter.

- Extend compassion toward yourself. This alone can open the velvet trapdoor to sleep. You might reflect on how hard you work and how good it would feel to lavish kindness and sweetness upon yourself, just as you do with your children.

- One of the hardest times to fall asleep is when you are mad at the person lying next to you. After focusing on compassion to yourself, you could try extending it to him. Compassion doesn't mean you agree with him or renounce your rights, but that you are aware of his distress and wants, and let yourself feel a basic kindness toward him. If you like, you could express that compassion through the form of simple statements in your mind, such as "May John be at peace" or "May John and I be at peace with each other."

- Try imagining that you are breathing love for your child in and out through your heart, or love for the child that still exists within you.

Minerals, hormones, herbs, and amino acids. Magnesium is needed for quality sleep, and it is often low in mothers. Its Daily Value (DV)* is 320 milligrams (mg) per day (360 mg if you are pregnant). As you'll see on page 122, we suggest that mothers consider taking somewhat higher levels of many nutrients than the DVs; we call these the Mother's Suggested Daily Values (MSDVs). (For general perspectives and guidelines on using supplements or herbs, please see the box opposite.) The MSDV for magnesium is 500 mg, and most busy mothers find it very difficult to get even the DV of 320 mg in their diet, so you could take a supplement in the form of magnesium glysinate, citrate, lysinate, or aspartate. Calcium is another mineral that can help you sleep better. Its DV is 1000 mg, and the MSDV is 1200 mg (1600 mg if you're pregnant or nursing). Calcium and magnesium are often combined in a single supplement.

Melatonin is a hormone secreted by the pineal gland that signals the body to sleep, and consuming a bit at night could help you get a good night's rest. (But before we say another word here, we need to make an important point: *Women who are pregnant, might become pregnant in the next few months, or are breast-feeding, should not take any hormones, herbs, or most amino acids without being in the care of a licensed health professional experienced in their use.*) Melatonin can be taken sublingually (beneath the tongue) for a quick effect if it's hard to fall asleep in the first place, or swallowed in time-release form if you are troubled by nighttime waking. Some mothers find that immediately taking a little sublingual melatonin if they wake up in the middle of the night puts them back to sleep. If you try melatonin, find the minimum amount that works for you. Dosages as low as 0.3 to 0.5 mg can be sedating; do not exceed 1 to 2 mg, and do not take any melatonin at all if you are using cortisone. Some studies, typically using high doses, have linked

I often feel a spiritual communion with all the other mothers who are feeding their babies in the still of the night. Having a baby makes me feel a general closeness with humanity.

—*Simone Bloom*

---

*The minimum amount a person should consume each day.

Using Supplements or Herbs

Used skillfully, supplements and herbs can be a boon to your health. But like any tool, they can be used to harmful effect. To minimize that risk, please consider these perspectives and guidelines.

- Herbs contain more types of molecules than most prescription drugs, so they often act in more complex ways. This may enable an herb to act through multiple pathways for a more comprehensive benefit, but it also increases the chance of unpredicted effects.

- The potency in herbal preparations varies widely, especially in raw herbs. This range means that you should generally try to use standardized extracts, start at relatively low levels, and if necessary, increase the dosages slowly. When you can't find standardized extracts, such as with many Western and Chinese herbs, you should take extra care. The range of potency also introduces more uncertainty into the question of whether an herbal intervention will work for you (see the discussion of levels of evidence for an intervention in appendix E).

- Some herbs and supplements have had standards established for their manufacture by the official U.S. Pharmacopeia, and these will have "USP" or "NF" (National Formulary) on their labels. Herbal formulas manufactured in certain European countries, notably Germany, are carefully regulated, which can increase your confidence in herbs from those sources. There are also numerous U.S. companies that are highly reputable, and a nutritionally oriented health professional can steer you in the right direction.

- Some herbs and supplements can interact with prescription medications or have side effects that complicate the diagnosis or treatment of an illness. Therefore, you should always tell the doctor who is treating you about the herbs or supplements that you are taking. (An easy way to do so is to bring them to your appointment.) In particular, we recommend that you do not take herbs (unless otherwise instructed by an experienced, licensed health care professional) if you are pregnant, nursing, have a liver disease, or think you could be allergic to the product. And, naturally, keep your supplements and herbs out of the reach of your children.

- At very high levels, nearly any herb or supplement can have harmful side effects, so you should not exceed the doses we describe unless you've been instructed to do so by a licensed health practitioner experienced in their use.

- But we suggest you not be needlessly alarmed about the risks of supplements or herbs. On rare occasions a news item about some tragedy appears, but these have to do with major overdoses or a tiny handful of herbs (none of which we suggest). To put the risks of supplements and herbs in perspective, consider that prescription drugs are the source of over 100,000 deaths each year (through side effects, interactions with other medications, or overdoses). Supplements, herbs, and prescription drugs are tools, and they require skillful use; if you use supplements or herbs sensibly, you should have nothing to fear.

How to Use Homeopathic Remedies

To take a homeopathic remedy, you typically place three to five of the little sugar pills under your tongue and let them dissolve. Do not eat or drink anything for fifteen minutes beforehand or afterward. Try not to touch the sugar pills with your hands; pour them onto a spoon or into the plastic cap of the vial the remedy comes in, and pop them into your mouth from there.

If you are using a remedy for an acute situation—such as a single sleepless night or a particularly upset stomach—a 30C remedy is a good place to start. Take the remedy every twenty or thirty minutes for a few doses; next spread the doses out to once per hour for a few hours; and then decrease to three times per day. If you are using a remedy for an ongoing problem—like chronic insomnia—you can still try a 30C dosage, three times a day for several weeks. A trained homeopath will probably be most helpful for an ongoing problem, as well as be able to give you a higher potency remedy (e.g., 200C), which you would probably take less frequently.

Most homeopaths feel that some remedies can be antidoted if you drink coffee, or eat or use menthol products, so these should be avoided if possible. Also, because of the potentially electromagnetic basis for the as-yet-unknown mechanism of action of homeopathy, remedies should not be stored near equipment (like computers) that puts out electromagnetic fields. Finally, do not use a remedy that has gotten wet or been placed in a hot place or in the refrigerator.

melatonin to increased allergies, depression, and sexual dysfunction; but in the range we suggest, Jan has never seen those problems.

Valerian and passionflower are Western herbs that can help bring on or deepen sleep, and they are often placed together in tinctures available in health food stores. Herbalists also use skullcap, oat straw, and lavender. As well, the Chinese formula Swan Zao Ren Tang, can aid your sleep. You can get it from an acupuncturist or some health food stores; see appendix B, Resources, for other sources.

Serotonin is a neurotransmitter that helps you sleep, and the body builds it from an amino acid, tryptophan. As an intermediate step, the body produces a chemical with the exotic name 5-hydroxytryptophan (5-HTP), and supplementing 5-HTP has been shown to be useful for sleep. Ironically, when you first start taking 5-HTP, you may need to consume it early in the day or it might cause insomnia. (A few people experience mild gastrointestinal distress with 5-HTP, which is usually resolved by increasing the dosage slowly, sticking with a minimum dose, and taking it just before meals.) After your body is used to it, you could probably take it before bed. You could start with about 50 mg, and increase the dose slowly if you need to (e.g., 50 mg every few days) up to 150 mg, settling at a dosage that helps you get good sleep, and before you start to feel groggy during the day or have overly intense dreams at night. Since serotonin is also involved in regulating your mood, 5-HTP may help with that, too (see discussion starting on p. 173).

Acupuncture. This technique consists of placing super-thin needles into specific points on a person's body, based on the Chinese theory of energy meridians. It has been used for several thousand years, and modern research has shown it to be helpful with many ailments, including pain, stroke, depression, and sleep. Since the emphasis in Chinese medicine is on healing ailments by balancing the whole body, you may find that acupuncture for insomnia provides other benefits as well.

Homeopathy. This method—originating in Europe several hundred years ago—dilutes a substance to an extraordinary degree. For example, a remedy that is "30C" means that the original substance was placed in a pure water and alcohol solution, diluted to one percent and shaken intensively, then that solution was diluted again to one percent, and then again and again for a total of thirty times; at this point, there cannot possibly be a single atom left of the original material. Paradoxically, the more times it's diluted, the more powerful a remedy is considered to be. It is unclear why homeopathy might work, yet some well-controlled studies have found significant effects (for a review, see Dr. Kenneth Pelletier's book, *The Best Alternative Medicine: What Works? What Does Not?*), and many individuals—including ourselves—have observed or experienced dramatic benefits.

Homeopathic remedies usually come in the form of small sugar pills upon which the remedy has been "inoculated." These are available in health food stores at dosages up to 30C (a person should generally use more potent remedies under the care of an experienced homeopath). Different kinds of sleep disturbance call for different remedies. See which overall pattern below best fits you; you might try the remedy before going to bed or in the middle of the night, and then see if it helps. (If you don't already know how to take remedies, please see the box.)

- *Sepia.* This is the classic remedy for a worn-out mother who has given it all for her children. She feels irritable, drained, worn out, or exhausted most of the time. She may be emotionally flat, or have become indifferent to those she loves the most. Regarding sleep, she may awaken around 3:00 a.m. and be unable to return to sleep; she's often still tired after a night's rest.

- *Arsenicum Album.* This is for a mom who is neat and fastidious no matter what is going on. She is anxious and restless during the day, perhaps with a sense of agitation. She could experience burning sensations in the hands or joints, perhaps comforted by applying warmth (like a hot water bottle). Regarding sleep, she often wakes in the middle of the night and is unable to stop worrying.

- *Nux Vomica.* This is a remedy for a hard-working, hard-playing, ambitious, take-charge mother. She may be very irritable, intense, or tense. She could drink alcohol or eat too much. Regarding sleep, it's hard for her to fall asleep, and she may awaken between 2:00 and 4:00 a.m., and not be able to go back to sleep. She may also have nightmares.

- *Coffea.* This is for the person who has lots of activities and lists of projects, and whose mind won't stop planning and problem solving. There is a zippy, buzzing quality to her daily life. She may feel like she's had too much coffee.

- *Cocculus.* This is for the mother who is used to being up at night, such as while taking care of a sick child. She could feel too tired to go to sleep. She may be irritable or giddy.

Ask Your Doctor

If these interventions don't help, you should speak with your doctor. Perhaps an illness is disturbing your sleep, such as hormonal disturbance, diabetes, or clinical depression. For example, a patient of Ricki's, Mary, came for her first visit since her baby was born, looking extremely pale, worn out, and depressed. She said: ***I'm just not sleeping. My head seems to bounce off the pillow when I lie down, my mind's in a whir, and there's a pounding in my ears like a drum beating.*** As it turned out, the mild anemia (shortage of iron) she had during pregnancy had worsened when she bled heavily after the birth. So busy with her baby and getting everything organized, Mary grabbed snacks on the run and didn't get much iron in her diet. But now her heart had to race—keeping her awake at night—because her blood was less able to carry oxygen. By eating iron-rich meats and taking supplements with iron, Mary soon felt—and was sleeping—much better.

Additionally, you may want to talk with your doctor about sleeping pills or certain antidepressants that aid sleep. These can help get your brain back in the habit of sleeping soundly, enabling you to stop taking them. But please ask about their potential side effects. In particular, if you are nursing or could be pregnant, you should not take any medication, including sleeping pills, without your physician's knowledge.

A Mother's Lullaby

Ask Dad to do his share at night.

Sleep when the baby does during the day.

Try sleeping arrangements that work for you.

Exercise routinely.

Have the last hour before sleeping be peaceful.

Thoroughly relax your body in bed.

Reschedule any worries to the morning.

Get enough calcium and magnesium.

Consider melatonin, herbs, acupuncture, or homeopathy.

Consult your physician if you continue to have trouble with sleep.

Eating Right

Without a doubt, the single most effective way to replenish your body is through good nutrition. Unfortunately, most of us currently have a diet that is vastly different from the one that we are adapted to through millions of years of evolution, which was mostly meats, vegetables, fruits, and nuts. Humans started eating dairy products and whole grains just ten thousand years ago—a blip on the evolutionary time scale. And it's only the last fifty years that have seen the widespread use of refined grains, sugars, and oils, as well as packaged foods, pesticides, and artificial ingredients.

It helps to look back in time just a few decades to appreciate how rapidly our dietary intake has changed. Prior to World War II, there were virtually no processed foods, with meals prepared mostly by stay-at-home mothers whose role identity was focused on the care and feeding of the family. Meals were made up of basic fresh ingredients, home-canned items, and breads baked locally.

But with the need for women in the workforce during the war, for the first time women came out of their homes in large numbers to work in industry and service jobs. This generated a demand for convenience foods and gave birth to a new industry of food processing to help busy, dual-role housewives. Canned foods were widely marketed as women no longer had the time to can their own. "Balloon breads," packaged baked goods, snack crackers, and chips made their way onto grocery store shelves for the first time.

Soon thereafter, with advances in refrigeration at home and on the trucking routes, frozen foods became increasingly a part of the average American household. By the 1960s, packaged and highly processed foods were commonplace in most American homes. With the rise of television advertising, sugar-coated cereals were being marketed directly to children. Quick, easy, and without a morning fight, they flooded our markets and kitchen cupboards. The percentage of total daily calories from refined sugar looks like the rise of the Dow Jones average over the years: up, up, and up! Meanwhile, fast-food restaurants have spread widely, emphasizing the same sorts of foods: quick, processed, and super-sized with fat, sugar, and man-made chemicals.

Although in the short run some people seem able to get away with this diet without too many bad consequences, the statistics on the explosion of cancer, heart disease, Type II diabetes, and obesity in children in the last century are cautionary for anyone. But in particular, your own needs now are special and specific: *bearing, breast-feeding, and rearing a child are physiologically demanding activities like no others,* and pulling them off while staying truly healthy requires that you honor the fundamental biology of your body and nourish it in ways that may have been less crucial before you had children. Which means eating a lot more like your great-great-Paleolithic-grandmother than having a bagel and coffee for breakfast, peanut butter and jelly sandwich at lunch, and something microwaved for dinner. It is not always easy, but mothers who have started eating better tell us that they soon experience more energy, a lift in mood, improvement in health conditions like dry skin or PMS, and an overall sense of greater health. It's fundamentally simple: you improve your body's balance sheet by eating more healthy foods and fewer worthless or toxic ones. At every meal, trillions of molecules at a time, you'll be literally rebuilding the tissues of your body.

For a snapshot of your current diet, please complete the self-assessment in the box. If you're already scoring high, great. But if not, in the next few pages you'll find our daily Mother Nurture recipe, designed specifically with a mom's nutritional needs in mind. It's comprised of only seven ingredients—though you need each one, just like the flour, salt, and baking powder in a recipe for biscuits. In sum, every day you should try to eat:

1. Eight to twelve ounces of protein
2. Five to seven servings of fresh vegetables, and one to two fruits
3. Unrefined oils and essential fatty acids instead of refined or hydrogenated oils, or trans-fatty acids
4. Two to five servings of unrefined, varied whole grains

Your Nutritional Self-Assessment

Put one or more points in the boxes that would describe your diet on a typical day in the past week. (A "yes" equals one point.) It is fine to make a ballpark estimate. Unless otherwise noted, a serving is half a cup.

Pluses:

[   ]   Number of pieces of fresh fruit (up to 2 points)

[   ]   Number of servings of fresh vegetables (count one point for every serving) (a serving of leafy vegetables is one cup)

[   ]   Number of servings of a whole grain—1 slice of bread from completely unrefined flour, 1/2 cup of brown rice or bulgur (up to 3 points)

[   ]   Drank four or more cups of water

[   ]   Number of servings of protein—meat, fish, tofu, eggs, cheese (up to 3) (a serving is 3 to 4 ounces)

[   ]   At least half of all foods were organic

[   ]   Oils used were mainly unrefined—virgin olive oil or oils labeled "unrefined"

[   ]   Ate foods rich in omega-3 essential fatty acids—salmon, mackerel, flax oil—or took an omega-3 supplement

[   ]   Took a good multivitamin/multimineral supplement

Minuses:

A food that is in two or three categories would be counted two or three times (e.g., a caffeinated soft drink has both caffeine and sugar, most potato chips are both processed and full of hydrogenated fats).

[   ]   Number of sweet desserts you ate—a soft drink, donut, candy bar, ice cream cone, piece of pie (if large, multiply by 2)

[   ]   Number of servings of processed foods—potato chips, canned soups, packaged noodles and cheese, TV dinners, or any product made with white flour

[   ]   Number of servings of foods with hydrogenated or partially hydrogenated fats—potato chips, margarine, most baked goods

[   ]   Had two or more caffeinated drinks—coffee, black tea, some soft drinks

[   ]   Had two or more alcoholic drinks—one "drink" is a beer, 4 ounces of wine, or shot of liquor

Add up your pluses. Add up your minuses (remember to count each serving of a sweet dessert or processed food). Subtract the minuses from the pluses. A score of 13 or above means you are doing well, 8 to 12 is pretty good but could be improved, and a score of 7 or below (including negative numbers) indicates a real need to make some changes in your diet.

5. Organic foods whenever possible

6. High potency nutritional supplements

7. Zero or very little refined sugar

There are basically two ways to shift your diet in a healthier direction: (1) make sweeping changes all at once, or (2) work your way into it. Whichever path you take, we urge you to stay on it until you end up with truly mother-nurturing nutrition. If you slip now and then, as almost everyone does, just get back on the path at your next meal. Optimizing nutrition often takes several tries, but each time something improves. Even small changes in the right direction add up as the years go by.

Since healthy nutrition usually involves trying new things and giving up some goodies (glazed donuts, etc.), a person needs to understand the reasons she's doing it, which is why we explain the health benefits of each ingredient in our recipe. You could also stay motivated by paying special attention to the ways eating whole-some foods helps you take good care of yourself, or even makes you feel part of a circle, offering the sustenance of maternal care and taking in the sustenance of the earth's great bounty. Eating in a healthy way provides a good model for children, too, and it helps their mother stay good-humored and patient with them, even when the oatmeal starts flying.

Ingredient #1: *Eight to twelve ounces of protein a day; protein with every meal, especially breakfast*

Why:

Because you lose protein during pregnancy and nursing, and your body uses more protein when it is chronically stressed, you need lots of protein, about 50 to 65 grams a day. Protein also helps stabilize your blood sugar and prevent insulin in-sensitivity and Type II diabetes.

How:

- Eat 3–4 ounces of protein (about the size of a deck of cards) at every meal.
- In particular, *eat protein at breakfast.* Rather than kicking off the day with wild swings in your blood sugar, try a breakfast with a serving of protein (e.g., two eggs, a piece of lean chicken, or a large handful of almonds). If

you make morning protein the foundation of your day's nutrition, you'll have less of an energy and mood crash in the afternoon.

- When you want something sweet, have some protein instead, like a hard-boiled egg, hummus on crackers, or a piece of turkey jerky. That will satisfy your hunger and keep your blood sugar on an even keel.

- You can get protein conveniently from these foods:

Eggs. These contain very balanced proteins. You may have avoided them because of concerns about cholesterol, but recent studies have found that eggs do not increase the risk of heart disease, and in fact they may raise the level of good, HDL cholesterol (but if your cholesterol is very high, check with your doctor about eating eggs). Try to get them from free-range hens on a healthy diet. If you're in a hurry, you can hard-boil eggs in advance and eat one or two at breakfast.

Fish. Salmon is an excellent choice because it contains high levels of the essential fatty acids (EFAs) every mother needs (see p. 116 for more on EFAs). Besides eating it fresh, you can find salmon jerky in many health food stores. Try to minimize fish at the top of the ocean food chain—like tuna, shark, or swordfish—because mercury and other toxins increase as you move up the chain.

Lean meat. Many mothers—especially when nursing or pregnant—seem to need animal-based protein (though some do fine with a vegetarian diet). Select lean cuts of meat (poultry without the skin, round steak, etc.) to decrease saturated fats and the toxins that concentrate in fat. For convenience, many health food stores sell different kinds of tasty "jerkies" made from beef or turkey, but without any nitrites or other preservatives.

Dairy products. Although milk, cheese, and yogurt are considered good sources of protein, they are best used in moderation because many people have an allergy to milk or cannot digest the lactose in it, and keeping the digestive tract in good shape is a top priority for a mother. If you have excessive mucus, sinus infections, gastrointestinal disturbance, or dark circles under your eyes, try experimenting with eating no dairy products for a couple of weeks, and see how you feel (see the discussion of allergies and food sensitivities on p. 160). If you have trouble with dairy, small amounts of goat milk products may be tolerable. If you're wondering about calcium, you can get a fair amount of it in cauliflower, broccoli, peas, and beans, but unless you're eating many cups of these vegetables every day (or several servings of sardines or canned salmon, which also contain lots of calcium), you'll want to make sure to take a calcium supplement if you don't eat dairy foods.

Nuts. Easy to take with you. Get a good trail mix or make your own (almonds are particularly high in protein); kids often like to help: just combine your favorite nuts with some nonsulfered dried fruit. Nut butters are also delicious; try almond or sesame butter instead of peanut butter if you are allergic or sensitive to peanuts. Almond butter on a rice cake topped with apple slices is a delicious and healthy breakfast.

Soy. Soybeans contain a high proportion of protein, and they may also help prevent cardiovascular disease and cancer. You can add soybeans to stews or soups, or toss tofu chunks into your stirfry or casseroles. In your baking, you could experiment with replacing half or more of the wheat flour with soy flour. Soymilk comes in many flavors, and you may be surprised to find that your children really like it. (But don't overdo the soy, since it's a common allergen, plus excessive amounts can suppress the functioning of the thyroid gland.)

Hummus. This Middle Eastern food is made from garbanzo beans and sesame seeds. You can buy it in most supermarkets or make your own, lower-fat version.

Protein shakes. Just put some protein powder into a blender with diluted juice, milk, or soymilk, and perhaps some fresh fruit, and voila!, you've got an instant high-protein meal. If you are going to use these regularly, alternate types of protein powder (such as whey-, soy-, or egg-based) to get a variety.

Combining vegetarian foods. If you're a vegetarian, as each of us has been at different times, you probably know about using food combinations (like rice and beans) for maximum protein. (*Diet for a Small Planet* or *Laurel's Kitchen* offer good introductions to this subject; please see the list below for other books on healthy nutrition.) Since meat is the only significant source of iron and vitamin B_{12} in the diet, a vegetarian should usually take these as part of a daily supplement.

Good Books for Good Nutrition

Staying Healthy with Nutrition by Elson Haas
Nutrition Made Simple by Robert Crayhon
Smart Fats by Michael Schmidt
Eat, Drink, and Be Healthy by Walter C. Willett
Diet for a Small Planet by Frances Moore Lappé
The New Laurel's Kitchen by Laurel Robertson, Brian Ruppenthal,
    and Carol L. Flinders
Diet for a New America by John Robbins

Ingredient #2: *Five to seven servings of fresh vegetables, and one to two fruits*

Why:

Vegetables are about the only thing that all nutritionists agree on, and they all agree that you should eat a lot. They're rich in vitamins and minerals, and they contain phytonutrients such as carotenes and bioflavonoids, as well as phytoestrogens, hormonelike substances that seem to help balance estrogen. The U.S. Department of Agriculture recommends that everyone has three to five servings a day (a serving is half a cup for most vegetables, and one cup for leafy greens). But since you have special needs as a mother, we recommend two additional servings, for a total of five to seven per day. So when you tell your kids to eat their veggies, that means you, too!

We recommend fresh vegetables because they have many more nutrients than ones that are canned, dried, or frozen; if you can't get them fresh, frozen is your next best option—and freeze-dried vegetables make great snacks. Fresh fruits are also nourishing, filled with vitamins, phytonutrients, and fiber. But most are also very sweet, so they are best eaten in moderation (please see the discussion of sugar on p. 124).

How:

- Eat a variety of high-quality vegetables, especially roots (carrots, beets), cruciferous vegetables (broccoli, cauliflower), dark greens (kale, collard, spinach), and sea veggies (kelp, kombu, nori).

- Eat raw vegetables when you can. Washed well, a couple of carrots, broccoli florets, or cauliflower nuggets are delicious and surprisingly sweet.

- Make several days' worth of vegetable snacks at a time, stored in plastic bags in the refrigerator. If you combine them with some whole grain rolls or pretzels, almonds, chunks of cheese, or jerkies, you can avoid prepackaged snack packs. (This is one way that Ricki survived her residency and long days at the hospital delivering babies.)

- With a sturdy juicer, you can have a vitalizing elixir in just a few minutes. If it's strong enough to make your hair stand on end and your toes curl— as some veggie tonics can—then you know it's good for you! And you can dilute it if you like.

- Enrich salads by adding grated carrots, beets, or dark leafy greens. It's also easy to make a little extra salad for dinner, refrigerate it in a plastic bag without dressing, and have it with lunch the next day.

- Try a "green drink" from your health food store for a serious blast of nutrients. (Pregnant or nursing moms should check with a health practitioner if the drink contains herbs, or find one without herbs; either way, start with a small amount of the drink and see how your body likes it.)

- Cooking can make vegetables easier to digest, but that takes some time, so we like to keep it simple. Try steaming four cups of veggies in the morning, and eat them throughout the day. A baked sweet potato with some protein (see the suggestions above) makes an excellent breakfast, Jan's morning fare for several years; if your oven has a delayed timer, you could pop it in the night before and wake up to a delicious smell. Substituting sweet potatoes or yams for regular potatoes provides variety, plus additional nutrients like tons of carotenoids.

  We like to make a big pot of hearty vegetable soup on the weekend that can last most of the week, perhaps adding some dark, leafy greens that may taste too strong for you when they're raw but are milder in soup. If you toss some protein (meat, beans, tofu, peas, lentils, etc.) into your soup, you've got a wonderfully nutritious meal (several, in fact!) in a pot. Please see the box for a recipe for our own Mother Nurture Stew.

- The best way to eat fruit is when it is fresh and whole, rather than canned, frozen, or in juice.

- Cooked fruits—like baked apples with a little maple syrup on them, or berries with a cobbler topping—make a wholesome, delicious dessert.

- Fresh fruits and vegetables are foods that are still alive. Every time you eat them, you can take a moment to sense that the living energy within them is entering your body, giving you a feeling of peace and a serving of stress relief with every meal.

Mother Nurture Stew:

Cook Once a Week and Eat Well Every Night

The plan is to make a giant stew—about ten to twelve quarts—that will last for most of a week. It will include tons of vegetables, lots of meat or other high-protein foods, and other goodies. When it's all cooked, put half of it in one or two containers in the freezer. The five or so quarts left will last your family about half of the week, depending upon everybody's appetites. Then you can unfreeze a different batch of stew from another week to get you through the rest of this week. This way, your family won't get sick of eating the same thing each dinner. And you or your husband will be able to cook dinner just once a week, but eat well every night!

Each stew is unique, depending on the particular ingredients on hand when it's made, but they all follow this basic framework:

In a big soup kettle, saute in olive oil:
   a couple of large onions
   and/or: some peeled cloves of garlic
   and/or: some peeled and diced fresh ginger
   and/or: some spices you like, such as basil, oregano, cumin, or rosemary

Add and sauté 2–6 pounds of protein:
   either cubes of skinless chicken
   or: very lean beef
   or: cubes of tofu (premarinated and/or baked, if you like)

When the protein is browned, add liquid up to about two-thirds of the pot:
   broth (chicken, beef, or vegetable)
   and/or: tomato sauce. Alternately, you could add coconut milk, plus lime and cilantro. You
                   may also add dry red or white wine if you like; cooking evaporates the alcohol.

If you've used stewing beef, you may want to simmer it for a couple of hours, until the meat is tender. Then, starting with the ones that take longer to cook, add many cups of chopped vegetables, such as carrots, beets, squash, broccoli, green beans, peas (organic frozen peas are fine), potatoes, whatever! (Since you are only cooking dinner once a week, it might be worth it to get the food processor out.) Include several cups of diced dark leafy greens, like kale, and try adding some dried seaweed, like kombu, arame, or nori for extra mineral nourishment.

(continued)

(continued from page 115)

Grains and beans: You could put grains (rice, barley, quinoa, pasta) or beans in the stew, or serve it over or alongside these foods. If you want to put them in, precook them or have enough extra liquid to allow for absorption. Check a cookbook for the beans you want to use since many must be precooked or presoaked; or you could use organic canned beans.

Regarding the kids: If there's no way in the world that they'll touch this stew, then you might as well have great meals for yourself and your husband while they eat macaroni and cheese, or whatever, every night. However, if there is a chance they can be wooed to it, you can make the meat and vegetables in bite-size chunks, and they can select the ones they want; many kids like broth and a lot of nutrients will have slipped invisibly into that liquid. If they like the broth but won't eat any vegetables, try pureeing some of the cooked vegetables in a blender and then adding them back to the soup. Sneaky....

Ingredient #3: *Unrefined oils and essential fatty acids instead of refined or hydrogenated oils, or trans-fatty acids*

Why:

The process of refining oils uses toxic chemicals to strip away good nutrients while often leaving behind potentially harmful, altered oils. When oils are hydrogenated—as they are to make margarine—or kept at high temperatures for long periods of time (as in deep fat frying), trans-fatty acids are formed, and these "bad fats" have been implicated in cardiovascular disease and other health conditions.

Essential fatty acids (EFAs) are "good fats" needed for the membranes of your cells and a healthy heart, and they comprise sixty percent of your brain. These oils are called essential because they cannot be synthesized by the body and must be consumed through foods or supplements. Unfortunately, they are often deficient in mothers since they are drawn on heavily to grow a baby during pregnancy and breast milk is loaded with them, and most women don't have anywhere near enough to start with. Increasing your intake of one type of EFAs—omega-3 oils found in fish and flax—can help prevent cardiovascular disease, rheumatoid arthritis, asthma, diabetes, and depression. It can also make your hair and skin more moist; dryness, including dandruff, is a potential sign of omega-3 deficiency. In general, Jan has found that a typical mom is likely to have a stronger response to supplementing omega-3 oils than to any other nutrient, probably because they are both so important and so commonly deficient in mothers.

How:

- Make virgin olive oil your everyday oil.

- Avoid trans-fatty acids. These are found in deep-fried foods, as in the hydrogenated or partially hydrogenated fats used in margarine, and in most baked or packaged foods. At home, use judicious amounts of butter or olive oil instead of margarine. At the store, check the labels and try not to get products with these oils.

- Balance the two main types of essential fatty acids, omega-3 and omega-6 oils. Most people are deficient in omega-3 oils yet have an oversupply of omega-6s. To put this point in perspective, throughout most of human history, people ate these oils in a ratio of approximately 1:1. But today, the average is about 20:1 omega-6s to omega-3s! That's completely out of balance with the way our bodies are built, and one of the results is a greater tendency toward inflammation—to which mothers are already vulnerable.

    The simple solution is to decrease the omega-6 oils in your diet and increase the omega-3s. The easiest way to eat less omega-6s is to stop using the oils that contain them: safflower, sunflower, soybean, and sesame oils; extra virgin olive oil is a tasty and versatile alternative. You can get more omega-3 oils by:

    § Eating omega-3 rich fish (salmon, mackerel, trout, or sardines); do not overcook, or the oils will be compromised.

    § Using flax oil in salad dressings and other nonfrying oil uses (essential fatty acids are degraded or destroyed at the temperatures oils reach during frying). You might like to mix it with olive oil for flavor. You can meet your daily needs with about 1 tablespoon of flax oil, which you can add to blended or juiced drinks, or simply take in a quick gulp; flax oil is also available in capsules at health food stores.

    § Grinding whole flax seeds in a coffee grinder and sprinkling them on cereals and vegetables, or adding to pancakes and baked goods. Make sure to drink one to two cups of water when you eat flax seeds since they are a major source of fiber. (It would take about five table-spoons of flax seeds to meet your daily needs for omega-3 oils, which is out of the question for most people, so you'll probably need other sources, too.)

§ Taking about 1000 milligrams of a fish oil supplement* that has been checked for purity, since fish (especially those at the top of the food chain) may have contaminants; usually, there will be someone at the health food store that knows about the purity of their supplements. For most mothers, this is the simplest way to consume adequate omega-3s. (Some people prefer flax oil to fish oil due to being a vegetarian. Unfortunately, a depleted person often lacks some of the enzymes or co-factors needed to convert flax oil into the long-chain fatty acids your body needs, which already exist in fish oil. If you do choose to use flax oil, make sure you're taking a good multi-vitamin/multi-mineral supplement as well, for the co-factors it contains.)

§ Using a gamma-linolenic acid (GLA) supplement if you have symptoms that suggest a deficiency, such as premenstrual tension, eczema, or arthritis. Even though GLA is an omega-6 oil, it's an exception to the general rule of minimizing omega-6 oils. The reason is that a person—especially if she's at all depleted—may lack the enzymes or nutrients needed to build GLA within her body. You can find GLA in supplements of primrose, borage, or black currant oil. Daily suggested doses are given on the labels.

• Do not using refined oils. Unless an oil specifically says "unrefined" (with the exception of virgin olive oil), it has been refined.

Ingredient #4: Two to five servings of unrefined, varied whole grains

Why:

Refining grains takes away the fiber and nutrients (B vitamins, etc.) present in the outer hull, but you need these to keep your GI tract running smoothly and meet the increased stresses and energy demands that come with children. Refined grains (e.g., white flour, pasta, white rice) also convert quickly to sugars in the body, further straining an insulin system that is already challenged by stress (for more on sugar, see p. 124).

Grains definitely have a place in well-balanced nutrition. But we don't think

---

*The blood-thinning effect of fish oils is usually good for the cardiovascular system, much like an aspirin a day. But if you are on a blood-thinning medication, or have a bleeding disorder, please consult with your doctor before supplementing fish oils.

they should make up as large a portion of a mother's diet as they do in the standard Food Pyramid, where they crowd out other kinds of carbohydrates and nutrients (plus, certain chemicals within grains called phytates can interfere with the absorption of minerals). It's also important to eat a variety of grains besides wheat, because different grains or sources of flour—such as rice, barley, millet, quinoa, corn, or soy—provide other nutrients, as well as complementary amino acids for maximum protein. Varying your grains also lowers the chance of digestive problems or inflammation, since wheat is one of the two foods that people are most often allergic or sensitive to (the other is dairy; please see p. 162 for how to test for allergies and food sensitivities).

How:

- Increase your carbohydrate intake from other sources, such as nuts, bananas, yams, other vegetables, etc.

- Try to get the majority of your grains intact, not ground up in flours. These could be fresh oatmeal for breakfast, a side dish of millet or quinoa at lunch, or a casserole with brown rice at dinner.

- If you have an allergy or sensitivity to wheat, try rice, millet, quinoa, soy, or corn flour products.

- Replace white flour with good-tasting whole wheat pastry, rice, or soy flours.

- Most of us do all right with having the occasional treat made from white flour, but try not to bring home white flour products in bulk (e.g., packaged noodle foods, pasta, white bread, frozen pizza, cake).

- Try pasta made from brown rice. It's delicious and can leave you feeling lighter than if you'd eaten wheat.

Ingredient #5: Organic foods whenever possible

Why:

Organic foods have fewer toxic molecules because they contain no pesticides or artificial fertilizers. The "safety" of these chemicals has usually been established through short-term studies using single substances, often on laboratory animals. But the experiment that counts is the one that is being carried out on human beings who consume many chemicals in combination for a lifetime—and the real-world findings over the past hundred years include a dramatic increase in cancer and autoimmune conditions. Anyone who is developing rapidly or is vulnerable—such as a child, or a pregnant, stressed, or depleted mother—is particularly likely to be affected by the mounting accumulation of potentially toxic molecules.

Organic foods also tend to have more nutritious molecules—especially minerals—because they come from richer soils. And besides being a two-part prescription for a mother's health—fewer bad molecules and more good ones—organic foods usually taste better: just compare an organic tomato with one that has been grown conventionally.

How:

- Avoid foods with artificial ingredients such as preservatives, colors, or flavor enhancers. (This will have the additional benefit of steering you away from packaged foods).

- These days, you can get almost any food product you want from organic sources, including meats, pasta, soup, macaroni and cheese, milk, catsup, or even wine (wines, especially red ones, have particularly high concentrations of pesticides if they weren't grown organically). Besides finding them in health food stores, they are increasingly available in regular supermarkets. Farmer's markets are another source, plus they can be an easier place to shop with young children. Food co-ops may have organic foods, and they're a good way to meet other parents. Organic foods sometimes cost a little more, but for a few pennies extra per meal, you'll be making a smart, long-term investment in your body.

- Nobody should drive herself crazy to eat strictly organic foods, since a single episode—whether it's lunch at McDonald's or a salad of organic greens—doesn't make a big difference either way. It's the accumulation over time that counts.

There's no way around it: preparing wholesome meals from fresh, mainly organic ingredients takes longer than popping a TV dinner into the oven or opening a can of stew. If you're reluctant to spend more time in the kitchen, the reasons may be nothing more than feeling too busy, or cooking bores you. But sometimes a woman has mixed feelings about walking too closely in the footsteps of her own mother or taking on some of the trappings of a traditional housewife. If that has a ring of truth for you, please take a look at the story in the box.

Kitchen Slave or Domestic Goddess?

Molly came to her gynecological appointment complaining of feeling run-down, and Ricki asked her what she was eating these days. Molly shrugged and said, ***We're loaded with baby foods, crackers, pretzels, and cereals. Or we get burgers or pizza at take-out. But the produce aisle and I are strangers. I just don't want to cook.*** Then she added pensively, ***My mom seemed to be in the kitchen all the time when I was a kid. She never worked outside the home, like a lot of women then, and I thought she was trapped in the kitchen, and when I got older, I think I looked down on her for that.*** She shook her head in an embarrassed way. ***I love her, but I never wanted to be stuck in the kitchen like her, with her kind of life, mostly washing and cleaning and cooking for her family. I'm leery of the classic role of being a housewife, becoming a kitchen slave, dependent on some guy. It's hard to make myself do any kind of meal planning or major grocery shopping. I'm afraid I'll get trapped, too.***

Ricki nodded and agreed with Molly that it's hard for many mothers to shift gears from career-type work to scullery work if they have a job, or from the prestige and money of paid employment to the low status of chief cook and bottle washer if they are a stay-at-home mom. It's hard to figure out how to keep the benefits of the feminist revolution while not throwing out the domestic arts with the dishwater.

But there's no reason a woman today can't have the best of both worlds. Ricki told Molly about a time when she baked gingerbread cookies for a meeting of women doctors at her house. One of the physicians smelled the great aroma and exclaimed, ***What an unusual juxtaposition. Here you're being a domestic goddess with an active oven while also hosting our women docs' group. I have never experienced these feelings together: happy domesticity and the medical profession!*** It became a topic of conversation in the meeting: how these professional women could let themselves be as nourished at home as at work, and as skillful in one sphere as they were in the other.

Molly went home, dusted off a cookbook, and began trying one new recipe a week. She started shopping on the edges of the supermarket and stayed out of the middle where the tempting convenience foods were concentrated. She even took a couple of cooking classes with her husband, and they enjoyed making dinner as a couple in the happy, relaxed atmosphere they had in their kitchen.

Ingredient #6: High-potency nutritional supplements

Why:

Certainly, the best sources of nutrients are usually fresh, whole, organic foods. But in real life, not some textbook, most mothers rely on quick snacks, meals on the run, and processed foods that lack even the Daily Values (DVs) of all the nutrients they need. Almost all women have some catching up to do since they already have significant nutritional deficits when they start their first pregnancy; it takes many months, and often years, of taking supplements to restore healthy levels of nutrients (especially minerals) to a run-down body.

Plus, we think you need more than the DVs, anyway! Growing and nursing a baby, as well as the hard work and stresses of raising a family, use up large quantities of nutrients. Building up reserves in your body is also a wise stockpile for future times of high stress or poor nutrition. And by their nature, micronutrients assist bodily processes in going well. These molecular helping hands may thus help protect a vulnerable mother from the widespread artificial chemicals that tend to make things go badly.

Further, the DVs are the minimum necessary to prevent diseases of nutritional deficiency, not necessarily what promotes long-term health and well-being. For example, the amount of vitamin C that prevents scurvy is less than that which brings the greatest cardiovascular health across a lifetime. A growing body of research has substantiated the benefits of above-DV levels of various nutrients for gastrointestinal dysfunction, depression, hormonal disturbances, and autoimmune diseases—for which women have an increased risk after children. (Of course, supplements are no substitute for a balanced diet or medical care.)

Finally, the risks of supplements are very low. If you stay within the range of the MSDVs presented in appendix D, about the worst thing that can happen is that your body will excrete any unused nutrients; those particular molecules will have been unnecessary, but since it is difficult to know exactly which nutrients will be fully absorbed and which won't, the money spent on supplements is a kind of insurance policy to give yourself the best odds, year after year, of filling the larder of your body with all the vitamins and minerals it needs.

How:

- Unless your doctor has instructed you otherwise due to a medical problem, take multi-vitamin, multi-mineral supplements whose dosages meet the criteria of our Mothers' Suggested Daily Values (MSDVs) listed in appendix D, pages 354–55. (If you are pregnant or breast-feeding, or have delivered or weaned a child in the past year, the appendix also gives modified amounts of nutrients.) We also list the Intensive Daily Doses (IDDs) that may help with certain health conditions. Do not exceed the IDDs unless you have been specifically told to do so by a licensed health practitioner. In particular, do not take more than 5000 IU of vitamin A if you are pregnant, planning to get pregnant in the next couple of months, or capable of conception (i.e., having sex without contraception).

Your prenatal vitamin/mineral supplements may be all you need, but check the labels; many have levels of important nutrients that are too low. Health food stores usually carry several brands of high-quality "multis" that meet most or all of our MSDVs. Whether you're taking an everyday multi or a more exotic nutrient, always be sure to get supplements with guaranteed purity and potency from reputable companies.

- Use a supplement whose minerals are chelated, which aids absorption. This is indicated when the name of the mineral is followed by a word ending in *-ate,* such as citrate, aspertate, malate, gluconate, or picolate. (Chelated minerals are also usually a sign of a quality product; magnesium ox*ide,* for instance, is cheap to manufacture, but it's not absorbed as well.) For iron, look for ferrous—not ferric—sulfate, fumorate, or gluconate.

- You will probably need to add calcium and magnesium to even the best multi in order to get the amounts of these minerals that you need.

- You may also want to take an additional B complex supplement. All the B vitamins help people deal with stress. For example, B_5 enables the body to make adrenal hormones. Vitamin B_6 helps balance the endocrine system; this vitamin often helps with PMS, morning sickness, and depression.

- If you are breast-feeding or have weaned your child in the past year, we suggest taking 500 mg of the amino acid taurine with your breakfast. (This is the exception to our general recommendation that you take no amino acid supplements if you are breastfeeding or pregnant, unless you've been otherwise instructed by a licensed health professional.) An infant is not yet able to make taurine, so it is drained from a mother's body if she is not getting enough in her diet. Taurine helps maintain proper mineral levels within your body's cells—particularly of magnesium, which is necessary for sleep, relaxation, and vitality.

- Expect to take a handful of pills each day, since there is no way that all the micronutrients you need can fit into a single supplement smaller than a hefty marble. It takes less time than brushing your teeth, and it's arguably more important for your overall health in the long run.

Ingredient #7: Zero or very little refined sugar

Why:

Probably the most important ingredient in a mother's recipe for long-term health has been saved for last. Sure, when we're blue or want some comfort, most of us like to have something sweet to eat. Or just to jump-start the day or allow us to finish the laundry after getting the baby to sleep. Initially, refined sugar does bring a blast of energy. But the spike in blood sugar triggers a big surge of insulin in the body's effort to get all that sugar into your cells. The wave of insulin does its job so well that your blood sugar levels quickly plummet. Suddenly you feel hungry, spacey, fatigued, jittery, shaky, short-tempered, or even panicky.

Clearly, these are not the desired effects of a sugar buzz! Even worse, our cells become less sensitive to insulin over time as a self-protective measure. That makes the pancreas pump out extra insulin, which makes our cells even less sensitive. It's a vicious cycle. If this process continues, at some point the pancreas just can't pump out enough insulin to get the cells to take notice, and now a person has Type II diabetes.

The average American today eats over 150 pounds per year of refined sugars—compared to zero pounds during most of human history. High consumption of sugar (and the elevated levels of insulin that come with it) is associated with Type II diabetes, weight gain, bloating, fatigue, arthritis, migraines, lowered immune function, gallstones, obesity, breast cancer, and cardiovascular disease. And sugar is depleting—the last thing a mother needs—draining (or disrupting the absorption of) the B vitamins, chromium, calcium, magnesium, and copper that she needs to manage her increased stresses. Rounding out the bitter aftertastes to all that sweetness, sugar force-feeds microbes in the digestive tract, which is already vulnerable to infection due to maternal stress, leading to impaired nutrient absorption, diarrhea, gas, or fatigue.

How:

- Sugar has an addictive quality: when you have a little, you want more. So for some people, cutting out sugar altogether is the way to go. If that's too radical, we suggest you set a personal goal of eating less than twenty grams of refined sugar a day (about two tablespoons). That's about what the average American ate a hundred years ago—and still more than the zero refined sugar our bodies are designed for. If you have any digestive problems, we think you should eat no more than ten grams a day. Food labels will tell you how many grams of refined sugar a serving contains, and it probably doesn't much matter if it's refined or "natural" (like fructose or honey).

- The easiest way of all to eat less sugar is to cut out soda and juice. Two soft drinks a day adds up to ninety grams of sugar: sixty-five pounds of sugar per year. Besides all that sugar, you'll be adding unwanted weight, since people who drink sugar-sweetened drinks tend to eat just as much as those who drink water. Instead, try carbonated water with a squeeze of lemon or lime, diluted juice, or delicious herbal iced teas. One way or another, you should drink at least eight cups of water or herbal tea a day.

- Check the labels on packaged foods like breakfast cereal, peanut butter, or spaghetti sauce, and try brands without any sugar.

- Think twice about extra sugar, like another packet in your coffee, tons of jam on toast, or a second helping of ice cream after dinner.

- By having fewer sweets around for your kids, it will be easier to avoid them yourself. Try not to let them get started on sugar in the first place, so they can still appreciate a juicy apple, bowl of strawberries, or handful of raisins.

- Avoid temptation by not having cookies, candy, ice cream, etc., at home. If you want something for your sweet tooth, purchase a single item. And if you do keep dessert around, try to have only one kind, since we eat more if there's a variety.

- Although the Food and Drug Administration (FDA) has judged aspartame (NutraSweet) to be safe, many people have still reported negative reactions, including headaches and depression; a large fraction of the nondrug complaints to the FDA are for aspartame. (Using artificial sweeteners doesn't seem to help people lose weight, either.) We're naturally cautious about man-made molecules for mothers, and an alternative is an extract of the plant *stevia rebaudiana,* which tastes intensely sweet in very small amounts, but without any calories. It comes in liquid or powdered form and you can use it just like sugar, including in baking (an advantage over aspartame). Like aspartame, there's an aftertaste, but you'll soon grow accustomed to it.

- If you are, like Jan, a chocolate addict, try high-quality unsweetened chocolate. Once you get used to it, it tastes very satisfying. You can melt it, add a couple drops of stevia and a handful of nuts, and make your own candy bar.

I can resist everything except temptation.

—*Oscar Wilde*

- Try to understand the forces that keep you hooked on sugar. For instance, Jan worked with a single mom who ate a huge, double handful of chocolate chips each day. She knew it wasn't healthy, but she said: *I know it's not good, but I work hard all day long, and this is about the only thing I do for* **me**. By finding better ways to nurture herself, she was able to cut down on this daily blast of sugar.

- Sugar is the ultimate comfort food, so it's really important to be nice to yourself while you reduce it. And try to think about all the wonderful things you are doing for your body by nourishing it in healthier ways.

Exercising Regularly

Samantha, a patient of Ricki's, came to her appointment concerned about her weight, which was still more than twenty pounds heavier than it had been before having her first baby, now three years old. Ricki asked about exercise, and Samantha smiled and quoted a saying: *Oh, I do get the urge sometimes. But I just lie down until it passes!* Then she became more serious and added, *I just can't find the time. My day is busy from 6 a.m. to 11 at night.* Ricki wondered about her husband, and Samantha explained that *He jogs from 6 to 6:45 every morning, then showers, bolts down his breakfast, and is out of the house by 7:30.* The gears began to turn. *You're right,* she mused, *he makes it a priority. Why don't I?*

They talked about how exercise has to be important, or it just won't happen. As a result, Samantha went home and had a long talk with her husband, Ben, and he agreed to take over child care and dinner preparation three nights a week. Samantha began jogging on a treadmill in the bedroom while watching the evening news. Ben enjoyed becoming more than a "microwave chef," and he liked spending more time with their daughter, who stood on top of a stepstool helping him with nightly lettuce tearing and salad tossing. In a year, Samantha lost twenty-two pounds, felt more energetic, and had a sunnier mood.

To motivate yourself, remember that exercise will improve your cardiovascular health, strengthen your immune system, and help prevent obesity and adult-onset diabetes. It brings vitality, energy, and relaxation, lifts depressive feelings, and keeps you trim. Think about your reasons for taking good care of yourself, like wanting to live a long and healthy life. None of us really "finds" time for self-care and exercise. We *make* time for these crucial activities because they are essential to our well-being and health.

You probably already have an idea of what kind of exercise you'd do if you only had the time. And if not, you can get loads of information about exercise in the books or videos listed below, or from personal trainers in your gym or health club. If you've recently had a baby, your OB/GYN can make recommendations about safe and gentle exercises to strengthen stretched-out abdominal muscles or tighten up the pelvic floor; of course, if you have any orthopedic or anatomic problems that interfere with exercise, please consult your doctor or physical therapist for specific suggestions. The real issue is how to shoehorn exercise into a day that's already crowded with work and family. That's our focus here, as we look at ways to fit fitness into everyday life with children.

Resources for Exercise

Strollercize: The Workout for New Mothers by Elizabeth Trindade and Victoria Shaw
Kinergetics: Dancing with Your Baby for Bonding and *Better Health for Both of You*
    by Sue Doherty
Strong Women Stay Young by Miriam Nelson (www.strongwomen.com)
Real Fitness for Real Women: A Unique Work-Out Program for the Plus-size Woman
    by Rochelle Rice

Getting Started

If you are just starting to exercise, take heart. It feels great simply to begin, to know that yes, you are really doing something wonderful for yourself. Set realistic goals that you know you can consistently attain, and perhaps write them down so you can see them every day and stay on track with your own care amidst attention-grabbing infant and child care. You can keep boredom at bay by doing a variety of things, like taking a brisk walk in the early morning on Monday while your husband handles the kids and breakfast, stopping at the gym on Tuesday and Thursday after work, and then going on a long bike ride with a friend over the weekend.

If you have a regular exercise partner, you can help each other stay motivated, and when she shows up at the front door, it'll be easier to extricate yourself from your housework or family. And if your resolve starts to sag, take a look at that picture of yourself as a child we mentioned in chapter 3 (p. 81); she is precious and beautiful, and seeing her sweet face can help sustain your positive self-loving energy. Once you build up momentum after a few weeks, it will feel odd not to exercise, and every step you take on your own behalf—whether baby-sized or big ones—will make you feel better and better.

If you haven't exercised for a few months or more, take it easy when you start up again. The old adage, "The road to hell is paved with good intentions" certainly applies to overzealous plunges into exercise. And if your body has become at all depleted, your muscles and connective tissue could be prone to strain, since they may have low levels of the minerals that keep them supple and resilient. So before you dive into a major program, we suggest you take a few days first to do ten to twenty minutes a day of gentle yoga or stretching. And try to do some stretches at the start of any workout; stiff muscles are like sleeping children: they need encouragement and a little time to wake up!

Aerobic Activities

Any good fitness program balances the development of aerobic capacity and strength. Your goal is to work up to keeping your heart beating fast (but not more than 140 times a minute) for at least twenty to thirty minutes, three or four times a week. No matter how out of shape you might be, or super-busy, there's always something you can do to get the blood moving and a sparkle in your eyes. Here are some suggestions we've seen work for mothers.

Go for a walk or a run. You can walk by yourself, grab another mom, or—courtesy of modern technology—use a cell phone with a headset to catch up with a friend. Bringing your child in a stroller or in a baby backpack will make it even more aerobic and eliminate the child care problem. Check out your community by asking friends, going through a local newspaper, or looking at bulletin boards: many have a group of moms who go for walks together; Jan joined one that took short hikes with little ones in baby packs. Or if you're ready to pick up the pace, you can go for a run; you could even bring your child, if you like, by using a baby jogger, a mommy-powered tricycle.

Ride a bike. Riding is great fun with a child. She can sit behind you in a kid seat, or you can get a cruiser-trailer that hooks on to the end of your bike, and she'll look like a queen in a carriage. If she's old enough to ride on her own, she can come with you, though you'll probably need to drop her off back home midway through your workout.

Take an aerobics class or use the equipment in a gym. Many gyms now have on-site child care, even for infants. We know mothers who joined a gym with high intentions, but it was so much hassle to get out of the house that they finally gave up—so try to work out a regular schedule with your partner that's truly feasible and not rushed.

Go for a swim. Swimming is especially good for mothers who have connective tissue problems and need low-impact exercise. If you're not thrilled about showing up in a bathing suit, you can tell yourself you've earned your body the hard way, and that most people are so self-conscious about their own appearance that they're paying hardly any attention to you.

In the comfort of your home. Many women like to exercise at home while watching a workout video tape. Or get your own treadmill, rowing machine, etc. For example, every morning Ricki reads the newspaper while riding a stationary bike at home. Beginning when Leah was in preschool, Ricki started getting up a half hour earlier to do this—and her only regret is that she didn't start a couple of months after her baby was born!

Exercise your mind as well as your body. For a double workout, how about combining aerobics with the stress-relief techniques described in chapter 2? For instance, try to imagine that a dark cloud of tension leaves when you exhale, and a lovely light of peace and happiness enters when you inhale. You could repeat affirming statements to yourself or listen to an inspiring tape. Or focus on "being here now" and let your attention rest in the sensations of your body or in what you see.

Strength Training

There's nothing like strength training to flatten a tummy, fortify an aching back, or get a grip on upper arm flab that seems like it has a mind of its own. The obvious option is to use the free weights or machines in a gym. But you might also be amazed at how much of a workout you can get while tending to children, running errands, or doing housework. During the tiny in-between times—such as when your baby is sitting in a high chair or walker, contented with a toy or a cracker—you could do some sit-ups or push-ups while leaning against a wall. You might try keeping a set of weights by the phone and working the free arm with bicep curls or tricep flexes. Carry your grocery bags by their handles, so you can either curl your biceps or stiffen your elbows and challenge your shoulders by seeing how high you can raise the bags; life is too short to worry about how it may look to others!

Just like with aerobics, there's always *something* you can do to become stronger.

Making a change is usually hard at first, especially when you're already fatigued from 3 a.m. wake-ups or long days at work. It's also a sad irony that guilt about not taking steps for yourself can make you feel so down and discouraged that it's even harder to get some exercise. But when women reflect back on their lives, it is the positive changes they have made and sustained that they feel best about. That's the very best way to show guilt the door: try some of the road-tested suggestions above, notice how good you start to feel, and go on to take another step toward your fitness improvement goals.

Keeping a Basic Balance in Your Life

The overall balance in your life does more than affect your emotions; it goes straight to the bottom line of your physical health. For example, you know how you feel when things start getting out of whack: you're running around, pouring out and not getting much back. Then, of course, you catch a cold.

So far, we've discussed your health mainly from the perspective of Western science and medicine. But as powerful as those approaches are, the idea of balance has been *vastly* more developed within an entirely different framework, that of Chinese medicine. Learning even a little about that system can lead to a far-reaching shift toward greater health. We'll apply its basic principles to three types of moms. See if one of these patterns fits you fairly well (it's the essence that matters, not all the details), and we'll tell you the Chinese herbal formula that could increase the well-being of each type.

The Classical Chinese View of Mothers

Chinese medicine—developed over five thousand years—is founded on the central idea of bringing harmony to the various forces inside and around a person. In your own life, these could include the interplay of systems within your body or the ebb and flow of your emotions. These forces all exist within the Tao, the mysterious, generative unfolding of the universe, considered to be itself the mother of all things:

> *The Tao is called the Great Mother:*
> *empty yet inexhaustible,*
> *it gives birth to infinite worlds.*

> —*Tao Te Ching* by Lao Tzu (English version by Stephen Mitchell)

A deep respect for mothering is woven into the fabric of Chinese medicine and culture. Traditionally, the Chinese mother is given great care around and after the birth of her child. Since she has poured out so much during pregnancy and childbirth, balance must be restored both by arranging for her to do as little as possible and by replenishing her through rest and nourishing foods and herbs. For at least a month, the woman and her baby are secluded from the rest of the world, and the mother is gently taken care of by others. Afterward, she is nurtured with good foods, exercise, herbs, and acupuncture.

The core elements of Chinese medicine are less mechanistic than the variables Western doctors study, like counts of white blood cells or transfer rates across cell membranes; rather than seeing the body as a machine, traditional Chinese doctors view it more as a dance of subtle energies. The more graceful the dance, the healthier the dancer.

The Mother with Depleted Yin

Two fundamental forces that waltz within a mother are called *yin* and *yang*. Yin is the receptive principle, with related attributes of earth, darkness, yielding, rest, passivity, cold, inwardness, pause, quiet, and decrease; it is sometimes viewed as feminine, although yin and yang are present in each person regardless of gender. Yang is the active principle, and its attributes include sky, light, firmness, activity, initiative, heat, outwardness, speed, noise, and increase; it can also be considered masculine.

The symbol of yin and yang is a circle, with one portion dark, for the yin, and one portion light, for the yang. But at the center of the yin is a spot of yang, and vice versa, which maintains the balance of yin and yang. Within each principle, the opposite one is blooming. For instance, inside activity there must be a center of quiet observation, and inside the darkness of the night sky there must be seeds of light.

Each principle has value: the sky is not better than the earth, and cold is not better than hot. But life becomes imbalanced when a person becomes stuck in one principle and lacking in the other, and this can lead to illness. If a mother is active, afterward she needs a period of rest. If she puts out love and attention all day long, she must receive it as well.

The balance of yin and yang that is harmonious will vary from person to person. To find the balance that is right for you, think about the following questions:

- What are the yin elements within your life? What are the yang ones?

- Does the yin principle seem to be lacking? Or does it seem excessive? How about the yang principle: lacking or excessive?

- How might it be healthy for you to build up the yin in your life? Or to limit it? The same for yang: increase or decrease it?

To put these questions in a larger context, consider the balance of yin and yang in our society. Modern civilizations are very yang, and that excess in combination with a lack of yin is a root cause of the stress- and lifestyle-related illnesses that plague us. It's as if we live inside a giant furnace, with the bellows of media, pagers, corporate culture, and all the rest fanning white-hot flames of excessive speed, activity, and clamor. To restore balance to her life, a mother typically needs to curb these too-powerful yang forces and foster more yin. Fundamentally, it is the principle of yin that mothers the mother. And within this context, a person will often benefit from boosting certain yang elements, such as asserting herself with her partner or taking initiative to find a better job.

Now let's apply these ideas to a mother with depleted yin. Laurie had always been sensitive and a little nervous, but she felt that way more than ever since becoming a mother four years ago. There was a background sense of being uneasy and frazzled much of the time, and seemingly little things could really upset her. It seemed hard for her to settle, and deep inside there was a longing for the nurturance of others, in part because it had become so hard to soothe herself. She felt frayed at the very root of her being.

Physically, Laurie sometimes felt a bit dizzy for no apparent reason, an irritating ringing in her ears came and went, and she often had low back pain. After each pregnancy, she went through many weeks of hot flashes and night sweats. She sometimes felt oddly dry no matter how much water she drank or lotion she put on. On occasion, she felt a sensation of heat, especially in the palms of her hands and the soles of her feet.

In Chinese medicine, depleted yin means insufficient calming, cooling, and nurturing. The body lacks the ability to absorb stress and return to equilibrium. In a sense, yin is embodied by the parasympathetic nervous system, which balances the sympathetic nervous system that is triggered during stress; without that regulating influence, the body is left in a continual state of "fight or flight" overdrive.

A formula for this pattern is called Zhi Bai Di Huang Wan (see appendix B for where to find all the Chinese formulas we name).* Its key herb is rehmania, known to the Chinese as Shu Di Huang. Rehmania is considered to be a richly moistening and nourishing herb—just what a mother with low yin needs.

The Mother with Depleted Qi

Qi—pronounced "chee" and sometimes spelled chi—is the "vital force" or subtle energy that flows in and around all life. In your body, Qi:

- Originates and accompanies all movement, from exercise to the gyrations of atomic particles
- Protects you, which links Qi, in Western thinking, to the immune system
- Provides for harmonious transformations, such as the metabolism of food into usable nutrients
- Holds things together; for instance, prolapse (dropping) of an organ would reflect a severe deficiency of Qi
- Warms; a person who often feels cold probably needs more Qi.

You get your Qi from the "prenatal Qi" you were born with (like a battery), and from breathing, food, and herbs (like freshly generated electricity). A person cannot replenish her prenatal Qi—the battery won't recharge—and in Chinese medicine, motherhood is considered to irreversibly drain a large portion of a woman's prenatal Qi. It is thus vital to make sure you are receiving a healthy influx of Qi and that it is flowing freely.

Megan was an example of a mother with depleted Qi. She felt tired all the time, and she hadn't gotten her energy back since she had Darrin, more than two years ago. She weaned him early, since it seemed like she couldn't produce enough breast milk. She still needed to nap when he did, even though she was sleeping eight or more hours at night. Megan had gained fifteen to twenty pounds over her prepregnancy weight, but she was too tired to do anything about it. She felt physically tired much of the time, and her body would break into a light sweat from even mild exertion.

Besides feeling weary, Megan thought her digestive system wasn't working very well anymore. She often felt bloated after meals, and she had noticed that a number of foods no longer agreed with her. Additionally, she frequently felt chilly and vulnerable, with few reserves inside to meet the day, and she caught just about

---

*To repeat an oft-made point, women who are pregnant or might be, or who are nursing, should not take any medication or herbs without the specific approval of the relevant, licensed health practitioner.

every cold her son brought home. She bruised easily, and she often felt dizzy when she stood up.

Simply eating nutritious foods and breathing deeply would increase Megan's Qi. But in cases of moderate to severe Qi deficiency, a classic Chinese formula— called Bu Zhong Yi Qi Tang—is worth considering. One of the key herbs in this formula is astragalus. In Western herbal practices, astragalus is used for its energy-boosting properties and to strengthen the immune system. (For more about astragalu, see p. 196.)

The Mother with Constrained Qi

Besides being insufficient (i.e., depleted), Qi can be dammed up or constrained. For example, Susan had a three-year-old son and an eight-month-old daughter. She often felt frustrated, edgy, and cranky. Her PMS was very intense, with bloating, sharp irritability, glum mood, sore breasts, and cramps. She noticed herself snapping at her husband and children when they didn't deserve it. Some days, she felt wound so tight that it seemed she could explode.

The Qi of this mother was not moving freely, and depression and irritability were among the results. Constrained Qi causes menstrual problems as well, including irregularities in the cycle, breast tenderness, cramping, and a sense of emotional turmoil. A mother with constrained Qi may have difficulty with lactation: the milk is present, but, like the Qi, it does not flow freely. She may have lumpy breasts or develop mastitis (breast infection).* Headaches are also common in individuals with constrained Qi.

You can unblock Qi simply by shifting your body into a more comfortable position, pursuing a creative interest, or expressing something you've been holding back. You could also try the Chinese formula Dan Zhi Xiao Yao San. If this is not available, a more general formula called Xiao Yao San could do the trick. Either of these formulas could be helpful for any mother under high levels of stress.

Avoiding Health Hazards

Of course, there's more to taking care of your body than sleep, good food, exercise, and staying balanced. It also means not exposing it to hazards like environmental toxins, smoking, alcohol or drug abuse, or excessive weight: these wear on your health at a time when you can least afford it, like trying to run a marathon while carrying a couple of bricks.

---

*If you have mastitis, please see a doctor; the formulas we mention will not treat your condition.

This section offers ways to drop those bricks, starting with the toxins that everyone is exposed to these days. If none of the three hazards that follow is an issue, just skip ahead to the part about detoxifying your body (p. 143).

Environmental Toxins

Each year, *billions* of pounds of toxic chemicals are released into our environment. If you've ever worked around high concentrations of these chemicals—such as in a beauty salon, bus terminal, dry cleaners, textile mill, manufacturing plant, cleaning service, or conventional agriculture—you are likely to carry an especially high load of them. These substances have been linked to numerous health problems, including endometriosis, autoimmune conditions, hormonal irregularities, and cancer.

We're not suggesting that you are about to turn green or glow in the dark.

Safer Household Products

- For surface cleaning, try citrus-based products.
- Deodorants, toothpaste, and cosmetics without artificial ingredients are available in health food stores and many drug stores.
- Ant traps with boric acid can replace death-spray aerosols (but keep boric acid away from young children).
- In the garden, lady bugs are natural predators of insect pests. You can also spray with a mixture of an insecticide soap and water.

But our concern about the toxins that could be entering your body comes directly from the basic principles of nurturing a mother: more good things and fewer bad ones. Avoiding toxins is more straightforward than changing a bad health habit, since there's no particular pleasure in them and there are many easy alternatives.

For example, simply by eating organic foods, you'll eliminate a major source of worrisome chemicals: pesticides. Wash conventionally raised produce carefully, and minimize strawberries and tomatoes since they have high concentrations of pesticides.

Make sure there's plenty of ventilation when you use household cleansers or insecticides, and step away frequently for some fresh air. Try to get pump-sprays rather than aerosols that diffuse more widely. Be sure not to mix chlorine and ammonia products, since they produce noxious fumes. By wearing rubber gloves, you'll prevent chemicals from slipping in through the skin of your hands. Maybe putting up with an oven that's getting a little gross is better than using an oven cleaner with a skull and crossbones on it. You can also replace most household cleansers or insecticides with equally effective but probably healthier, natural products.

When you can, store food in glass containers, because plastics contain artificial chemicals that slowly leach into foods. And try not to microwave foods in plastic containers, even ones that are supposedly microwave safe: why take the extra risk when it's easy not to?

The quality of tap water in the United States varies, depending on the location, and impurities that have leached into wells or from old pipes can add further traces of chemicals to the water you and your children drink, so we suggest using a high-quality bottled water or water filters on a regular basis.

Air pollution can build up indoors, so open the windows each day, even for just a few minutes if it's nippy. You could also get more indoor plants, and consider buying an air filter or ozone machine.

Outside your home, try not to stand right next to the pump when you're putting gas in your car. We ask our dentists not to use amalgam for our fillings; even though the research on this potential hazard is still unclear, why put a substance that contains a toxic metal, mercury, inside your head when there's a good alternative? If you've got a job in a known toxic environment, see if there is any way possible to find other work or shift to a different department in the company.

Smoking Tobacco

We've all heard of someone who smoked two packs a day throughout her life until she died peacefully in her sleep when she was eighty-eight. But that's playing Russian roulette with one bullet in five chambers, since 20 percent or more of the people who smoke will die from it. Despite all the warnings, one woman in six smokes, and over 150,000 women die from tobacco-related causes every year. Even if it doesn't kill you, smoking weakens your immune system, and it contributes to diseases of the heart and lungs, stroke, osteoporosis, and early menopause. It also harms children. A baby whose mother smokes is twice as likely to die of SIDS, and her older children are more likely to have asthma, pneumonia, and bronchitis; secondhand smoke causes 150,000 to 300,000 lower respiratory tract infections annually in American infants and toddlers.

If you smoke, you already know you should quit, and if you've tried to do so, you know how hard it can be. Thankfully, there has been tremendous research on changing the habits that aren't good for your health. Let's go through the keys to success.

Change the thinking. In a sense, the part of your mind that wants to smoke tricks you into doing it in three ways. First, it makes you overestimate the immediate pleasure; for example, your mind says that a cigarette would be good right now, but in reality, by the fifth puff your mouth is already starting to taste bad once again. Second, it underestimates the future costs: who wants to think about cancer when she has a cigarette after lunch? Third, it downplays the rewards of doing something that's healthier, like breathing regular air instead of tobacco smoke.

Once you understand these tricks, the solution is straightforward. First, notice how unpleasurable most of the moments spent smoking actually are, maybe even writing a note to yourself about them. Then, the next time there's the impulse to smoke, really remember what it's going to be like, seeing it clearly, without any rosy-smoke-colored glasses. Second, before lighting up, look squarely at the horrible risks of smoking. If you really want to stop, you could make yourself imagine the moment when the doctor says you've got lung cancer, the chemotherapy, your hair falling out, having to tell the kids about your disease, getting weaker and weaker, going to the hospital for the last time, saying good-bye to your children . . . we're sorry, but you only help yourself if you, frankly, twist the blade. If that's just too intense, remember how your mouth feels after you finish a cigarette, the wheezing as you go up a flight of stairs, the extra coughing by your children. If your partner doesn't smoke, consider what it's like for him to kiss you: *Like licking an ashtray,* a famous actress once said, after filming her love scenes with a leading man who smoked. Third, imagine how good it will feel to do something healthier, such as going for a walk in the fresh air to get an energy boost instead of using nicotine. Perhaps write yourself a note describing how you'll feel after a month without tobacco, or glue a picture of a vibrantly healthy woman to your pack of cigarettes. Think about the nice things you could have with the money saved by not buying cigarettes.

Change the context. Smoking, or any bad habit, occurs in a context; change that, and you disrupt the habit. For example, if you normally smoke in the house, go outside, preferably to an unpleasant place like the garage or tool shed. If you normally have a cigarette with your morning coffee, try having a cup of black tea. Spend time with friends who don't smoke, and stay out of bars or other places people smoke. Instead of having your lunch outside, eat inside a restaurant where no-smoking rules apply. Put your cigarettes in a different, out-of-the-way place where you have to think twice before getting one.

Since the context of smoking includes the routine physical behaviors of lighting up, holding the cigarette, and so on, try varying those, too, even if it seems a little silly, like smoking with gloves on; or try this: the next time you feel like smoking, take a few big breaths and hold the inhalation on each, then light a match, blow it out slowly, and crush the match in an ashtray while imagining it's

Tobacco use is . . . the single most important preventable cause of death and disease in our society.

—Centers for Disease Control and Prevention

a cigarette. Take advantage of disruptions in your routine: if you can't smoke while visiting the relatives, do you really need to start up again when you get home? At the end of a long plane flight, you could capitalize on the fact that you're already six hours into quitting smoking. Sometimes the disruption is dramatic. Jan's mother, Dorothy, had a very serious stroke, and when she was leaving the hospital (happily, after a remarkable recovery), she asked her doctor if she could still smoke. *Sure,* he said, and paused for effect: *If you want another stroke.* Dorothy chose right then and there to stop cold turkey, and she said later, *It was the easiest decision I ever made.*

Replace the pleasure of the bad habit with one that's more positive. If you smoke for a jump-start, make sure you're eating well (especially protein), try a cup of coffee or tea, splash cold water on your face, or get some exercise. Many people smoke to manage their nervous energy; instead, get up and move around, take big breaths, or use the other relaxation techniques in chapter 2. If cigarettes provide oral stimulation, you could chew gum, munch popcorn, or press a knuckle against your lips.

Get support. It's much easier to quit smoking, or any risky behavior, when someone who cares about you is on your side. You could tell your husband or a friend that you're trying to—going to!—stop smoking, perhaps by naming a "last day" and going public with your intentions. Look into Nicotine Anonymous (NA) and see if that twelve-step approach speaks to you; NA and its close cousin, Alcoholics Anonymous (AA), have been profoundly helpful for millions of people. You can find local meetings by calling NA or AA in your phone book. (There are other support groups, like Rational Recovery, that take a generally similar approach but without referring to a "higher power.") Your doctor may be able to help you quit through a combination of a nicotine patch and a low dose of an antidepressant.

Be good to yourself. Besides the psychological stress of changing a familiar habit, there could be symptoms of physical withdrawal such as a craving for tobacco, feeling jittery, or fatigue. So try to be nice to yourself during the withdrawal phase. Eat extra well, especially fresh fruit and leafy green vegetables. Get lots of sleep. Dial back your commitments at work and try to minimize stressful activities at home: it's probably not the moment to reorganize the garage. Try to do more pleasurable activities than usual, especially those that preclude smoking, like going to lots of movies.

Avoid relapses. Most smokers have "quit" several times before they finally, truly do so. To make this time the last one, look back on any previous attempts at quitting and study the reasons why they failed—and then target those factors to stop them from controlling you and undermining your health.

You can ask people not to smoke around you, or stay away from the places you used to smoke in (other than, obviously, your own home), until it doesn't affect you. Notice that if you let yourself really feel the craving to smoke, without trying to suppress or resist it, it always passes within a few minutes. Watch out for those tricky little voices in your mind: *There's nothing wrong with just one. I'll only take a puff. No one will know.* If you feel like you're getting close to smoking again, tell someone who cares about you and ask for his or her support; maybe go to more NA meetings. If you slip and have a cigarette, you don't have to assume it means you're smoking again: tell yourself that cigarette was just part of quitting and get right back onto your program. Every day, remind yourself of the many benefits of not smoking: from being able to taste food fully to living to see your grandchildren. Acknowledge yourself for succeeding at one of the hardest things a person will ever do.

Abusing Alcohol or Drugs

Each of us drinks alcohol, and we enjoy it when we do. But it's also true that drinking is a calculated risk, and the healthiest thing a person could do is to have little or none.

Other than the antioxidants found in red wine, alcoholic beverages do nothing good for your body (and it's easy to supplement antioxidants through vitamin E and other nutrients). They're empty calories that convert quickly to sugars, taking your metabolism through a slump, and leaving you with a hangover of unwanted weight. A single drink—one beer, four ounces of wine, or a one-ounce shot of liquor—kills neurons by depriving them of oxygen: you feel that rosy glow because cells in your brain are drowning. Women metabolize alcohol more slowly than men, so its nasty effects last longer. Drinking weakens the immune system and increases the risk of heart disease, diabetes, cirrhosis of the liver, and cancer. If a mother drinks too much, it's no good for her children, either: among other problems, it feels to them like she isn't really "there" even though her body is in the room.

And, of course, drug abuse has similar consequences, whether it's something illegal—cocaine, amphetamines, marijuana, etc.—or an overuse of a prescribed medication, such as Valium, sleeping pills, or diet pills. In particular, using drugs during pregnancy—even unwittingly, before you realize you're pregnant—can harm the baby.

The keys to stopping smoking apply to alcohol and drug abuse as well. We'll review them more quickly here.

Change the thinking. You could notice that the third—or fifth—drink/joint/line doesn't add much to your buzz. You could remind yourself of the costs of abuse, both to your body and to your children. If you're willing to take off the kid gloves, you could write a letter to yourself from your children telling why they want you to stop drinking so much or using drugs. And you could focus on the benefits of acting differently. The next time you don't drink, etc., ask yourself at night if it wasn't really a better day because you didn't: notice that you feel more alert, more yourself, less edgy, and less likely to have lost your temper with the kids.

Change the context. If you like getting high on long walks, exercise in a gym.

Replace the pleasure of the bad habit with one that's more positive. If you drink when you get home from work because you're stressed, try taking a shower first, perhaps followed by some relaxing stretches. Replace your favorite drinks with similar ones without the alcohol: Virgin Marys, nonalcoholic beer, or soda water with lime. Do some hard thinking about why you drink or use drugs, and maybe talk with a friend about it. Very often, people self-medicate with alcohol and drugs in order to cope with depression, being abused, or overwhelming stress—and there are much better methods than getting drunk or stoned! Self-medication is a crutch that prevents a person from dealing with her issues in a real way, through therapy, support groups, or making changes in her lifestyle.

Get support. If you want to cut down or quit, tell a friend or your husband; for example, if a drink (or toke) with your husband gets you started, ask him if he'd be willing to unwind with you without it. Try Alcoholics Anonymous, Narcotics Anonymous, or other support groups. Your doctor could also help you stop drinking through prescribing Antabuse, which makes a person nauseous if she consumes alcohol.

Be good to yourself. Cutting back or stopping the use of alcohol or drugs means letting go of a familiar pleasure. Plus, if a person is dependent on any chemical, her brain wants that molecule. One of Rick's clients shook her head in amazement as she said: *My husband can drink half a beer and leave the rest on the counter. I've been sober for six years, and I still can't really understand how anyone can do that. There's no way I could drink just half a beer.* So be sure to get plenty of rest, fill your day with pleasurable activities that don't allow the use of your drug of choice, and hang out with people who support your sobriety.

Avoid relapses. Try to avoid the situations or people you associate with alcohol or drug use. If you feel the urge to use again, go back to or increase your support group meetings. And redouble your efforts to see the ways that using isn't really that great, to face its true costs, and to imagine the benefits—for yourself and your family—of staying sober.

Carrying Excessive Weight

Excess weight is associated with many health problems, including diabetes, heart disease, breast cancer, colon cancer, and gallbladder disease. About one woman in three is considered, by current medical standards, to be overweight. While there is such a thing as taking weight management to an extreme—one need only think of super-slender models—maintaining a reasonable weight is very important for your health. Besides, being overweight can make you feel embarrassed around others, uncomfortable making love, and bad about a fundamental aspect of yourself.

Fad diets come and go, but the best way to get to and then stay at a healthy weight has always been the same: get regular exercise—the key to losing weight—and eat sensibly. If you simply exercise every other day for half an hour straight and reduce your daily calories by five percent or so, you'll lose about two pounds a month, or twenty-plus pounds in a year. Plus it will be easier to maintain your weight since now you've got more muscle mass, which uses up more calories, and your overall metabolic rate—how fast your body burns calories—will be greater.

If you can dive into and sustain an intense exercise regime and a serious diet—and then keep the gains without your weight yo-yoing up and down—fantastic. But for many of us, the big push is followed by the big flop. Instead, it's really all right to think small: get relatively brief (thirty minutes or so) sweat-generating exercise three or four days a week and make little omissions of fat, sugary, or white-flour foods every day. And whatever approach you take, drink at least eight glasses of water a day; besides filling you up, water helps eliminate the toxins in fat cells that are released when you lose weight.

Women who treat themselves kindly reach their weight-loss goals with less of a struggle than women who are mad at themselves for "being fat." If you take a little side trip from your personal program—or a major detour through the forbidden continent—don't be harshly self-critical (which makes diet-busting comfort foods more appealing than ever), or keep on stuffing down the wrong foods while thinking something like: *Oh, well, I already blew it for today. I might as well go whole hog and load up on my forbidden items.* Be self-loving, not self-punishing!

The basic methods of losing weight are straightforward, and almost everyone can use them. The crux, therefore, is—as usual—motivation. By now, you're getting familiar with the steps.

Change the thinking. The brain sees the cookie on the tray and thinks, *Oh boy, that's really going to be delicious,* but in fact, when you actually put it in your mouth and chew and swallow and feel it in your stomach . . . oh well, it's pretty ho-hum, even disappointing. So when you're faced with a choice—eat this or not—remember the fundamental unsatisfyingness of overeating. Second, tell yourself the price you'll pay later from that chunk of unnecessary calories: sluggishness, pants that are too tight, feeling unhappy about what you see in the mirror, or the health risks down the road. Third, mainly, think about how great you'll feel and look if you eat more of the foods that are really good for you and less of the ones that are not. Eat to live, instead of living to eat!

Change the context. If you're always tempted by the pastries at a diner, eat somewhere else. If you nibble snacks in the kitchen, sit down in another room and munch a couple of carrots or handfuls of popcorn.

Replace the pleasure of the bad habit with one that's more positive. Books on losing weight often have delicious low-calorie recipes. If you eat to relax or to give yourself a treat, do something else, like read, knit, take a quick walk, or make some special tea. If you eat to feel full, drink lots of water—or another cup of that tea! This may sound odd, but you can breathe deeply for a few minutes and imagine that your body is being fed by the energy in the air. Or look at art, flowers, or your child's sweet face, and imagine that your eyes are absorbing all that beauty, which is filling and nourishing you.

Get support. You could tell a close friend or your husband that you are going to lose some weight. Overeaters Anonymous could also be a good source of support. You might like to check out Weight Watchers or other companies like it. Some have inexpensive home programs combined with telephone support that are convenient for a busy mom.

Be good to yourself. Eating less, or differently, can bring up feelings of boredom, deprivation, or even panic, sometimes reaching all the way back to childhood. So you'll need more kindness than ever, both from others and yourself. Try to increase the nice things in the nonfood parts of your life, like more cuddles with your kids, a fantastic new novel, or a deepening of your relationship with your husband. Give yourself rewards along the way, like permission to linger in the shower or a new pair of pants that fit great.

Avoid relapses. Rebound weight gain is very discouraging; a friend of Jan's once said, sighing, ***I've lost two hundred pounds, but it was the same twenty, over and over again.*** Once you've gotten to a weight you like, you could write a letter to yourself—to be opened if you're tempted to overeat—that talks about how good you feel and look when you're trim. If you use a program like Weight Watchers, find out what its success rate is with helping people maintain their weight loss. If

At the end of a
meal, your
stomach should
contain one-third
food, one-third
water, and one-
third air.

—Sufi saying

Approximate KCal burned per 20 minutes of exercise

Aerobic dancing	105
Bicycling (12 mph)	188
Cross-country skiing	205
Dancing	74
Downhill skiing	169
Hiking (average slope)	174
Ice skating	100
Jogging (6 mph)	160
Roller skating	171
Rowing machine (400 strokes)	206
Running (7 mph)	245
Skipping rope	245
Standing	23
Swimming (800 yds.)	152
Walking fast (4.5 mph)	100
Watching TV	18

you start down the slippery slope of eating the wrong things, try to have the warning bells ring loudly inside your head; tell someone if you're starting to slip, and go back and do the things that worked for you the last time you lost weight.

Detoxifying Your Body

Reducing or eliminating your health hazards—whether it's environmental toxins, smoking, drugs or alcohol, or excessive weight—will make a significant difference in your health. You can also accelerate the improvement in health by actively detoxing your body, in large part by supporting the functioning of your liver.

The liver works twenty-four hours a day to cleanse your body of substances that can harm you, including the waste products of normal metabolism, food preservatives and additives, solvents in household cleaners, pesticides and herbicides, alcohol, drugs, toxins excreted by microbes in the digestive tract, and heavy metals (e.g., mercury or lead). Your blood continually circulates through the liver, which filters out these harmful molecules and converts them into a form that can be readily excreted.

Studies have linked poor detoxification to several diseases, including fibromyalgia, chronic fatigue syndrome, Parkinson's disease, and cancer. The ability of the liver to do its work varies from person to person, and you could find out about the strength of your own detoxification processes through a liver detoxification panel offered by several medical labs (see appendix B). Meanwhile, you can help your liver through lifestyle choices and by taking certain nutrients. You've already learned about several actions that will support the liver: getting good nutrition (particularly cruciferous vegetables) from mainly organic foods, limiting your exposure to toxic chemicals, and taking supplements containing the MSDVs (notably the B vitamins, vitamins E and C, and magnesium, selenium, and molybdenum).

In addition, your body produces a peptide called glutathione that strongly aids liver detoxification. Vitamin C and selenium support glutathione production, and you could take their Intensive Daily Doses (see appendix D). Whey protein also boosts glutathione, and you could try to eat a daily serving of this food (available at health food stores as a protein powder—which could be part of an easy breakfast). Additionally, you could take a precursor to glutathione, N-acetyl-cysteine, with a dose of 500–1000 mg/day, or take glutathione directly, at 100–400 mg/day (although there is some question about how well the body assimilates glutathione in an oral supplement).

Other amino acids, including taurine, methionine, glutamine, and glycine can also be helpful to liver detoxification. Try supplementing any one of these, at 200–500 mg/day; start at a lower dosage if your body is particularly sensitive.

Numerous herbs promote liver detoxification as well. Perhaps the best known is milk thistle, also known as silymarin, which functions as an antioxidant and prevents depletion of glutathione. The standard dosage is 70–210 mg, three times per day.

In some cases, using supplements or herbs to aid detoxification can put the body into a temporary state of discomfort (as toxins are being processed at an accelerated pace). If this happens, reduce the dosages and see if that helps. If the discomfort continues after a day or two, stop taking the supplement or herb. If detoxification has strong side effects, that suggests a need both to detoxify your body and to do so carefully while working with an experienced, licensed health practitioner. Finally (as usual), we don't think you should take supplements or herbs for detoxification if you are pregnant or nursing.

Having Regular Checkups

Depletion starts at the molecular level in your body, and it can go a long way before becoming really obvious. To stay healthy, you've got to catch little things before they get big: putting off checkups until you're ill is like searching the stable for clues after the horse has run away. For instance, Margie brought her two-year-old to the pediatrician and mentioned, only in passing, that she was four months' pregnant but had not yet seen her obstetrician (Ricki) because she had been unable to "organize" the appointment. Margie lost her train of thought a few times, but she reassured the doctor that she was only tired, due to still getting up at night with her daughter. Nonetheless, he was concerned about Margie, and he prodded her to see her obstetrician within the week. Based on Margie's fatigue, sluggish reflexes, and swelling in the skin of her lower legs, Ricki ordered blood tests for thyroid, which showed dangerously low levels. Margie immediately began taking a thyroid supplement; within eight weeks she felt fine, and at twelve weeks, follow-up testing showed normal amounts of thyroid.

In another case, Carolyn came to see Jan for help with her nutrition. Flustered about arriving twenty minutes late to her first appointment, she made an off-hand remark about feeling *like there's no insulation anymore on the wiring in my brain.* She had previously managed a high-powered career with aplomb, working as a senior editor on a major newspaper. But now, small hassles looked huge, and she always felt both tense and exhausted. In addition to receiving a routine physical from her family doctor, Carolyn had seen a knowledgeable endocrinologist, but that assessment had found no problems with Carolyn's hormones. Jan suggested testing her amino acids, and indeed, two important ones—tyrosine and taurine—had become seriously depleted. Jan arranged for Carolyn to get a balanced amino acid formula, and she began feeling much better after a couple of weeks. Looking back on what had happened, she said: *I don't think I would have let things go so far before I had Chianna. You're coping with something new every day, and you're so tired that you just hold on and figure it'll get better. But, you know, I think I also sort of expected to feel not-great, so when I started feeling worse and worse, I thought it was normal for moms, or at least this one. If I had it to do all over again, I'd seek help for my health much sooner.*

Most mothers see a physician for themselves just once a year, if at all, during their annual appointment with a gynecologist. And lab studies other than pap smears are not routinely done unless you mention a problem or something of concern is found during the exam.* So it is important to take a moment before a doctor's appointment to reflect on how you are feeling, especially if you have changed providers since your last checkup. No one likes to complain. But health care providers can figure out what is going on and lend a helping hand only if they know how you are doing. So here are some suggestions for getting the most out of an appointment with your gynecologist, or another doctor.

Keep a personal health file. If you're concerned about a symptom or possible health condition, try to make a brief note about it in a daily diary. You could describe what you felt, the severity, how it changed during the day, and what seemed to make it better or worse (e.g., your menstrual cycle, supplements or medications, diet, stress). This information will be clarifying to your doctor or other health professionals, and it will also help you make sense out of how you're feeling. We aren't suggesting that you catalog every ache, pain, or blue moment. But it's important not to downplay physical or emotional problems.

In addition, keep copies of laboratory test results, notes from previous office visits, patient handouts, and so on together in a secure place. Along with your symptom diary, these will give you a highly useful personal health file.

Be organized for the appointment. Bring your personal health file and a list of questions you want to address. Take notes during the appointment (or right afterward), so you can be sure about key points later on.

Be brave. Acknowledging the problems or sense of frailty you're experiencing can take courage. But your doctor can't know that you, let's say, are losing urine with coughing and sneezing unless you mention it. Similarly, if you feel worn out but it doesn't seem serious enough to mention, please remember that it really *is,* since fatigue is a symptom of many illnesses; be clear with the nurse or attendant when he or she interviews you that this is an important item to address with the doctor.

Tell your doctor about your history and any risk factors. For example, a family history of problems with the reproductive, endocrine, gastrointestinal, or nervous sys-

---

*Or if you had certain health problems during a recent pregnancy.

tems increases your risk for depletion. Heavy and frequent menstruation may drain iron or suggest an imbalance in your hormones. Difficult pregnancies or miscarriages challenge a woman's body. A postpartum depression triples the risk of another one, and it may indicate underlying instabilities in the endocrine system. Past experiences of clinical depression, anxiety, trauma, or drug or alcohol abuse can suggest a vulnerability to the stresses of motherhood.

Share how you've been feeling. Let your doctor know how you are managing emotionally while taking care of your children, home, work, and other obligations. He or she will want to know about the stressors in your life, like a child with health problems, or marital conflict. You can ask for a referral to other professionals or to agencies that might help, such as a therapist, a psychiatrist for possible medication, or a parenting resource center.

Bring all your medications and supplements. The easiest way to let your doctor know what you're taking is to bring it all in a bag. That way, he or she can be aware of any interactions or side effects.

Perhaps make a special appointment. If you need to, make another appointment besides your annual physical to discuss your health concerns, since they deserve adequate time for reflection, not the hurried type of "roller skates" doctor visit that has become so common with managed care schedules. Most doctors will be sympathetic and helpful. But if little interest is shown, you may need to look around for another physician.

Follow up if necessary. Examination and history taking alone may give your doctor enough information to make an initial assessment of your health status. Based on the findings, the doctor could recommend a course of action, and if it works, then that would tend to confirm his or her initial diagnosis. For example, if you feel run-down and have been eating poorly, a reasonable first step is to improve your diet and find ways to get more rest; if that restores your sense of vitality, there could be no need for further investigation.

But if the initial assessment raises nagging questions, the first round of intervention has mixed results, or you simply want a thorough review of your health, then we encourage you to pursue further testing; as a guide, the next chapter summarizes how to assess the gastrointestinal, nervous, endocrine, and immune systems of your body. If you take this step, please be sure to look at appendix E for an insider's view on how to advocate for yourself in the modern health care system, and how to think clearly about the assessment results and your doctor's recommendations.

Unfortunately, some health care organizations resist assessment because it costs money, and you may have to stick up for yourself to get the tests you need. At worst, you could have to pay out of pocket for some testing. As difficult as that can be, an investment in your health usually comes back tenfold in decreased long-term medical costs. Additionally, there is the intangible but precious benefit of feeling good in your own body.

Of course, the purpose of assessment is to understand what *action* you could take in order to feel better. In the next chapter, we will describe how to reverse the process of depletion and restore greater balance to your body's systems.

What to Do If You're Getting Depleted

*Y*OU CAN PREVENT DEPLETION by maintaining a low level of stress and following good wellness practices (discussed in the previous chapter). But if you find that there's just no way to have a low-stress life, or you entered motherhood with a physical vulnerability, or you—like most mothers—have already undergone a year or more of serious outpouring with little replenishment, there's a good chance that you're already getting depleted—perhaps to the point of having Depleted Mother Syndrome (DMS). In this chapter, you'll learn about physical interventions that can reverse that process and restore:

- The nutrients that keep you healthy
- Balance to the systems of your body

This chapter is different from the others. Basically, it's a repair manual full of detailed information about four key systems in your body: gastrointestinal, nervous, endocrine, and immune. (A person could have a health condition in another system, such as musculoskeletal or cardiovascular, but we've selected the four that, in our experience, are most commonly depleted by motherhood.) As with any repair manual, it makes sense to focus on the sections that deal with the problems you're facing and skip the ones that don't (unless you have a particular interest in health, especially from a holistic perspective). And if you're feeling very well in general, you could go on to the next chapter.

The check-up described at the end of the last chapter may already have identified a health issue and made it clear which section(s) of this chapter you should look at. Additionally, see if any of the following symptoms apply to you:

- *Gastrointestinal* (p. 159): Overfullness or gassiness after eating, heartburn, indigestion, stomach or abdominal pain or cramping, blood or mucus in the stool, food sensitivities, frequent vaginal yeast infections, overproduction of respiratory mucus, constipation, diarrhea, irritable bowel syndrome, fatigue

- *Nervous* (p. 169): Depressed mood, chronic anxiety, feeling reactive, problems sleeping, worsened concentration and memory, tremor, frequent headaches, any sudden change in cognitive function

- *Endocrine* (p. 176): Fatigue, PMS, feeling chilled or hot (including hot flashes), vaginal dryness, change in sexual response, dry skin, unusual hair loss, depression or anxiety, feeling hyper, heart palpitations

- *Immune* (p. 189): More frequent or longer bouts of cold, genital herpes, or cold sores, new allergies or heightened reactions to known allergens, new or heightened autoimmune reactions, chronic inflammation (e.g., painful joints).

You can find out more about the state of these systems, including the extent of any depletion, through the assessments described in this chapter.

When your body is humming along, you can simply maintain your wellness practices and leave it at that. Yet if it starts getting depleted, you've got to give it serious attention, which requires knowledge and skills you probably never expected to need as a mother. If you persist in caring for your body, health problems (such as those listed above) often improve. But our focus here is on replenishing and balancing the gastrointestinal, nervous, endocrine, and immune systems rather than treating any particular ailment. If you have (or suspect you might have) an illness, you should see your doctor immediately. Additionally, we recommend that you try the interventions we describe only in the context of an ongoing professional relationship with a knowledgeable, licensed health provider—ideally one who is familiar with holistic methods (see appendix E).

Since Jan developed problems in all four systems she'll start by telling her story, which illustrates how health conditions are often intertwined, and how to address them *in combination.* Then we will describe the spectrum of conventional and alternative methods you can use for your own health; in consultation with your providers, you can select the interventions that make the most sense for you. Next, for each system, you'll learn about:

- The system in general
- How motherhood can affect it

- Common symptoms when it's drained or dysregulated
- Tips for assessing it
- Ways to replenish and balance it

Because long-term maternal health has received fairly little attention, our suggestions are essentially a first draft of a protocol for reversing depletion; as new information comes in, there will be more sophisticated and integrated approaches. We've also chosen to be conservative, generally mentioning only those interventions that have received support in the research literature and with which we are familiar (see www.nurturemom.com for the references); other practitioners may suggest different methods. You'll probably find that there is an intuitive wisdom inside that lets you know which methods will be best for you. To your health!

Jan's Story: "I'm Going to Get Better!"

Before having children, I had always been a healthy, basically happy person with an even-keeled disposition. That's why it was so shocking when I became increasingly depleted, even as I was feeling joyously fulfilled by motherhood. Although I've spoken with many moms who had experiences that were similar in some ways to my own, every mother's story is different; please see what fits for you in mine.

Drains and Stresses

I was thirty-two when I became pregnant for the first time, but after twelve weeks, I miscarried in a night of intense labor, and I was very upset at this loss. After a few months, I got pregnant again. I enjoyed my size; having always been a little overweight, it was now okay to be so! Because my baby was in a breech and oblique position, we scheduled a C-section, our son Forrest was born without complications, and I quickly bounced back.

I feel committed to a very nurturing style of parenting. But it sure is a lot of work! I responded to Forrest quickly if he wanted something, and I nursed him whenever he was hungry. Rick loved taking care of Forrest and was very skillful at it. But since he was the sole provider while also going to graduate school, Rick wasn't around much. And no one else seemed to be around, either. Our relatives all lived far away, and our circle of friends—none of whom had children—gradually evaporated. I felt isolated for the first time in my life. Meanwhile, I went back to work part-time at home, doing a form of deep-tissue bodywork called Hellerwork. Taken as a whole, I was pouring out a lot and handling a fair amount of stress with very little replenishment. But so far my health had remained good, and Rick and I felt eager to have another baby.

I became pregnant with Laurel soon after Forrest turned two, and I continued breast-feeding because I felt it was the best thing for him. But the nursing, which had always gone well, started to get physically uncomfortable, a warning sign—which I ignored—that something was out of balance. I kept working—and looking after a rambunctious two-year-old—until one month before Laurel was born.

Another warning sign: my relationship with Rick began to deteriorate during this pregnancy, for the first time in our long relationship. I was worn out, busy with Forrest and work, and queasy most of the time, so my marriage was at the bottom of my priorities. Rick saw how much I was dragging and worried about me. He encouraged me to take more time for myself, but I just couldn't: it seemed like such a hassle to organize, and it was hard to be away from my son. When we went to the hospital to deliver Laurel via C-section (same breech problem), I became painfully aware of the gulf that had grown between us. Rick was very sweet with me while we waited to begin the surgery, and I hadn't felt that connection to him for so long. It made me deeply sad.

Laurel was a really easy baby. Nonetheless, with a single child you occasionally get relief, but two of them never seem to sleep at the same time! Each day became a long sprint of work leading up to an exhausting night. On top of that, I was now nursing both children. My body seemed to cry "no" at the thought of breast-feeding Forrest as well as Laurel, but I felt I couldn't refuse him. He would have been devastated if he lost his nursing along with having to share his mother's love and time with his sister.

Amidst all this outpouring, the stresses continued to add up during that first year after Laurel's birth. My body had undergone its second surgical procedure (the C-section) in a few years. Sleep was constantly interrupted. When Rick and I argued about raising the kids, there was an intensity that had never been present before in our fights, because the issues had never been as serious. Our quarrels would rattle me for many hours afterward.

I wasn't getting replenished and the resources in my body were low from extensive nursing and three pregnancies in three years (counting the miscarriage). I ate whatever I could on the run, and when a well-meaning friend told me she got all the nutrients she needed from her foods alone, I followed her lead and stopped taking any vitamins. As to psychological resources, I had almost no time to myself. Our marriage had also grown cooler. We kept loving each other, and there were nice times together, but it was getting all too easy to feel quite disconnected.

This one-two punch of growing demands and shrinking resources was wearing on me right where I was most vulnerable. I was thirty-six when Laurel was born, and my body lacked the pep and resilience it had had ten years before—let alone twenty years before, the age when women in earlier generations typically began having children. Second, as I would later discover, my gastrointestinal tract had already been disturbed by years of taking antibiotics for teenage acne, and by even more years of a hefty diet of sweets.

The Crash

Trouble had been headed my way long before I saw it, like a tidal wave starting a thousand miles offshore. Unbeknownst to me, microscopic changes in my body were accumulating, and when they finally crashed into plain view, the consequences were serious. As we approached Laurel's first birthday, I acquired a chronic, daily headache that no amount of ibuprofen could eliminate, and I began to experience ongoing pain in my shoulders and back. I routinely awoke in the middle of the night and was unable to return to sleep. My whole body started feeling reactive; small scares would get my heart pounding, and it felt like my nerves were frayed and raw. I became uncharacteristically forgetful, I was rarely happy, little things that had never bothered me before now sent me into tears, and it took longer to recover emotionally.

Gloomy, pessimistic circles of thought captured my attention, and I became preoccupied with the alarming and inexplicable collapse in my mood and health: *What is happening to me?!* I am a very analytical person and it was completely frustrating not to be able to figure out what was going on.

The Realization

Finally, the first breakthrough occurred a few months after Forrest turned four. A chiropractor examined my loose connective tissue, sagging muscles, and gaunt appearance. She asked soberly, *"What do you hold your baby up with, your will?"* It was a great moment. I realized that instead of being a wimp, I was doing my best within a deteriorating body. Rick and I talked a lot and he began to understand what was going on with me in a new way. Rather than seeing me as someone who, unaccountably, just couldn't get it together to keep the house straight while he was working hard to make a living as well as studying for his licensing exams, he now realized that I was struggling with a *physical* condition.

A second breakthrough soon followed. I had arranged for a baby-sitter to watch Laurel while I went to the mall with Forrest. This was supposed to be a fun time when I got to do three of my favorite things: be with my son, window shop, and have something sweet to eat. But I walked around the mall with absolutely no interest in shopping, and when I bought Forrest and myself some ice cream, I just stared at my cone numbly, with no appetite. I was stunned at my reaction and looked inside myself. What I found was a big dark blah. I had little interest in Forrest or life altogether. For his sake, I tried to put a good face on our time together, but when I came home, I immediately called Rick. *Honey,* I said, *I think I'm depressed.* The lightbulb went on for him too, and we had one of our best talks in years.

Because we were starting to realize that I had a health problem—not just the so-called "normal" fatigue of a mom with young kids, or some kind of character flaw—Rick became much more supportive. Nonetheless, we still did not know what to *do,* nor did the doctors we consulted. Meanwhile, my health was getting worse, not better. Soon after Laurel's second birthday, I developed chronic diarrhea, which was so serious that it sometimes called me out of bed in the middle of the night. I started to have a tremor in my hands, more intense memory problems, and a sense of "roaring" under my skin. I weaned Laurel, which helped me feel a little less drained, but my chronic back and shoulder pain still got worse.

Then came the third breakthrough, around the time Forrest turned six. One day, while talking with a friend about how poor our diets had become since we had kids, I had a brainstorm that my pregnancies, breast-feeding, and stress might have taken something out of my body. I asked a physician to run a series of blood tests, and the results finally brought some clarity to what I'd been experiencing. All of my minerals were far below the normal range. Deficient minerals can compromise every system in the body—including connective tissue and muscle fiber (thus my chronic back pain)—and that is exactly what had happened to me.

These findings prompted me to assess my endocrine system, and there, too, I was running on empty. My hormone levels were generally at the low end of the so-called normal range. My doctor, a good general practitioner, reassured me that these findings were nothing to worry about, but years later, more specialized physicians concluded that my health probably would have been improved if we had addressed my endocrine system when I was first tested.

The fourth breakthrough came several months later when a holistically oriented doctor suggested that I make sure there wasn't an infection in my digestive tract. Testing revealed that I had developed a serious case of gastrointestinal dysfunction. I had contracted digestive parasites: *entamoeba hystolytica,* one of the causes of amoebic dysentery. I had never traveled outside the country, so I must have acquired them on a stray leaf of lettuce or something similar. A healthy person's bodily defenses would probably have gobbled those parasites up and ended the invasion right there. But my vulnerable immune system was worn down by years of stress, and it was soon overrun. The results were nasty. Gastrointestinal pathogens (i.e., parasites, and some bacteria and viruses) disrupt the digestive tract and impair the body's ability to absorb the nutrients in food. Some also excrete toxic substances, and these can disrupt the subtle balance of brain chemistry, increasing depression, anxiety, and a sense of mental fog.

The Diagnosis

Now I finally had an accurate diagnosis. I had entered motherhood with low nutritional reserves due to years of a mediocre diet and a digestive tract that was far from optimal because of antibiotics and sugar. These reserves were drained further by several pregnancies, five years of continuous breast-feeding, and lots of hard work. The impact of maternal stress on my GI tract made it less able to absorb nutrients, so I became even more depleted. Nutrient shortages and stress had weakened my immune and endocrine systems. Gastrointestinal pathogens had exploited these vulnerabilities and infested my body. The results were digestive problems, tremor and other neurological symptoms, fatigue, muscle tension and pain, depression, and anxiety. In short, I had developed a severe case of Depleted Mother Syndrome.

The Treatment

With this clarity, I was able to pursue a course of treatment that has enormously improved my health, although it took time and there were many ups and downs. Because my problems were complex and severe, I used many approaches over a number of years. It is unlikely you will need to do anything as elaborate.

In sum, I took the following actions:

- I started taking multiple rounds of antibiotics and herbs to treat the digestive pathogens.
- I switched to a diet low in sweets (to stop force-feeding the pathogens) and high in vegetables and protein.
- I introduced a daily regimen of minerals and vitamins (for better general nutrition), as well as beneficial bacteria for my digestive tract.

- I used Chinese herbs and acupuncture.
- I took iodine to support thyroid function (initially, my body could not tolerate hormones given directly).
- I tried biofeedback for tension and tremor, and with some reluctance took antidepressants for chronic pain, insomnia, and low mood. After two years, I tapered off and I doubt I'll need antidepressants again. I am now aware of natural methods that might have been as useful, but the medications were an effective bridge to healthier functioning, and they gave me a clearer head with which to make decisions about my overall care.

These days I can still get thrown off by overstress or poor nutrition (such as sugar binges over the holidays, alas), but now I usually have decent energy, normal digestive functioning, no pain, no tremors, and a positive mood. I feel very grateful that the methods above worked.

In retrospect, though, probably my most useful intervention of all was intangible: acquiring a greater understanding about maternal health. Knowledge gives you choices and a sense of direction, which is why there's so much detail in this chapter. Feel free to skim the parts that don't seem relevant to you, and talk with supportive professionals about the parts that do.

The Spectrum of Care

In our experience, generally the best way to replenish and settle a person's body is to combine Western medicine with sensible, alternative techniques, all resting on a foundation of basic wellness practices (as discussed in chapter 4). This integrated approach is increasingly accepted, and its methods form a *spectrum of care** (see Figure 3). There are a number of advantages to drawing from the entire spectrum of care—not just Western medicine—for reversing maternal depletion:

- Alternative methods excel at treating the core characteristics of depletion: nutritional deficits, imbalanced bodily systems, and a chronic, subclinical course. (Subclinical conditions are clear departures from health that are not severe enough, or sufficiently well defined, to be considered an illness.)
- Your body is like a fragile house of cards when it's depleted, and alternative methods are gentler and less likely to disturb it.

*Aryuvedic medicine is an additional option within the spectrum of care, but none of us has any experience with it, so it is not included; if you'd like to explore that modality, you can find experienced practitioners in every major city.

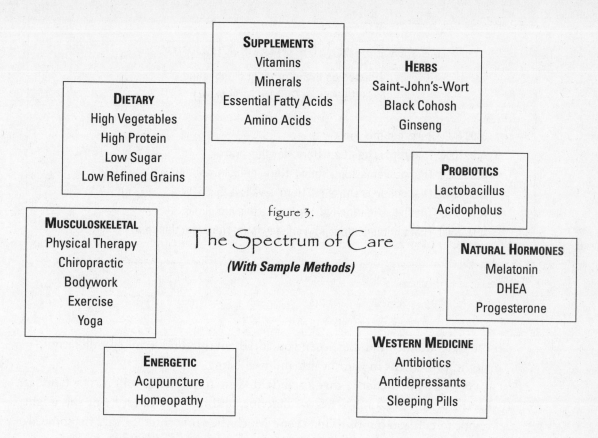

figure 3.

The Spectrum of Care

(With Sample Methods)

SUPPLEMENTS
Vitamins
Minerals
Essential Fatty Acids
Amino Acids

HERBS
Saint-John's-Wort
Black Cohosh
Ginseng

DIETARY
High Vegetables
High Protein
Low Sugar
Low Refined Grains

PROBIOTICS
Lactobacillus
Acidopholus

MUSCULOSKELETAL
Physical Therapy
Chiropractic
Bodywork
Exercise
Yoga

NATURAL HORMONES
Melatonin
DHEA
Progesterone

ENERGETIC
Acupuncture
Homeopathy

WESTERN MEDICINE
Antibiotics
Antidepressants
Sleeping Pills

- Depletion has multiple causes and consequences that usually call for several kinds of interventions.

- Different methods work for different people—but you don't always know what will succeed until you try it. Therefore, if you come at a problem with several approaches, if one doesn't help, chances are that another will.

- Different types of interventions often work together synergistically, so that the whole is greater than the sum of the parts.

- A comprehensive approach brings together professionals with different perspectives, which means a check on each other's assumptions.

- The spectrum of care allows a mother to select methods with which she is comfortable; for instance, you could want to treat a depressed mood through antidepressants, or you might prefer first trying regular exercise.

In sum, we recommend that your health care start with a Western medical doctor in order to rule out or treat any serious medical condition. But we also suggest that it not end there, because of the benefits of alternative methods. Individually, some of

A Brief History of Medicine

(Posted on the Internet and published
in the *Family Therapy Networker*)

2000 B.C.: Here, eat this root.
A.D. 1000: That root is heathen. Here, say this prayer.
A.D. 1850: That prayer is superstition. Here, drink this potion.
A.D. 1940: That potion is snake oil. Here, swallow this pill.
A.D. 1985: That pill is ineffective. Here, take this antibiotic.
A.D. 2000: That antibiotic doesn't work anymore. Here, eat this root.

those gains will be mild, but when you add them up, mild + mild + mild + mild = major improvement in your health and well-being.

There is a good chance that a standard Western physician will not be familiar with the alternative approaches we describe, and in some cases, he or she might attempt to talk you out of trying them. Much the same could be said for some alternative practitioners with regard to Western medicine. We think any intervention for your health should be judged on its merits, not tradition or dogma. For help with discerning the strengths and weaknesses of different approaches, finding competent professionals who understand the spectrum of care, and getting the most out of any assessment, see appendix E, the Insider's Guide.

As you look at the options within the spectrum of care in the rest of this chapter, please don't be overwhelmed by all the possibilities: the point is that there are *lots* of things that could help you feel better if you've become depleted. Start with something that makes sense for you, try it for a month or so, and if it doesn't seem to make much difference, try something else. It probably took a year or two for you to become depleted, and it will take a while to turn that around. It's more important to keep plugging away at a broad and sensible effort to replenish and settle your body than to seek one hypothetical magic bullet that might make everything better.

So let's get down to business, starting with the primary pathway to replenishing your body, the gastrointestinal system.

Your Gastrointestinal System

If your gastrointestinal system (GIS)—housed mainly in the stomach and intestines—is not in good working order, you will get fewer of the nutrients you need to handle the demands and stresses that come with being a mother. That means you need to take care of three important elements:

- *Membranes.* The surface area of your small intestine would cover an entire tennis court if all the millions of microscopic folds in its walls were laid out flat. This forms a membrane between the contents of the digestive tract and the rest of the body that absorbs food and filters out damaging substances.

- *Enzymes and hydrochloric acid.* Enzymes in your mouth start the process of digestion, and hydrochloric acid in the stomach breaks food down further. Enzymes secreted into the upper end of the small intestine cut these particles into even smaller pieces, and then they are absorbed in the small and large intestine.

- *Microbial ecology.* Your intestines are home to vast populations of microorganisms. For example, bacteria normally comprise about forty percent of the dry weight of stool, with roughly 400 billion bacteria per gram (456 grams = 1 pound). These include several hundred species of bacteria, both benign and harmful, as well as yeast and perhaps some parasites. The beneficial microflora aid digestion, make vitamins, and help keep the harmful microbes in check.

What Can Disturb the Gastrointestinal System

The GIS is easily disturbed by stress—but that's part of a mother's daily diet! As we saw in chapter 1, stress causes the mouth to produce less saliva and the stomach to secrete less hydrochloric acid. It also leads the small intestine to stop necessary contractions, and blood flow to decrease to the stomach and intestines. If the demands of raising a family give a mom more headaches, increased use of nonsteroidal, antiinflammatory drugs (NSAIDs) such as aspirin or ibuprofen, can irritate and inflame the lining of the gut. Nutritional shortages, accumulating over several years, may deplete the intestinal walls of the bricks and mortar that keep them in tip-top shape. In order for digestion to proceed properly, things have to keep moving along, but pregnancy often makes the GIS sluggish, and the effects can linger after the baby is born if you've been eating a diet that's low in vegetables, whole grains and fibers—which is widespread among busy mothers.

Maternal stress can disrupt the delicate balance of the microbial ecology in the digestive tract, leading to a condition termed *dysbiosis*. As well, a mother's reliance on quick foods—which usually contain lots of white flour and sugar—can foster a population explosion of harmful microorganisms (especially if her immune system is already taxed), worsening the dysbiosis. A healthy GI tract requires the beneficial microorganisms to outnumber pathogenic ones many times over. It's like a lawn: a few weeds are inconspicuous and easy to pull, but if the crabgrass takes over it damages the whole yard, and it's really hard to remove. Dysbiosis has been linked to numerous symptoms, including constipation, diarrhea, cramping, and inflammation in the digestive tract.

Further, these factors may lead to what is called a food sensitivity, in which the immune system "thinks" there is something threatening about a particular food and produces high levels of antibodies to it.* Why would this happen? When your GIS is disturbed, the membranes of the digestive tract may become inflamed and compromised, allowing food molecules that have been incompletely broken down to pass through into the bloodstream; this condition is termed intestinal permeability or "leaky gut syndrome." The sentinels of the immune system know what a thoroughly digested bit of steak is supposed to look like, but these oversized, only partially processed "macromolecules" are strange: they could be a threat, so the body's defenses are mobilized to protect you.

In a vicious cycle, a food sensitivity causes the immune system to attack that food in your GIS, which creates more inflammation and makes it even easier for incompletely digested food particles to enter your bloodstream, leading to more sensitivities. Clearly, it pays to keep the GIS humming along at peak efficiency so that it can fully digest the foods that come down the hatch.

Motherhood can also impact the GIS indirectly, through its effects on the nervous, endocrine, and immune systems. For example, disturbances in neurotransmitters such as serotonin can trouble your digestive tract. Irregularities in thyroid hormone (more likely after children) can lead to constipation or diarrhea. And if the immune system is weakened by maternal stress, it is less able to protect the digestive tract against infection.

Of course, factors unrelated to motherhood could be impacting your gastrointestinal system, such as work stress or overuse of laxatives. Therefore, we suggest

---

*This theory is somewhat controversial, but we think the research and clinical evidence for it is persuasive; see the Reference Notes at www.nurturemom.com for more information.

that you discuss any GI symptoms with your doctor. (This point applies, as well, to the nervous, endocrine, and immune systems.)

Signs and Symptoms of Disturbance in the GIS

In our experience, many mothers have some kind of disturbance in their gastrointestinal systems. You might experience indigestion, a feeling of overfullness or gassiness after eating that may include heartburn. There could be pain in your stomach, intestinal cramping, or a general sense of discomfort throughout your abdomen. Or nausea, constipation, diarrhea, or gas. Any one of these symptoms feels bad, plus it makes it harder to give your full attention to your children or work.

GIS dysregulation can also lead to problems in other parts of the body. Poor absorption in the digestive tract causes shortages of nutrients elsewhere. More speculatively, there is some evidence that food sensitivities can lead to an overactive immune system in general, which would tend to increase inflammation (and perhaps the likelihood of developing an autoimmune condition). Some health professionals have observed an apparent association between vaginal yeast infections and an overgrowth of yeast in the digestive tract.* And the toxins excreted by pathogenic microbes may lead to fatigue, inflammation, depressed mood, or poor memory.

Gastrointestinal Assessment

The first consideration in gastrointestinal assessment is evaluating whether there is an illness, such as an ulcer, Crohn's disease, or cancer. To find out, start with your doctor, who may refer you to a specialist called a gastroenterologist. And when you assess *any* system of your body, it is important to rule out other possible causes of health problems. For example, fatigue might be due to a GI disturbance, but it could also be a result of thyroid disease, autoimmune disorders, anemia, malnutrition, lupus, or alcohol abuse.

Next, we suggest you consider innovative and specialized laboratory testing. Unless your doctor focuses on nutritional medicine or holistic health, he or she

---

*Low levels of yeast are normally present in the digestive tract, usually without apparent harm. Yet high levels, particularly in terms of your own body and its needs, can cause constipation or diarrhea, increase the likelihood of vaginal infections, and produce microtoxins that can weaken your immune system. Additionally, in our experience, when populations of intestinal yeast are reduced, there is usually an improvement in energy and overall well-being.

may be unfamiliar with these tests. In order to find a professional who is, see appendices B and E.

What might these tests reveal? You can find out if you have any nutrient shortages through analyzing your blood or urine, and your symptoms will guide the focus of testing. For example, dry skin and hair suggest a lack of essential fatty acids, while fatigue, shortness of breath, or a pale complexion may be due to insufficient iron. (While an iron panel is a routine test, other minerals—as well as vitamins and essential fatty acids—require a specialized assessment, ideally of the levels of these nutrients within red blood cells.) Amino acids can be assessed through a urine or blood sample; we encourage many mothers to have this test since amino acids are so often depleted in them. These various tests can identify specific nutritional deficiencies. Additionally, multiple deficits may point to overall GI dysfunction, especially if you have a reasonably good diet and take a multivitamin/mineral supplement.

Pathogenic microorganisms can be assessed through stool tests. The byproducts of these tiny organisms will also be revealed in a urine test for organic acids; this test is particularly useful for assessing anaerobic bacteria, which are nearly impossible to detect in a stool test (since they die on contact with oxygen). Finally, beneficial bacteria such as acidopholus may be cultured to see if there are good quantities of these helpful bugs in your digestive tract.

Allergies and food sensitivities are assessed through skin and blood tests. Skin tests detect foods (and other substances, like airborne molds) that you have an immediate, strong reaction to, like getting hives after eating shellfish. Blood tests measuring the immunoglobulim G (IgG) antibody can identify responses to foods that build more slowly, which means these tests are more likely to reveal immune system reactions that you were unaware of. Because your immune system reacts to food in multiple ways, no one test is perfect, and arguably the most effective method for finding out if you are sensitive to a food is to eliminate it and observe the results (please see the box opposite). You could also keep a daily diary of what you eat and any symptoms; when you look back at your notes, you can sometimes see definite patterns.

In general, any one of the tests above may miss a genuine problem (called a "false-negative" error; see appendix E for more on this error). If you have GI symptoms but testing doesn't seem to identify a specific cause, keep persisting and looking at your gastrointestinal system from different angles, perhaps with other professionals. Meanwhile, even without clear assessment findings, you could intervene cautiously, using modalities that have little chance of harm, such as Energetic, Dietary, or Probiotic.

Possible Indications of
Gastrointestinal Disturbance

Overfullness or gassiness after eating

Heartburn

Indigestion

Diarrhea

Constipation

Stomach or abdominal pain, burning, or cramping

Blood or mucus in the stool

Food sensitivities

Fatigue

Frequent vaginal yeast infections

Overproduction of respiratory mucus

Balancing Your Gastrointestinal System

Here are some options within the spectrum of care for bringing greater balance to your GIS.

Energetic. Promoting gastrointestinal health has long been a cornerstone of Chinese medicine, and there is evidence that acupuncture could help your GIS. We've also seen homeopathy be useful for strengthening a mother's overall constitution—benefiting the GIS indirectly—as well as for specific gastrointestinal symptoms. Proper homeopathic diagnosis is based on a precise analysis of an individual patient, which usually requires an experienced homeopath. But on your own, you might like to experiment with one of the remedies below, listed with their identifying characteristics (see p. 104 for how to take homeopathic remedies); it is all right to try a remedy even if some of the details about it don't fit you.

- *Nux Vomica.* This is a remedy for a hard-working, hard-playing, ambitious, take-charge mother. She may be very irritable, intense, or tense. She might drink alcohol or eat too much. Regarding GI disturbance, the intensity and indiscretion with food and alcohol may cause an upset stomach. She could crave sweet or fatty foods, and she may be constipated.

- *Lycopodium.* This remedy is for someone with considerable rumbling in the stomach and gas. This person may sit down to a meal feeling very hungry, but is full after only a few bites. She tends to constipation, and her symptoms often seem worse between 4 p.m. and 8 p.m.

- *Sulfur.* This is for those suffering from burning pains in the stomach, intestines, or other places in the body. This person may tend toward diarrhea, particularly in the early morning. She may have smelly flatulence, with an odor of rotten eggs. She could feel bloated, and is usually the worse for drinking milk. She tends to be messy.

- *Arsenicum Album.* This remedy is for the mom who is neat and fastidious, no matter what is going on. She is anxious and restless during the day, even with a sense of agitation. She could experience burning sensations in the hands or joints, perhaps comforted by applying warmth (like a hot water bottle). Regarding GI disturbance, there are likely to be sensations of burning throughout the digestive system, and perhaps burning diarrhea.

Musculoskeletal. One simple way to reduce the effects of stress on the digestive tract is to do a minute or two of deep breathing before meals. If your child is old enough, see if you can get her to join you—and maybe she'll be more willing to eat her peas!

Dietary. Follow the nutritional approach described in the previous chapter (p. 107), with these additions:

- *Sugar.* If there is a significant imbalance in the microorganisms in your GI tract (i.e., dysbiosis), you should starve the microbes by completely eliminating sugar, refined carbohydrates, and alcohol (which converts quickly to sugars). Once the coast is clear—indicated by an end to symptoms and laboratory testing—you can usually return to the sugar guidelines in chapter 4.

- *Fiber.* Try to consume about 35 grams of fiber each day. In part because fiber-rich foods often require more preparation time, mothers tend to eat too few of them, but fiber both aids the movement of food through the digestive tract and supports beneficial bacteria. High-fiber foods include whole grains, legumes, beans, and many fruits (especially pears and apples) and vegetables. You could make a big pot of rich, high-fiber soup (split pea, lentil, bean, etc.) over the weekend. If you can't get your daily dose of fiber from foods alone, you

Common
Food Allergens

Wheat
Corn
Eggs
Milk
Soy
Chocolate (sorry . . .)

Assessing Possible Food Sensitivities Through Elimination

Eliminating a particular food can be difficult, since it is often the foods we desire most that give us the greatest trouble. Nonetheless, trying an experiment for a week or so can often tell you a lot.

Select the food (or foods) that you want to evaluate, and *completely* eliminate it for seven to ten days; for instance, with dairy this would mean no milk in your coffee, no butter, no pesto with parmesan cheese, etc. Meanwhile, make no other changes in your health practices so that the impact of the elimination will be as clear as possible.

Notice if any symptoms of GIS dysfunction (p. 161) have gotten better. If they have, that suggests a food sensitivity. For extra confirmation after the elimination period, challenge your body with a large serving of the food in question while making no other changes; if symptoms return, it is even more likely that you are sensitive to that food. But do not perform this challenge with foods that you have had a strong reaction to—particularly anaphylactic shock—unless you are doing so under a doctor's supervision.

Unfortunately, eliminating a food to which you are actually sensitive may not always lead to an improvement within ten days, particularly if your GIS has been compromised by multiple factors. For some people, a period of elimination up to six weeks may be necessary, and even then, other factors besides food sensitivities may continue to give you trouble. Therefore, a lack of improvement in your condition following a period of elimination does not necessarily prove that you are *not* sensitive to a food. That's why assessing potential food sensitivities through both blood tests and elimination is often most informative, combined with a common-sense analysis of whether other factors may also be disturbing your body.

can take it as a supplement, but then be sure to drink at least eight cups of water a day.

- *Food sensitivities.* Eat as few foods as possible to which you know you are sensitive. In particular, if you have any GI symptoms, try eating no gluten* or milk products for a couple of weeks, and you might be amazed by the results. A mild sensitivity can frequently be managed by eating a food only once every few days, but a moderate to severe sensitivity usually requires total elimination for at least six months; sometimes it is possible to reintroduce the food sparingly, but often it will remain something you'll

---

*Foods high in gluten include wheat, rye, oats, and barley.

never do well with. Cookbooks are available with delicious recipes for foods that can replace the ones that disturb your digestion (please see the suggestions below). Diet is largely a matter of habit. After getting through the phase of "withdrawal" and shifting to other foods, we bet you'll be quite content with your new diet, especially with the rewards of feeling so much better.

Selected Cookbooks if You Have an Allergy

The Allergy Self-Help Cookbook by Marjorie Hurt Jones (Rodale Press)

Special Diet Solutions by Carol Fenster (Savory Palate)

The Allergy Cookbook and Food Buying Guide by Pamela Nonken and
    S. Roger Hirsch (Warner Publishers)

Cooking for People with Food Allergies by USDA Human Nutrition Information
    Service (U.S. Government Printing Office)

Baking for People with Food Allergies by U.S. Department of Agriculture
    (U.S. Government Printing Office)

Allergy Recipes by American Dietetic Association

Going Against the Grain: Wheat-Free Cookery by Phyllis Potts (Central
    Point Publishing)

The Complete Food Allergy Cookbook by Marilyn Gioannini (Prima
    Publishing)

Food Allergy Field Guide by Theresa M. Willingham (Savory Palate)

Supplements. At a minimum, take the MSDVs of the nutrients listed in appendix D. Going one step further, intensive daily doses (IDDs) of one or more of the nutrients just below could provide additional benefit to your GIS, particularly if there is a functional deficiency in that nutrient. For example, essential fatty acids are needed for the walls of your intestines, plus they may help with serious GI disturbances, such as ulcerative colitis. While some studies and practitioners have found benefit in even higher doses, we recommend that you not go beyond our IDDs unless you are working with a licensed professional who has experience in doing so. (All of the IDDs are listed in appendix D.)

Hydrochloric acid is required for proper digestion, particularly of proteins and minerals. Although TV commercials make acid stomach sound like an epidemic, in fact *low* acid is a more common problem. Supplements containing hydrochloric acid are available at most health food stores. Try taking one or two pills at the end of a meal, in order to allow your body to produce as much of its own acid as possible before reinforcements arrive. Don't use them if you already have a sense of burning in your digestive tract or if you experience discomfort afterward; pregnant or breast-feeding women should take them only under the care of a health practitioner.

To mobilize the enzymes in your GIS, start by following the advice you may have heard as a child: "Don't wolf your food!" Yes, sometimes you've got just eight minutes for lunch, but whenever you can, take your time between bites—at least enough to set your fork down. And during meals drink liquids in moderation so as not to dilute your enzymes.

Additionally, taking enzymes as supplements can assist your digestion. There are two types: plant- and animal-based. Generally, plant enzymes are taken at the beginning of a meal, based on the theory that they are more able to survive the acid in the stomach, while animal-derived enzymes are typically taken at the end; for dosages and other details, look at the label on the bottle.

Herbs. Many Chinese herbal formulas "tonify the spleen Qi," which is metaphorical shorthand for strengthening the digestive tract. Two formulas mentioned in chapter 4 (p. 134) may be particularly beneficial. Bu Zhong Yi Qi Tang is believed to strengthen the digestive tract and immune system, and Dan Zhi

NUTRIENT	INTENSIVE DAILY DOSE (IDDs) FOR THE GASTROINTESTINAL SYSTEM
A	50,000 IU for several days, then reduce to MSDV levels; do not ever exceed 5000 IU per day if you are pregnant (or might become pregnant) or are nursing
C	5 grams to bowel tolerance (the maximum dose that does not lead to diarrhea), divided into at least two separate doses, and buffered if you have an ulcer or experience stomach irritation
E	800 IU
Zinc	50 mg (after a few months, stay at about 30 mg)
L-glutamine	1–10 grams
Essential fatty acids	2000–4000 mg of omega-3 fish oil containing 500–1000 mg of DHA; or 2 tablespoons of flax oil

Xiao Yao Son may be useful for individuals whose digestive tracts are especially vulnerable to becoming disturbed by stress. Each formula is meant to be used over several months, rather than as a quick fix. They can be purchased from Chinese herb pharmacies (see appendix B), www.nurturemom.com, or an acupuncturist (who can also make you a customized formula).

Numerous Western herbs could benefit your GIS. Licorice root—in the form of deglycyrrhizinated licorice (DGL)—has a soothing effect, and studies have shown that it can reduce gastric pain and even help heal ulcers; the dosage ranges from 250 to 750 mg, three times a day.

In particular, several herbs can suppress the populations of pathogenic microorganisms, including garlic, goldenseal, and oregano (this last one is best used when it is emulsified or enteric coated). With mild GIS symptoms, you could try one of these herbs on your own for a month or so, and see if it gives you some relief. It's generally best to start at the low end of the range of dosing given on the label, and increase gradually, if at all. Sometimes a "die off" reaction happens, in which symptoms get worse for a few days, presumably because the microbes are releasing toxins as they die. If your symptoms are moderate to severe to start with, the herbs don't help much, or you have a strong reaction to them—please seek out the care of an experienced practitioner. And after you've finished a trial of antimicrobial herbs, you should supplement probiotics to restore healthy populations of beneficial bacteria.

Probiotics. These beneficial microorganisms crowd out pathogenic ones as well as aid digestion in general. Lactobacillus bacteria (such as acidophilus) occur naturally in yogurt, and you can also get a much more concentrated supply of probiotics in supplements from a health food store, including lactobacillus strains and bifidobacteria (i.e., bifudus). Probiotics should be refrigerated both in the store and after you bring them home, and check for a guarantee of viable organisms on the label of the bottle. There are several schools of thought about the best time to take probiotics, but in general, we suggest you do so between meals.

Western medicine. As we've said, if your GIS is disturbed you should tell your doctor. The treatment options include antidiarrheal agents, antispasmodics, and low doses of antidepressants. You could also try over-the-counter drugs for indigestion, constipation, or diarrhea. But these interventions are aimed at reducing symptoms or treating a specific condition, not at replenishing and balancing bodily systems *as a whole*—and those are the primary goals when you are reversing depletion. While antidirrheal drugs or Pepto-Bismol might provide temporary relief, the underlying causes of disturbed digestion will persist until they are addressed through reducing stress, following general wellness practices, and taking the steps discussed above within the spectrum of care.

Similarly, you could use antibiotics to treat an infection in your digestive tract, but these are a double-edged sword, disturbing your GIS while attacking bacteria or parasites. If an infection is not yet deeply entrenched—let's say you just returned from a trip overseas and some microbes hitched a ride back with you— then antibiotics could be a silver bullet. But we've known numerous people, including Jan herself, for whom one or more rounds of antibiotics were unsuccessful in eradicating intestinal pathogens. For this reason, some professionals use a combination of drugs and herbs, since the herbs (though less potent) can be tolerated for much longer periods. Meanwhile, in order to care for your gastrointestinal system as a whole, you should starve the pathogens by eliminating sugar and refined flour products, compete with them by adding probiotics, and repair their damage to the linings of the digestive tract (see the IDDs on p. 167, especially the essential fatty acids and L-glutamine). Microbes have had a three-billion-year head start over multicellular organisms like ourselves; they are tough adversaries if they infect your digestive tract, and we recommend working with professionals experienced in holistic approaches to treatment.

Your Nervous System

Let's start with a little experiment. Think about your child giving you a hug, and imagine the emotions and body sensations you'd feel. Now let all that go, and try thinking about her screaming in a store, and imagine your emotions and body sensations.

In each case, whatever you experienced involved the workings of your nervous system. To accomplish this extraordinary feat, your nerve cells—called neurons— are organized in a fantastic network that is arguably the most complex object yet known in the universe. Your brain has about 1.1 trillion neurons, and 100 billion of these comprise the "gray matter" that is principally involved in thinking, feeling, and acting. A typical neuron will connect with 10 to 10,000 other nerve cells at junctions called synapses, which look a little like the painting in the Sistine Chapel of God reaching out to Adam: two fingers almost touching. Neurons communicate with each other by shooting chemical messengers known as neurotransmitters across the gap. A typical neuron can fire ten to one hundred times per second, which means that somewhere between a billion and a trillion or so synaptic events involving neurotransmitters have occurred in your brain in the time it took to read this sentence.

So you can see why neurotransmitters are important. In order for you to feel good—or to have anything function very effectively in your body—the system of neurotransmitters must be in top working order. Of course, so must the rest of the brain. Because the nervous system contains such complexity, we'll focus mainly on neurotransmitters. And within that part of the nervous system, our emphasis will be on the factors that affect emotional well-being, since depressed mood is so common among mothers.

What Can Disturb the Nervous System

Of all the bodily systems, the nervous system is the one in which there is the most intimate connection between lived experience and physiology. It's a two-way street. On one side, frequent feelings of sadness, helplessness, and irritation can alter your neurochemistry to the point that a drug, such as Prozac, that increases the saturation of serotonin in the soup between your synapses can help you feel dramatically better. On the other, the effects of motherhood on your body can send ripples—sometimes shock waves—through your mind:

- *Stress.* Whether you're intervening in sibling quarrels or worrying about a sick child, recurring everyday stresses can change the balance of neurotransmitters in your brain, creating a biochemical highway to depressed mood, and poorer concentration and memory.

- *Nutrition.* Pregnancy, breast-feeding, and the work and stress of raising a family can lead to deficits in nutrients that either are neurotransmitters—such as the amino acids taurine, glycine, and GABA—or are needed to build them. For example, taurine has a calming, soothing function in the brain, but as mentioned in chapter 4, there's a high demand for it during breast-feeding, and without an excellent diet, low taurine can result.

- *Other bodily systems.* Raising a family can affect your brain indirectly, through its impact on other systems in your body. In the endocrine system, fluctuations in estrogen or progesterone—whether following childbirth or due to chronic stress—can disturb neurotransmitter systems, leading to depression, anxiety, or a poorer memory. Thyroid dysregulation after childbirth,

---

Possible Indications of Disturbance of the Nervous System

Depression

Anxiety

Insomnia

Poor concentration or memory

Chronic headaches

Any sudden change in cognitive function

Tremor

or due to an autoimmune condition related to motherhood (see p. 179), can lead to depression. And as cortisol rises due to stress, DHEA declines, which has been linked to depressed mood.

In the immune system, allergies and inflammation (which increase after children) can lower your mood. Gastrointestinal dysfunction due to maternal stress can have a similar effect, both by impairing the absorption of nutrients needed for serotonin, and by causing upsetting symptoms.

Signs and Symptoms of Disturbance in Neurotransmitters

Fleeting, everyday experiences of sadness, fatigue, or anxiety do not in themselves suggest a fundamental change in your brain chemistry. But chronic experiences of this sort just might. (As might other symptoms that are unrelated to motherhood, such as ringing in the ears, tremor, or a sudden change in cognitive functioning; any one of these should prompt an immediate call to your doctor.) For example, consider the effects of imbalances in these neurotransmitters:

- Serotonin: Depression, irritability, anxiety, and insomnia
- Norepinephrine: Depression and fatigue
- Dopamine: Depression and fatigue
- GABA (Gamma-aminobutyric acid): Anxiety and insomnia

Brain chemistry is intimately involved in your fundamental sense of "me," and it can be very troubling to experience an unpleasant change within your own mind. But you can get a good assessment of your nervous system, and there are many effective ways to replenish and balance it.

Assessment of Neurotransmitters

There are two levels to assessing neurotransmitters: your subjective experience (symptoms), and the objective status of these chemicals in your body (signs). For example, most evaluations for depression—and prescriptions for antidepressants—are based on the first level alone, using questions such as *How long have you felt this way? How frequently, within a typical week? How intense does it get?*

But you can also get laboratory tests that assess the second level. Some can reveal shortfalls in the amino acids that function as neurotransmitters or the building blocks from which they are made. You can also test for vitamins and minerals needed to build neurotransmitters. Other tests measure the breakdown products of serotonin, dopamine, and norepinephrine—which is like estimating the number of animals in a meadow by counting their scat. (See appendix E for how to find a licensed health professional familiar with these various tests.)

Balancing the Neurotransmitters of Mood

Whether you're just feeling a little blue or slipping into a mild depression, here's how to intervene within the brain (focusing on neurotransmitters) to nudge it in the direction of more positive mood. Our emphasis is on balancing neurotransmitters in general rather than treating any specific psychological condition. If you have moderate to severe depression, these methods might help somewhat, but they will probably not resolve it completely, and you should be sure to see a therapist or doctor. (Also see the section on depression in chapter 3.)

Energetic. Acupuncture can lift a mildly depressed mood, and we have seen several homeopathic remedies help as well:

- *Sepia.* This is the classic remedy for a worn-out mother who has given it all for her children. She feels irritable, drained, worn out, or exhausted most of the time. She may be emotionally flat, or have become indifferent to those she loves the most.

- *Ignatia.* This is for someone who feels quite sad and often has a sense of loss and silent grieving. She could sigh a lot, be quite nervous, or be moody and changeable.

- *Natrum Muriaticum.* This is for the mother who is sad and depressed, but does not want to be consoled or receive sympathy. She likes to be alone. Even if she is upset, she may not cry, especially if around others. She may feel dry, with cracked lips and a frequent sense of thirst, often craving salt.

- *Nux Vomica.* This is a remedy for a hard-working, hard-playing, ambitious, take-charge mother. She may be very irritable, intense, or tense. She could drink alcohol or eat too much. Regarding mood, this mother may be angry, and find fault with everyone around her.

Musculoskeletal. Regular exercise (p. 126)—particularly aerobic—often provides a strong boost for mild depression, sometimes working as well as an antidepressant.

Dietary. Since shortages of specific nutrients can affect how you feel, it's important to eat nourishing, well-rounded meals. And please don't go on a low-protein diet if you tend toward a drop in mood, since it could plunge you into a bout of depression.

On the other hand, one food can lower your mood when present in *excess*: sugar. Studies have found that eliminating sugar can improve mood; in fact, significant changes in brainwaves have been documented in some individuals after saying good-bye to sweets. Eliminating caffeine and alcohol can help as well.

Supplements. Studies have shown that deficits in the nutrients listed in the table below—especially omega-3 essential fatty acids and vitamin B_6—are associated with depressed mood; for example, shortages in B_6 reduce the metabolism of tryptophan into serotonin. Supplementation, especially when there is a deficiency, could improve your mood. (Add individual B vitamins only if you are already consuming MSDV levels of B vitamins in general.)

Amino acids also play an important role in your mood, and supplementing one could lift your spirits if it is deficient in your body and the neurotransmitter it supports is the principal source of the slump in your mood. *Tyrosine,* for instance, is the basis for the neurotransmitters norepinephrine and dopamine, which are involved in the regulation of mood. If you are deficient in tyrosine or its amino acid precursor, phenylalanine, supplementing one of these may help improve your mood. A commonly used dose of tyrosine or phenylalanine is 500–1000 mg, and it's best taken in the morning on an empty stomach for good absorption and to avoid insomnia.

Another amino acid, *taurine,* can also help take the edge off of irritability or

NUTRIENT	INTENSIVE DAILY DOSES FOR THE NERVOUS SYSTEM
Omega-3 oils	500–1000 mg DHA (from 2000 to 4000 mg fish oil supplement)
B_6	50–100 mg pyridoxine; or take 50 mg of pyridoxal-5-phosphate an hour before eating breakfast or taking supplements containing minerals
B_{12}	Try sublingual tablets, 2000 mcg, 1–3/day; severe deficiencies may require B_{12} injections
Folic acid	800 mg
Iron	If lab test shows deficiency, 30 mg, twice daily between meals; try to avoid taking it at the same time as calcium
Zinc	50 mg; or 100 mg for one month, then decreasing to 50 mg
Magnesium	800 mg, ideally as magnesium glycinate; decrease if there is soft stool or diarrhea

tension. You could try 500 mg, taken in the morning; to optimize its effect, make sure you're also taking at least 400 mg/day of magnesium.

Methionine is an amino acid that becomes *S-adenosyl methionine (SAMe)*, which in turn helps the body with a process called methylation that is required for the production of many neurotransmitters. Low levels of SAMe are associated with depressed mood, and several well-controlled studies have found that supplementing SAMe is often quite effective in relieving depression (and it also seems helpful for joint pain). Taking methionine or SAMe is likely to be most successful if an amino acid test has indicated that you have low levels of methionine (but you could experiment with supplementing either of these without testing). The most commonly used daily dosage of SAMe is 400–800 mg, and it should be taken in special enterically coated capsules on an empty stomach. We suggest starting at 200 mg—especially if you are sensitive to medications—or at 100 mg if you have a history of panic attacks; a person with manic-depression should take SAMe only under medical supervision. Since SAMe is several times more expensive than methionine, you may prefer to use that nutrient; the typical daily dose is 500–1000 mg, but our suggestions and cautions about dosing with SAMe apply to methionine as well. If you use methionine, take at least 400 mg of magnesium per day for optimal benefit. Also be sure you're getting the MSDVs of vitamins B_6 and B_{12}, folic acid, as well as 125 mg of betaine; methionine and SAMe metabolize into homocystine, a compound linked to cardiovascular disease, and these B vitamins convert homocystine into benign substances in your body.

Tryptophan is used to make serotonin, and studies have shown that supplementing it or *5-hydroxytryptophan* (a metabolite of tryptophan that is closer to serotonin) is often successful in the treatment of mild depression. For suggestions about taking 5-HTP, please see page 104 in the previous chapter. Although the dosage of 5-HTP commonly used in studies of depression is 200–300 mg/day, we recommend starting at 50 mg and then increasing by 50 mg every few days, depending on how you feel; do not exceed 150 mg per day, and do not take 5-HTP along with Saint-John's-wort, antidepressants (especially MAO inhibitors), or any psychoactive drug or herb, unless you are doing so under an experienced doctor's supervision.

Herbs. The most common herbal treatment for depression is Hypericum perforatum, also known as *Saint-John's-wort.* Many studies have found it to be helpful for mild depression about fifty to eighty percent of the time, though it does not appear to be an effective treatment for severe depression. The dosage commonly used is 900 mg per day of "standardized extract" (containing 0.3 percent hypericin, one of the active ingredients), divided into two or three doses. Although some people may feel it in the first few days, it often takes several weeks for the full effects to be apparent.

As with any herb you take, use Saint-John's-wort that is produced by a reputable botanical company to ensure that you are getting both high quality and the correct dosage. About two to twenty percent of people taking Saint-John's-wort suffer side effects (which may diminish after a few weeks), such as mild gastrointestinal disturbance, sedation, dizziness, or sensitivity to sunlight. Do not use Saint-John's-wort with 5-HTP, antidepressants, or any psychoactive drug or herb. If you are on *any* prescription medication—in particular for contraception, blood pressure, or HIV—ask your doctor before trying Saint-John's-wort.

Kava has been long used by South Pacific islanders to promote a relaxed and peaceful state of mind, and in several studies it was as effective in relieving anxiety as benzodiazepines (valium, etc.), but without their drawbacks (e.g., impaired mental activity or addiction). The dosage typically used is 45–70 mg of kavalactones, three times per day; we recommend starting at the lowest dose and using the minimal amount to get the effect you desire. Do not take kava in conjunction with alcohol, antianxiety medications, or sedatives (including valerian; see p. 104); if you have Parkinson's disease; if you already feel de-energized by depression; or while you are driving. At high doses over several months to a year, kava may cause dryness and scales; these side effects can usually be reversed by reducing or eliminating this herb.

Natural hormones. From a practical standpoint, hormones come in three varieties:

- *Natural or bio-identical.* Whether they are extracted from natural sources or manufactured, these hormones are identical to their form in your body, and some are available over the counter (i.e., melatonin, DHEA,* progesterone).

- *Natural or bio-identical, but available by prescription only.* These include thyroid, estrogen, and testosterone.

- *Manufactured, modified versions of the hormone, available by prescription only.* These molecules are similar to hormones and have hormonelike effects. Examples include progestins such as Provera.

The natural molecule—the one your body is adapted to—generally has advantages over a near copy (though there may be a specific reason that your doctor rec-

---

*Technically, DHEA is often not considered a hormone, since there are no specific receptor sites for it. But it is a crucial building block for many other hormones, and for simplicity, we will discuss DHEA as if it were a hormone.

ommends the manufactured version). But beware: The fact that you can walk into your local drugstore and buy several kinds of natural hormones may give the impression that there's little to worry about; yet just because something is "natural" or available without a prescription doesn't mean it's harmless. Hormones are powerful substances, so we must repeat this point: you should *always* consult with a licensed health practitioner about their use—especially if you are pregnant or breast-feeding.

Supplementing DHEA may help lift a depressed mood, particularly if there is an "adrenal insufficiency" (you can find out by testing; see p. 187); in some cases, it also seems to boost a woman's sex drive. But there are also risks in supplementing DHEA, since it is the basis for numerous hormones, including estrogen and testosterone, and unnaturally high levels in those hormones can be problematic. We suggest you discuss the pros and cons with your doctor before trying DHEA.

Western medicine. Antidepressants have been one of the great medical success stories in this century, and millions have used them to good effect. They are most often prescribed by physicians in general practice; if the first choice works for you, fine, but if not, we suggest you consult with a psychiatrist who specializes in them.

Compared to the natural alternatives (such as 5-HTP or Saint-John's-wort), antidepressants are stronger and more likely to help with moderate to severe depression. On the other hand, they are also more likely to have significant side effects, including emotional blunting, dry mouth, loss of libido, or inability to climax. (Pregnant or breast-feeding women need to be particularly careful about the use of antidepressants.) One strategy is to start with a natural remedy, and if that is not powerful enough, consider moving on to an antidepressant.

If the root cause of feeling blue is physiological, a biochemical solution—whether it's Serzone or Saint-John's-wort—may be all you need. But if a depressed mood is due to psychological, interpersonal, or circumstantial (e.g., sleep deprivation) factors, a purely physical intervention could allow the real causes of your suffering to remain unchecked, as well as rob you of an opportunity for learning and personal growth. In many cases, a biochemical approach is best used as a short-term intervention to lift a smothering cloud and thereby free a person up to take action—psychologically, interpersonally, and materially—to improve her well-being over the long term.

Your Endocrine System

Similar to the multitasking mother, hormones manage a wide range of vital business, from the essentials of survival to keeping a smile on your face. You hear so much about estrogen and progesterone because of their role in menstruation and menopause, but there are many other hormones involved in every bodily function, including reproduction, digestion, sleep, emotion, and thought. They travel around the body like little boats launched by various glands—such as the ovaries, pituitary, hypothalamus, or adrenals—carried by the tides of blood and other fluids, and then docking at their destination in receptor sites perfectly designed for the shape of their hull.

Sometimes a hormone goes off to work on an organ, such as estrogen preparing the uterine lining to play loving hostess to the embryo. Other times the destination of a hormone is the brain itself; as a result, hormones affect memory, self-control, and mood. And sometimes the target organ is another endocrine gland—like when the pituitary sends a message to your adrenals to secrete cortisol to handle a new stressor. Hormones thus affect each other in intricate feedback loops of extraordinary complexity and dynamism. Some even turn into other hormones, such as progesterone to cortisol. Adding a further layer of complication, one hormone may have many functions; for instance, estrogen plays an important role in memory and in promoting rapid immune responses to invading microbes.

For the endocrine system to function well, several kinds of things have to work properly:

- Correct amounts of hormones; for example, too little thyroid leads to lethargy and too much may lead to the protruding eyes and speedy buzz of Grave's disease
- Sufficient numbers of correctly formed and available receptors that can receive the hormones circulating in your body
- A well-regulated system; small changes in the proportion of one hormone to another can make a large difference: for example, it is the changing ratio of estrogen and progesterone—not their absolute quantities—that is an important factor in determining whether you'll suffer from PMS
- Effective detoxification of the waste products of hormone metabolism, so that they do not accumulate in and harm your body

What Can Disturb the Endocrine System

Conception, pregnancy, childbirth, breast-feeding, and the deepest instincts to nurture a child are all guided by your hormones. Whenever so many hundreds of complex and intertwining molecular processes are set in motion, it doesn't take much to disturb that dance—and leave the dancers reeling and out of place. For example:

- After a child is born, progesterone and estrogen crash, dropping to a hundredth of their previous levels. Most women recover in a few weeks from the "baby blues," but progesterone and estrogen levels may end up settling down to somewhere other than an optimal point, even after the baby's first birthday.

- And of course, a new roommate has moved into your home: stress. Everything from sleep disturbance to quarrels with your partner tends to rattle your progesterone, estrogen, insulin, cortisol, and thyroid hormones.

- The thyroid gland seems to be especially vulnerable postpartum. One possibility is that the immune system—which has to be "turned off" in certain ways in order not to attack the developing fetus—may go to the other extreme in some cases when it is "turned on" after childbirth, and start attacking the thyroid gland. Whatever the causes may be, about one woman in ten will develop an autoimmune disease of the thyroid gland in the postpartum period. In general, the risk of thyroid problems increases three to four times after a woman has children.

Common Signs of Endocrine System Imbalance

Fatigue

Feeling of chilliness

Dry skin

Hair loss (but some hair loss postpartum is normal, with regrowth over the next few months)

Depression or anxiety

Hyperactivity

Heart palpitations

Feeling hot

Marked premenstrual symptoms of irritability, water retention, breast tenderness

Hot flashes

Vaginal dryness

- Your body is designed to return to menstruation within a few months after childbirth if you are not breast-feeding, and by six months or so if you nurse. But sometimes this restoration of normal cycling does not occur smoothly, especially if you were prone to menstrual irregularities, or are now eating poorly or under a good deal of stress.

- The impact of motherhood on the GI, nervous, and immune systems can also affect the endocrine system. Digestive imbalances can throw off the delicate rhythms of the hormonal dance, and deficiencies in key nutrients can weaken the dancers. Several endocrine glands (such as the pituitary) are located within the brain, and ups and downs in the neurotransmitters that regulate mood affect your hormones as well. Disturbance in the immune system can trigger autoimmune reactions that attack endocrine glands such as the thyroid or pancreas.

Signs and Symptoms of Disturbance in the Endocrine System

Although the complexity of hormonal interaction can make it difficult to point to a single hormone as the culprit, these are some symptoms that might indicate hormonal imbalances:

- Fatigue, feeling of chilliness, dry skin, hair loss,* lack of menstrual periods, or a glum mood are signs of *low thyroid.*

- Hyperactivity, racing heartbeat, tremor, bulging eyes, feeling hot, or anxiety could indicate *high thyroid.*

- Marked premenstrual symptoms of irritability, water retention, breast tenderness; irregular bleeding; or depressive feelings suggest rapid shifts in or low levels of *progesterone.*

- Hot flashes, vaginal dryness, or depressed mood are signs of *low estrogen.*

- Waking around 4 a.m. and being unable to return to sleep, overreactions to stress, or daytime fatigue could mean *disturbed cortisol.*

- Lack of menstrual periods or continued milky discharge from the nipples may indicate *high prolactin.*

- Jitters or sweating may be caused by too rapid a fall in blood sugar due to an *overproduction of insulin.*

- Low energy or mood may be a sign of *low DHEA.*

---

*Since hair loss postpartum may be a side effect of the normal drop in progesterone after birth, ask your doctor about significant hair loss.

Assessing the Endocrine System

There are various ways to assess your hormones; we'll discuss the methods most relevant to reversing depletion. Hormone assessment is typically conducted by an endocrinologist, and assessing sex steroid hormones (estrogen, progesterone, etc.) is often done by a specialist in gynecological endocrinology.

- *Thyroid.* As an initial screening, you could take your basal body temperature. If it's low and you also have symptoms of low thyroid, that's good evidence you need further testing (and that taking steps to improve thyroid function may be beneficial even if lab results are "normal").

   Formal thyroid testing is commonly done through blood tests that measure thyroid stimulating hormone (TSH), which tells the thyroid gland to pump out more thyroid. (Blood tests can also measure two types of thyroid hormone, T3 and T4.) High TSH is a sign that thyroid levels are low enough that the body needs more, while low TSH means there is too much thyroid hormone, so the gland is being asked to cut back its production.

   Urine tests can reveal how much thyroid is actually being *used* by your body, even if normal amounts are being produced. There is a gray zone between high and low thyroid that requires clinical judgment that considers what might be high or low for *you.* Even with seemingly "normal" levels of TSH or thyroid hormone, you may benefit from increasing the amount of active thyroid in your body through the interventions that start on page 185.

- *Progesterone and estrogen.* These hormones can be assessed through blood and saliva tests. (If a blood test is performed, your physician will ask you to take it at a particular time if you are having menstrual cycles, when progesterone and estrogen are peaking.) Saliva tests are a sensitive measure of the "free," unbound hormones that are available for use by your body. Some labs can test your hormones during the entire menstrual cycle, providing quite a clear picture of your hormonal rhythms over time. Finally, taking your basal body temperature can also shed light on the status of your progesterone (see the box).

- *Adrenal hormones.* Cortisol and DHEA levels can be tested in saliva, blood, and urine. Since cortisol normally rises and falls over the course of the day, this hormone is generally best assessed four times during a twenty-four-hour period, which is easily done with saliva samples.

Taking Your Basal Body Temperature

• *The right thermometer.* Basal body temperature is your resting temperature without the influence of activity. To measure it, you'll need a highly accurate "basal" thermometer with two-tenths-of-a-degree increments between 97 and 100 degrees; mercury is best, and you may have to check a few pharmacies to obtain a proper thermometer.

• *Taking your temperature.* Shake down the thermometer before you go to sleep and set it on a bedside table. When you awaken in the morning, put the thermometer in the middle of your armpit with minimal movement and lower your arm. Leave it there for ten minutes, resting as deeply as possible. Then remove the thermometer and record the reading.

• *Checking thyroid.* Take your basal body temperature for three to five days during your menstrual period, while progesterone and estrogen are relatively low; if you are in menopause you can do it at any time. The ideal reading is between 97.8 and 98.2 (the familiar temperature of 98.6 is an orally measured temperature that we have when we are active). The further above or below that range you are, the more likely it is that thyroid is out of balance. If your temperature is four-tenths or more out of range, we encourage you to discuss further testing with your physician.

• *Checking progesterone.* Take your basal body temperature daily, throughout a complete menstrual cycle. The sign of progesterone is an increase of a couple of tenths of a degree in the middle of your cycle when you ovulate, and your temperature should stay at this slightly higher level until just before your period begins. If you do not find this rise in temperature, further evaluation of your progesterone could be useful.

• *Insulin.* Glucose was probably assessed during your pregnancy to make sure you were not developing gestational diabetes. If it was high at that time, that suggests increased risk for adult-onset diabetes and more reason to limit your sugar (another reason is a family history of diabetes). The standard tests for adult-onset diabetes are glycated hemoglobin and a fasting test of blood glucose; other tests may also be ordered by your doctor to assess additional details of how your body handles sugar.

Once you have a good understanding of the current state of your hormones, you can start nudging them toward greater balance. Let's see how to address three disturbances in the endocrine system that are frequently suffered by mothers: menstrual irregularities, low thyroid, and "adrenal burnout."

Balancing Your Menstrual Cycle

Menstrual imbalance often reflects a broader dysregulation in a woman's hormones. By using the spectrum of care to bring more harmony to your menstrual cycle—usually indicated by an improvement in the symptoms of PMS—you can replenish and settle a major part of your endocrine system.

First, a bit of background. PMS has many different faces, and no single solution. Its potential symptoms include anxiety, depression, irritability, carbohydrate craving, or bloating, but these can vary from woman to woman, or even from month to month in the same person. The fluctuating hormones involved in the various types of PMS—such as estrogen and progesterone, and perhaps prolactin, cortisol, the androgens, or thyroid—also vary. The ways in which your body is using and metabolizing hormones probably play a role as well. Further, imbalances in various neurotransmitters have been implicated in PMS. All this complexity means that the package of interventions that will work best for you has to be individualized.

Now, some practical suggestions. Your overall well-being is the root of hormonal health, so probably the greatest improvement in your menstrual balance will come from following the wellness program in chapter 4, supporting detoxification in your body (p. 143) so that hormones can be properly metabolized, and decreasing your stress. Based on that foundation, let's see how you could use the spectrum of care to settle your menstrual cycle and relieve PMS.

Energetic. In our experience, acupuncture can sometimes be quite helpful with PMS. These homeopathic remedies may also be useful:

- *Sepia.* The classic remedy for a worn-out mother who has given it all for her children. She feels irritable, drained, worn out, and exhausted most of the time. She may be emotionally flat, and might feel indifferent to those she loves the most. Regarding endocrine imbalance, this mother is chilly, and she may have darkened patches of skin at the upper crests of the cheekbones under her eyes. She wants sweets or perhaps salty foods; she has little or no sex drive. She may have a sense of being pulled down, perhaps of organs about to fall out. This remedy could be useful for a woman with adrenal exhaustion (see p. 187).

- *Calcarea Carbonica.* This is for the mother who is tired and lacks energy. She may be overweight, and perhaps clumsy; her breasts are swollen and painful, and she may crave sweets or eggs.

- *Nux Vomica.* This is a remedy for a hard-working, hard-playing, ambitious, take-charge mother. She may be very irritable, intense, or tense. She could drink alcohol or eat too much. Regarding endocrine imbalance, her period may be heavy, with achy and crampy pains in the lower back. She may be cold, and crave sweet or fatty foods.

- *Lachesis.* This is for a mom whose symptoms are worse first thing in the morning; her breasts may be painful. She probably doesn't like constriction, particularly around the neck. She may be talkative, even loquacious.

- *Natrum Muriaticum.* This is for the mother who is sad and depressed, but does not want to be consoled or receive sympathy. She likes to be alone. Even if she is upset, she may not cry, especially if around others. She may feel dry, with cracked lips and a frequent sense of thirst, often craving salt. Regarding endocrine imbalance, this mom has fluid retention and swollen breasts.

- *Magnesium Phosphoricum.* This is a specific remedy for menstrual cramps, particularly those made better through warmth, such as by curling up in bed with a hot water bottle, or taking a hot bath. Take the remedy at a 30C potency every fifteen minutes for three dosages, then every hour for several hours.

Musculoskeletal. In general, regular exercise promotes production of carrier proteins—tugboats guiding your body's fleet of hormones—which helps keep hormone levels more even. More specifically, exercise often has a clear benefit for PMS; for example, one study showed that women who participate in sports experience less PMS than those who don't. Regular massages can help as well, perhaps swapping with your partner or a friend.

Dietary. You are likely to have less PMS if you consume less (or no) sugar, salt, refined carbohydrates, caffeine, alcohol, and dairy products, and if you increase your intake of fruits, vegetables, and other fiber-rich complex carbohydrates.

Two types of foods are worth your special attention. The first is the cruciferous vegetables, particularly broccoli, Brussels sprouts, and cabbage. These have a compound called indole-3-carbinol (I-3-C), which has been shown to affect the metabolism of estrogen in a positive way; some of the metabolites of estrogen have been implicated in the role this hormone might play in a woman's health problems, and indole-3-carbinol appears to help protect the body from some of the effects of these metabolites. As a result, you should make sure that cruciferous vegetables are a regular part of your diet. Additionally, supplementing I-3-C may help ease PMS, but since this compound is still relatively unstudied, the most conservative approach would be to get it from your veggies alone.

Soy foods contain phytoestrogens, molecules that are close cousins of estrogen. In the body, they seem to function like a very weak estrogen, slipping into the estrogen receptors but producing a milder effect. If your estrogen levels were too high, the "competitive binding" of phytoestrogens to the receptors would be beneficial, gentling the impact of estrogen on your body. On the other hand, if your estrogen levels were too low, the phytoestrogens would activate some estrogen receptors, giving your body a needed boost. (This capacity of a single substance to moderate both high and low characteristics of a bodily system is termed "adaptogenic," and it appears to be a property of several other herbs, such as Siberian or *Panax* ginseng.) Of course, as with any other food or nutrient, you shouldn't consume extreme amounts (like soy with every meal). If you're not allergic to soy, you could have one serving of soy foods each day or so, and see if that helps.

Supplements. On top of a generally healthy diet—and the MSDVs of essential fatty acids, vitamins, and minerals (especially calcium)—supplementing intensive daily doses of one or more of the nutrients below may bring greater balance to your menstrual cycle, particularly if that nutrient is lacking in your body:

NUTRIENT	INTENSIVE DAILY DOSES FOR THE MENSTRUAL CYCLE
Vitamin B_6	100 mg pyridoxine; or take 50 mg of pyridoxal-5-phosphate an hour before eating breakfast or taking supplements containing minerals; in either case, supplementing magnesium as well may have a synergistic effect
Vitamin E	800 IU
Magnesium	800–1000 mg, ideally as magnesium glycinate; decrease if there is soft stool or diarrhea

Some women also seem to experience benefit from the essential fatty acid GLA found in evening primrose oil, especially for breast tenderness.

Herbs. A number of herbs or herbal formulas may be useful for PMS, such as the Chinese formula Dan Zhi Xiao Yao San (see p. 167). The single herb Dong Quai is found in most Chinese formulas for women's health problems, and you can try it individually (in a 1:5 tincture, 1 teaspoon 3 times a day), although it's generally best in a formula. You could also see an acupuncturist and have a formula custom made for your individual pattern of PMS.

The Western herb Vitex agnus-castus (chasteberry) has been shown to be helpful for PMS, but do not take it if you are using oral contraceptives. Try a standardized extract containing 0.5 percent agnuside, taking 175–225 mg/day.

Natural hormones. The research evidence is mixed for using progesterone to reduce PMS, perhaps because this hormone is a factor for a subgroup of women. Jan has worked with mothers who experienced symptom relief with progesterone, used either as an over-the-counter cream or as a prescription through a compounding pharmacy. If you explore this option, we recommend you do so under the care of a licensed health care provider, and that you stop if you get uncomfortable symptoms signaling too much progesterone.

Western medicine. If you try some of the suggestions above and your PMS remains moderate to severe, you might consider two options within Western medicine (each one requires the care of a medical doctor). The first is oral contraceptive agents (OCAs)—a.k.a. "the pill." OCAs can impose an artificial balance on your menstrual cycle, but they also interfere with the metabolism of some vitamins (including B$_6$, which helps *reduce* PMS) and increase your long-term risk for heart disease, especially if you smoke. Second, fluoxetine (Prozac, Serafem)—and perhaps other antidepressants—can often relieve the depressed mood some women have with PMS, and sometimes other discomfort as well.

Balancing Thyroid Hormone

Your thyroid gland—about the size of a pair of fingertips on either side of the base of your throat—produces hormones that determine the pace of many of the processes in your body. When these hormones are disturbed, you can experience one or more of the symptoms noted on page 179.

After a woman has children, it's more common to see thyroid levels that are too low than are too high—particularly mildly to moderately low (termed hypothyroidism), so that will be our focus in this section. Nonetheless, an overactive thyroid gland is a serious medical condition, and you should speak with your doctor immediately if you are concerned about that possibility.

Energetic. Jan has seen the homeopathic remedy *Sepia* appear to relieve the symptoms of low thyroid, and some practitioners of Chinese medicine use acupuncture for hypothyroidism. If your case is mild, an energetic shift might help, but if you have moderate or severe symptoms, other forms of care will probably be needed.

Supplements. Iodine combines with tyrosine to make thyroid hormone; in spite of the addition of iodine to salt, deficits are still widespread, and they can cause hypothyroidism. You could try supplementing this mineral, which is usually well assimilated in the form of kelp tablets; 150 mg is the DV, but some practitioners go as high as 600 mg. Or you could supplement tyrosine, which is best taken in the morning to avoid thyroid activity keeping you awake at night; start at 500 mg and increase the daily dose up to 1000 mg. A third possibility would be to supplement phenylalanine, the amino acid precursor of tyrosine, which is often more easily absorbed by the body (use the same dosing as tyrosine). Supplementing tyrosine or phenylalanine is particularly worth considering if testing has found low levels of either amino acid. If you try one of these three options, start with a low dose and increase it slowly, if at all, in order to avoid pushing the pendulum too far in the other direction, toward overstimulating thyroid production.

Selenium and zinc help activate thyroid hormone in your body, and it's important to make sure you are getting enough. The DV of selenium is 55 *micro*grams, and you could try 200–400 micrograms. The DV of zinc is 8 mg, but most women can easily use 30–50 mg a day.

Herbs. The preeminent symptom of hypothyroidism is low energy, and numerous Chinese herbs or herbal formulas could help you feel more vitality, perhaps through pathways that, at least in part, affect your thyroid. We've already mentioned one widely used formula for increasing energy and tonifying the Qi, Bu Zhong Yi Qi Tang. Other formulas directed at boosting your Qi are Su Jun Zi Tang and Ba Zhen Tang.

Natural hormones and Western medicine. Thyroid hormone is available only by prescription, either in the form of a natural extract of the thyroid gland of cows (bovine) or pigs (porcine), or as a synthetic product (e.g., levothyroxine); some professionals consider thyroid extract to be more effectively used by the body. If your thyroid is low, supplementing it can feel like a not-so-minor miracle, and a variety of ailments can disappear over a few months. (At the same time, you should reduce or eliminate any other supplements directed at boosting thyroid, particularly tyrosine, so that the results of the hormone trial will be clear.)

On the other hand, supplementing thyroid carries the risk that your body will "turn off" this gland, since now there is plenty of available hormone floating around without the thyroid gland having to do anything (this concern does not apply if your body has already stopped producing thyroid hormone). In order to minimize this risk, your doctor may increase the dose slowly, or maintain a low dose, and keep checking to see that your body is still producing the hormone on its own.

Balancing Your Adrenal Hormones

The adrenals, two little walnut-shaped glands that sit on top of your kidneys, release hormones—notably cortisol, epinephrine and norepinephrine*—that play key roles in guiding your body's responses to stress. With an acute stressor—let's say you're at the park with your preschooler and she trips, scrapes her knee, and starts crying loudly—the hypothalamus tells the pituitary gland to signal the adrenals to send epinephrine and norepinephrine into your bloodstream, soon followed by cortisol. Ideally, when the stress is over—your daughter's recovered and playing happily again—both your knowledge that she's OK *and* the rising flood of stress hormones signal your hypothalamus and pituitary to tell the adrenals to settle back down. But with *chronic* stress, three bad things can happen:†

- Your hypothalamus and pituitary could become so used to high levels of stress hormones that it takes increasing amounts to get these glands to stop ordering the adrenals to release more cortisol, etc. As a result, your mind may know that everything is all right—you see your daughter laughing happily in the sandbox—but your hypothalamus and pituitary glands, and thus your adrenals, aren't getting the message. Consequently, increasingly high levels of stress hormones could become the status quo in your body, even when no actual stressors are present: now you feel routinely "stressed out."

- The normal rhythm in your cortisol—low during the night so you can sleep, and higher in the morning to help you be active in the day—could be disturbed, making cortisol peak around 4 a.m. and drop by lunchtime: now you've got insomnia, and no pep at all in the afternoon.

- Your adrenal glands could become desensitized or exhausted, so that they produce insufficient hormones even when the alarm bells are ringing: now it feels harder than ever to kick into gear, and you may be more prone to allergies and joint pain (since cortisol inhibits inflammation); this state is sometimes termed "adrenal burnout" or "adrenal insufficiency."

If you are experiencing any of these conditions, we suggest you do a relatively inexpensive, twenty-four-hour salivary test of your cortisol and DHEA; your doctor or an endocrinologist can advise you about whether it makes sense to do addi-

---

*Epinephrine is another term for adrenaline, and norepinephrine is noradrenaline.

†These are simplified summaries of extremely complex processes that involve other aspects of the body as well, such as the hippocampus (a part of your brain).

tional assessments. Based on these findings, try one or more of the options in the spectrum of care below; many of them will not be specific to the three conditions above, but will have a balancing effect in general. But the first step of all has got to be reducing your stresses; otherwise, any intervention will be like trying to fill a bucket with a hole in the bottom. Also take a look through the spectrum of care applied to other conditions for any suggestions that have a relaxing effect, such as exercise, 5-HTP, or kava. And get as much sleep as possible; even one night of poor sleep leads to elevated cortisol levels the next day.

Energetic. Numerous studies have found that acupuncture can affect the hypothalamic-pituitary-adrenal (HPA) axis, often lowering the levels of circulating cortisol and other stress hormones.

Musculoskeletal. Yoga is a well-researched and powerful method of stress relief that can have specific impact on the adrenal hormones. If you can arrange it, a good time for yoga is in the late afternoon or when you get home from work: it helps release the stress from your day and move you into a relaxed mindset for the evening. Yoga classes are available in nearly every community, or you could watch a TV program, use a videotape, or read a book. Sometimes children like to get in the act as well—at least for a few minutes—giving them some relaxation of their own.

Dietary. We tend to self-medicate when we're under stress—using caffeine, alcohol, or illegal drugs. Besides the long-term problems this causes (see p. 139), it can mask a growing disturbance in the HPA axis. Try eliminating caffeine, alcohol, or other drugs for a few days and see how you do; the results could be a wake-up call that you need to make a more serious effort to manage your stresses or tend to your adrenals. At a minimum, do not exceed a couple of cups of coffee and/or two of drinks of alcohol a day.

One potential source of cortisol rising at night and waking you up is low blood sugar (which stimulates cortisol secretion). For a week, eliminate or radically reduce sugar and refined carbohydrates, eat more protein, and see if that helps.

Supplements. A shortage of pantothenic acid—vitamin B_5—can weaken the adrenal glands; try the intensive daily dose of 500–1000 mg. Vitamin C increases adrenal function, but chronic stress depletes it. The intensive daily dose for vitamin C is to start with 5000 mg and increase slowly up to bowel tolerance (the amount just below that which causes diarrhea).

The amino acid tyrosine is the precursor to norepinephrine, and numerous studies have shown it to improve the adaptation to stress. A reasonable daily dosage would be to start with 500 mg, taken before noon, and increase slowly to about 1 gram. On the other hand, Jan has found that women who tend to be sensitive or nervous often don't like tyrosine—they find it too stimulating; check in with yourself, and don't push something that doesn't feel right.

Another nutrient that might help balance the stress feedback system in your body is phosphatidylserine (PS), in doses of 100 to 200 mg per day.* (PS has also been shown to be effective in slowing the cognitive decline associated with aging.)

If stress has thrown off your sleep clock, try methylcobalamin, the active coenzyme form of vitamin B$_{12}$; it is particularly effective when used in combination with twenty minutes or more of bright light between 6 and 8 a.m. See if you can get out for a brief walk at that time, which will be relaxing in its own right!

Herbs. Siberian and *Panax* ginseng appear to have an "adaptogenic" effect on the adrenal glands, both lifting low levels and decreasing high levels. Unfortunately, the dosage required for this function is poorly researched, in part because the potency of ginseng varies greatly, depending on the source and the preparation. We suggest starting with 500 mg/day of dried herb from a reputable company and perhaps increasing slowly up to 2000–3000 mg/day; it's generally best not to take ginseng in the evening to avoid an overly stimulating result.

Licorice binds to the hormone receptors of cortisol, creating a cortisol-like effect. In the context of supporting the HPA axis, licorice would generally be most appropriate for conditions of "adrenal burnout." Initially try 100–300 mg/day, and perhaps increase slowly to 1000 mg. In about a fifth of the population, high doses of licorice lead to hypertension, so you should take this herb under the supervision of a licensed health care provider, and check your blood pressure frequently when you first start using it.

Natural hormones and Western medicine. To restore a normal sleep cycle, try melatonin, 0.5 to 1 mg taken sublingually 30 to 60 minutes before bedtime.

In cases of severe adrenal exhaustion, hydrocortisone can be given in dosages that approximate the body's normal production of cortisol. If you need it, this treatment can feel life-changing, but it should only be initiated by a doctor who is familiar with such a protocol.

Your Immune System

Day and night, the immune system works to destroy cancer cells and to keep bacteria, viruses, parasites, and toxic chemicals from invading your body and causing disease. It is the primary defender of your health and it has two arms:†

---

*Some studies used 800 mg, but we have no experience with that dosage.

†This description of the immune system is simplified, focusing mainly on elements that will be discussed further.

- *Nonspecific.* This includes your body's soft armor (the skin and mucus membranes), large cells (such as macrophages) that engulf microorganisms and toxins, and chemicals that kill or disable microbes.

- *Specific.* This part of your immune system "learns" to recognize and attack microbes, diseased cells, or foreign substances, sometimes using parts of the nonspecific immune system to assist it; its elements include:

  § Antibodies: molecules that mark an antigen (the molecular fingerprint of a microorganism, cell, or chemical) and guide an attack

  § B-cells: white blood cells that produce antibodies

  § T-cells: the three types of these white blood cells kill diseased cells, or activate or inhibit other parts of the immune system

  § Thymus gland: transforms immature T-cells into mature ones that can tell the difference between "self" and "non-self," and secretes hormones that help guide the immune system

When your immune system goes into action, the results can include inflammation (enabling your defenders to get to the battlefield), mucus production, fever (which helps kill heat-sensitive microbes), and fatigue (so you'll rest and your body can heal). But they could also include misguided assaults on neutral substances (allergies) or the body's own tissues (autoimmune disease).

What Can Disturb the Immune System

The key to a healthy immune system is *balance,* so that it is vigilant and powerful, yet also discriminating and controlled. Let's see how bearing and rearing children can wear down and disturb your immune system, making it like a weary soldier lurching into battle, too depleted to defend herself and too rattled to distinguish friend from foe.

Stress. Your stresses make your immune system both weaker and more prone to overreact. First, stress stimulates the release of corticosteroid hormones, and these suppress both arms of your immune system—so it's less able to ward off viruses, bacteria, or parasites. Second, a woman's immune system is more active than a man's, so it's easier for stress to make it *over*reactive. For example, stress increases the release of histamines within your body, causing inflammation signals to be sent out at a shout instead of a whisper. As a result, an allergen that would once give you no more than a few sneezes could now lead to hives or asthma. Stress also seems to play a role in the development and severity of autoimmune illnesses, which are more likely in women after they have children.

Nutritional deficits. Like an army at war, your immune system consumes resources at an amazing rate when it fights an infection. For example, an activated B-cell will produce about a thousand antibodies per second before dying in a day or two. Therefore, the immune system needs a big stockpile of nutrients; consequently, if your body is depleted, a lack of protein or a deficit in any one of a number of nutrients will lower its resistance to disease.

Weakened thymus. Stress is linked to a shrinkage of the thymus gland and a drop in its immune-regulating hormones. Nutrient shortages—especially antioxidants—make this gland more susceptible to the effects of aging. Additionally, surges in estrogen—such as those during pregnancy—inhibit the thymus and may have lingering effects.

Fetal tissue. Long after you've given birth, some cells from your baby will normally remain within your body. It is possible that the immune system may interpret those fetal cells as "foreign," putting it on red alert, now more likely to overreact and develop an autoimmune disease.

Other systems of the body. Disturbed digestion can decrease the absorption of the vital nutrients your immune system needs. Additionally, GI disturbance increases the chance of developing food sensitivities, which activate your immune system needlessly.

Similarly, changes in the nervous system due to motherhood can reduce the potency of your immune responses. Depression, for instance, is associated with a slower rate of recovery from illness and less effective white blood cell activity.

Common Signs of Immune System Imbalance

More frequent, severe, and lingering:
  Infections
  Colds and flu
  Cold sores
  Genital herpes
Increased response to known allergens
Increased autoimmune reactions
New allergies or autoimmune reactions

Hormones bind to immune cells throughout your body, sometimes telling them to hit the gas and other times the brakes. For example, low estrogen can reduce the effectiveness of your immune system. On the other hand, healthy levels of estrogen, progesterone, oxytocin, and prolactin help control overzealous immune function. Rapid fluctuations in these hormones—from stress, weaning, new pregnancies, etc.—can lead to hair-trigger immune responses, increasing the chance of an autoimmune disease.

Signs and Symptoms of Disturbance in the Immune System

Reduced response. If your immune system is weakened, you are prone to suffer more frequent, severe, and lingering diseases, from the common cold to serious infections.

Allergic reactions. As we've seen, an overly reactive immune system can intensify your body's response to allergens.

Autoimmune disease. When the body is attacked by its own immune system, the general symptoms typically include fatigue and inflammation. The specific symptoms vary, depending on the illness.

Assessment of the Immune System

Routine office visits with your doctor do not usually detect subtle abnormalities in the status of your immune system. These are diagnosed with tests that doctors usually order only if you mention some of the signs and symptoms described above. Basic tests of immune function include a complete blood count (CBC), white blood cell count (WBC), or sedimentation rate (a general index of inflammation). Additional tests can check specialized elements of the immune system, such as helper T-cells. And you can assess for allergies and food sensitivities, as we discussed on page 162.

Strengthening and Balancing Your Immune System

Probably the most important things you can do for your immune system are mental, not physical: a positive outlook, social support, and low stress will nurture the healing powers of your body. Since angry quarrels depress immune system function, you'll also benefit from finding positive ways to work out issues with your partner (covered in the next three chapters). Second, promoting your overall wellness will support the immune system in numerous ways. In particular, try to get lots of deep sleep, since that's when your brain and body produce several substances that enhance immune function. Good nutrition, a balanced digestive tract, and effective detoxification (see p. 143) are also vital allies to a potent immune system. Third, you'll want to keep the overall load on your immune system as low as possible—by minimizing your exposure to toxins, allergens (including foods to which you are sensitive), or infection—so that it is not already burdened when new challenges come along.

On this foundation, let's look at the options within the spectrum of care for strengthening and balancing your immune system. (An additional option is to use hypnosis or guided imagery, which have been shown to enhance immune function.) Some of these are preventive, while others help the immune system when it is being attacked or disturbed. (Please see the box on page 194 for specific suggestions for reducing the chance of developing an autoimmune condition.)

Energetic. Acupuncture can increase T-cells and other white blood cells. As to homeopathy, there is evidence that this method—through mechanisms that are not yet understood—can strengthen the immune response; for example, studies have found that homeopathic remedies seem to reduce respiratory infections. Additionally, homeopathy appears to help balance the immune system, decreasing both allergic and autoimmune reactions; various studies have successfully used remedies to control the symptoms of hay fever, asthma, and rheumatoid arthritis. While a remedy is most likely to be helpful when it is selected by an experienced homeopath, based on your individual profile, you could try *Oscillococcinum* on your own. This remedy is used at the beginning of a flu or cold, and it seems to strengthen the immune system response to viral infection. It typically comes in small vials, each of which may be divided into three to four doses. Take one dose every hour at the onset of the flu or cold, and after three or four doses, decrease to about three doses per day.

Musculoskeletal. Moderate exercise raises the levels of several kinds of white blood cells, but strenuous exercise—like running a 10K race—briefly lowers lymphocytes, natural killer cells, and antibodies in your respiratory and digestive tracts. If you're interested in something a little more relaxed, massage and even affectionate touching have been shown to increase immune system function.

Dietary. You really can turbocharge your immune system with every bite you eat. Lots of vegetables and a reasonable amount of fruit will give you immune-boosting carotenoids and flavonoids. A solid serving of protein at every meal will also keep your immune system humming along. And it's critical to minimize sugar and refined flours: besides wearing on your body in general and thus affecting the immune system indirectly, sugars have direct effects as well. For instance, studies have found that consuming about two sodas' worth of sugar knocked down the effectiveness of white blood cells by roughly fifty percent within one hour, with residual effects lasting for several more hours. Finally, a low-fat diet with minimal caffeine has also been shown to improve immune function.

Supplements. The immune system requires a full cupboard of nutrients, so we'll repeat our recommendation that you take high-potency multivitamin/mineral supplements every day. Depending on what your supplements contains, add one or more of the nutrients listed on the next page.

How to Lower Your Risk for Autoimmune Disease After Children

Autoimmune diseases are the fourth leading cause of disability among women in America. Their exact causes of autoimmune disease are still unknown, but what is clear is that the risk of developing one increases after a woman becomes a mother. These strategies are no guarantee that you will avoid such a condition, but we think they'll improve your odds.

1. Reduce chronic activation of your immune system: Lowers the chance of misguided reactions, including cross-reactivities in which an antibody to a pathogen or allergen (or white blood cells that have "learned" to attack those antigens) mistakenly targets some part of your own body. Here's how:

• Lower the chance of developing food sensitivities, through getting good nutrition, minimizing caffeine and alcohol, and keeping a good balance of microorganisms in your digestive tract

• Treat chronic infections (including intestinal dysbiosis); for example, researchers have found associations between strep throat and rheumatic fever

• Minimize exposure to allergens and foods to which you are sensitive; for example, aggressively target mildew on surfaces and use an ozone machine or air filter to sweep molds from the air in your home

• Minimize exposure to toxins (p. 135)

2. Settle inflammation: Reduces the possibility of errors in the communication of information among the cells that regulate inflammation, as well as the likelihood of developing food sensitivities. Here's how:

• Use the spectrum of care to lower inflammation in the digestive tract (p. 163).

• Balance your essential fatty acids (p. 116). Increase your intake of omega-3s up to the intensive daily dose (p. 167). Take 240–480 mg/day of GLA (found in supplements of primrose or borage oil). Eliminate trans-fatty acids, and reduce saturated fats.

• Take the IDD of vitamin C, divided into two or more doses, ideally in combination with 1000–2000 mg of mixed bioflavonoids such as rutin or hesperidin.

• Try quercetin, which has been shown to regulate allergenic and inflammatory reactions. A standard dose is 500 mg, three times a day, taken before meals.

3. Support the thymus gland: Enables it to continue to "train" immature T-cells to target foreign invaders, rather than your own body. Here's how:

• Take the intensive daily doses (see opposite) of antioxidants, notably zinc, selenium, carotenoids, and vitamins C and E.

• Consider glandular extracts (p. 196).

- *Antioxidants.* These nutrients aid your immune system in numerous ways. They are generally most effective in combination with one another, but you can also use them individually:

  § Vitamin A plays an essential role in nourishing the skin and mucus membranes, your primary barriers against infection; the micellized form is easily absorbable. It also stimulates white blood cell activity and antibody response. As long as you are not pregnant (or could become pregnant) and do not have a liver disease, you could take 5,000 IU per day, or as much as 50,000 IU for a few days at the onset of an illness.

  § Vitamin C supports many aspects of the immune system, including white blood cells, interferon, and secretion of thymic hormones. For maximum immune support, you could try the intensive daily dose, taking increasing quantities of vitamin C up to the point that you develop diarrhea, and then lowering the dose until normal bowel function is restored.

  § Vitamin E helps the immune system in several ways; the intensive daily dose is 800 IU.

  § Carotenoids are best consumed through eating five to seven servings of vegetables each day. If you use supplements, take a product with mixed carotenoids, since high doses of beta-carotene alone may be harmful in some cases.

  § Quercetin is useful for settling the immune system and reducing the symptoms of allergies and food sensitivities; take 400–500 mg, three times a day, ideally before meals.

- *B vitamins.* A deficiency in nearly any B vitamin will weaken the immune system, and vitamins B_6, B_{12}, and folic acid are particularly important. The levels of the B vitamins in the MSDVs will support proper immune function. For an extra boost, increase them up to the intensive daily doses listed on page 173.

- *Minerals.* Several minerals have a striking ability to support your immune system:

  § Iron deficiency (even when minimal) lessens the effectiveness of several parts of your immune system. Unfortunately, low iron levels are widespread among women in general, and mothers in particular can have a shortage of iron due to the lingering effects of pregnancy, which typically drains about 700 mg of iron from your body. Getting more iron is best accomplished through eating liver; however, since toxins concentrate in the liver, it's important to get this meat from beef or chickens raised on organic foods and no artificial chemicals. The next best source of iron is a chelated supplement, such as iron glycinate, ferrous succinate, ferrous sulfate, or ferrous fumarate.* If you are already taking the MSDV of iron and testing shows that your body is still deficient, try an intensive daily dose of 30 mg twice a day, between meals. (But don't take more than the MSDVs of iron unless your body is clearly lacking in this mineral, since *high* amounts of iron can lower immune function.)

§ Selenium shortages weaken many aspects of the immune system. Even when blood levels of selenium are normal, taking 200 mcg per day has been shown to help the immune response.

§ Studies have found that zinc deficiency decreases immune system activity, while supplementation enhances it. For purposes of preventing illness, take 50 mg of zinc citrate, picolinate, or gluconate for one to two months, and then decrease to 30 mg. If you feel a cold coming on, zinc lozenges can be helpful (about 25 mg every two hours up to about 250 mg per day); in one study, this dosing shortened the duration of colds by 64 percent.

• *Glandular extracts.* These are concentrated extracts from animal glands that contain many of the substances and cofactors used in human organs. Some studies have indicated that thymus extracts can restore or enhance immune function. Glandular extracts are best tried while working with a practitioner who is experienced with them.

Herbs. Astragalus is used in Chinese medicine as a long-term immune tonic and for active viral infections, and you can usually buy it in health food stores; for dosing, follow the instructions on the package. Echinacea has been shown to boost the immune system, particularly when used at the beginning of a cold, flu, or respiratory infection. It should be taken in small doses, about an eighth of a teaspoon of a 1:5 tincture, every few hours, for at most six weeks; do not use this herb if you are prone to allergies or have an autoimmune disease since it might overstimulate your immune system.

Probiotics. By helping balance the microbial ecology of your GIS, probiotics can support your immune system indirectly. Additionally, there are intriguing in-

---

*Be sure to keep iron supplements out of the reach of young children.

dications that certain probiotics, such as lactobacillus, can stimulate the nonspecific immune system, making it more active in fighting off invading microbes. Giving probiotics to pregnant or breast-feeding women has also been shown to decrease allergic eczema in their babies, suggesting a balancing effect on the child's immune system.

Natural hormones. DHEA appears able to buffer the impact of stress on the immune system as well as provide general support. As with any hormonal intervention, we recommend that you explore this option only while working with a licensed practitioner experienced in its use.

Motherhood is startling in its sheer physicality, from the first swelling in your belly or the crick in your neck while holding your baby perfectly still so she won't wake up again—to the long-term depletion many women experience after having children. Those so-tangible effects can take you by surprise and make you feel vulnerable. They're humbling, and they fly in the face of the perfectionistic expectations many women have for themselves.

Everyone has frailties, yet sometimes it's hard to acknowledge your own to others, or even within your own heart. But that's what's needed for compassion—for yourself and for your body: you're both hard-working, weary, and deserving of loving care. A clear-eyed respect for your body's needs can help you feel that it's right to ask for and receive support from others for any health problems. In the next three chapters, we'll explore how to cultivate a supportive, loving marriage—for its own sake, and as an important resource for your lasting health.

PART FOUR
Nurturing Your Intimate Relationship

A marriage has two fundamental aspects—a practical partnership and an intimate friendship—and children can't help but challenge each of them.

Regarding the first one, kids bring hard questions that good-hearted and otherwise like-minded partners can disagree about, from the best way to get a baby to sleep through the night to how to pay for college. The total workload jumps dramatically, yet you can probably no longer call on the village of "helper moms" that would have supported your family in past generations. Chances are, much of what would once have been carried by many has now shifted to one, your partner (which is hard on him), but if he doesn't shoulder that burden, it all falls on you.

Regarding the intimate parts of your relationship, it's hard to find the time or energy for fun together, good conversation, or sweet lovemaking after children arrive. Issues from the practical partnership—such as arguments over how to parent the kids or divide the workload fairly—tend to reduce intimacy. And issues from the intimate friendship—whether it's the depth of conversation or the frequency of sex—spill over onto your practical partnership, adding heat and smoke to subjects that are tough enough already.

As a result, even with the best of intentions, it is common for a mother and father to have conflicts about some matter of childrearing or sharing the load, and to experience a loss of intimacy. Besides making you feel bad, these can lower your health. For example, quarrels increase blood pressure, wear down the immune system, and disturb your hormones. Additionally, the way spouses treat each other when the children are little shapes their relationship for many years, and in the extreme, it can tear a marriage apart. If the couple stays together, an atmosphere of tension and emotional distance increases the chance that their children will feel insecure and develop psychological problems.

Therefore, it is vital for parents to be strong partners, and the next three chapters are designed to give you the tools you need to keep your relationship moving in a good direction, or to get it back on track it if it's been derailed. Chapter 6 covers skillful communication, chapter 7 addresses the practical partnership, and chapter 8 focuses on the intimate friendship. Ideally, your husband will read these. (If you are living apart from the father of your children, or with another person who is helping raise your kids, you can adapt them to your situation.) But we know that may not happen, so we wrote these chapters to be used either together or by you alone. Used alone, they should help you see more clearly what you have a right to ask for and how to do so more effectively. And you can learn how to be a more skillful partner yourself in order to draw out the best in him, reduce his complaints about you and take your stand—with or without him—on the moral high ground.

Of course, it may feel doubly burdensome to have to learn new skills in order to get your husband to do what you think he should have done in the first place. But the alternative is to feel immobilized and resentful while matters stay the same or get worse. If you make an effort, things are likely to improve. It will help you feel better to be active, rather than passive, in your relationship, and it is better for your children to see you sticking up for yourself. Even in the saddest scenario—if your marriage was already in the intensive care unit and nothing could revive it—the skills you learn by trying will help you with both your ex-husband and any future partners.

But it's *much* more likely that your efforts will help increase or bring back the good feelings you and your husband have had for each other. Over and over, we've seen that just a few small changes in a marriage—a little more understanding, a little more skill in communicating, a little more support—can make a huge difference in the quality of a relationship.

Communicating with Your Partner

It is an amazing but true thing that practically the only people who ever say mean, insulting, wounding things to us are those of our own households.

—Dorothea Dix

Sometimes talking about the simplest thing is like walking through a minefield. For example, imagine a father coming home from work to his wife who has been alone with their young child much of the day; they've grown so irritated with each other that this dialogue is fairly typical:

HE: (*walks through the door, sees some clutter, and mutters to himself*) What a mess.

SHE: (*stung at the criticism after having spent many selfless hours with their child*) There you go, always criticizing when you first get home.

HE: You're so messy it drives me crazy.

SHE: I don't see *you* lifting a finger to help.

HE: (*walks over and puts a toy on a shelf*) There, I helped. Now are you happy?

SHE: (*under her breath*) Such a jerk.

HE: Well, there *you* go again, losing control. You can't talk without getting hysterical.

SHE: Your mother spoiled you rotten, but I don't have to take your crap.

HE: (*yelling*) Once and for all, stop talking about my family. Or I've about had it!

203

A Civil Tongue

Thirty years of research have shown that the key to a loving and lasting marriage is how the spouses *interact* with each other. Positive exchanges build up an emotional bank account of trust and warmth, and they make it easier to get through a conflict without losing your temper. In strong couples, positive interactions outnumber the negative ones by three or more to one.

An interaction is like a rally in tennis, and civility is what keeps the ball in bounds. Each time it is your turn to "hit the ball," you have choices about how you hear what was said and how you respond. First, you could focus on the most useful or accurate aspect of the other person's communication, which helps you see the best in him and feel more hopeful and calm. Or you can fix on the parts that are exaggerated, inaccurate, or inflammatory, making you feel misunderstood, attacked, hurt, and angry. Second, you could send back the most constructive communication possible—given what came at you—which preserves your dignity, puts you in a good light, and gives your partner something positive to work with. Or you can fire back with some nasty topspin, losing your cool, clouding the issues, and motivating him to retaliate in kind. In sum, you each can build on the positive, or go negative on the negative.

Besides feeling awful, negative interactions stress your body and deplete you further. An atmosphere of marital conflict worries children, and it's a risk factor for them developing depression, anxiety, and behavior problems. Frequent quarrels also wear down marital bonds. Every ugly, nasty little exchange makes each person more sensitive to the next one, the same way repeated chafing of the skin makes it increasingly tender to the touch, so even a light bump feels harshly abrasive. Then partners can trigger each other in runaway chain reactions. But civility interrupts the cycle of negativity, even if just one person does it.

Disagreements are natural in any relationship, and they usually increase after children. Civility does not prevent you from speaking your mind. It just helps you make your point better and be listened to more receptively.

How to Make a Conversation Go Badly

Let's look first at what went wrong in the interaction that opened this chapter, and then at how it could have gone better.

- *Leading with the negative, making no emotional connection* (What a mess!). If the very first statement is negative, the other person will feel jolted and attacked. There also needs to be some stage setting that makes an emotional connection and finds out if this is a good time to talk.

- *Overstatement* (There you go, always criticizing when you first get home). The speaker makes it sound like *you do this entirely bad thing all the time in every way* if she uses words like *always* or *never,* or if she does not use qualifying, softening language such as *often, around bedtimes,* or *when you're watching TV.*

- *Blaming* (You're so messy it drives me crazy). These attacks are shaming and hurtful. Intended to make the listener realize something about herself, instead they just push the button for an angry defense. Blaming also assumes that the listener is the cause of the speaker's actions or experience, and that's just not true. *He* is responsible for how his brain or body reacts, not her.

- *Counterattack* (I don't see *you* lifting a finger to help). This both escalates the conflict and introduces a new topic. When multiple topics swirl around in an argument, nothing gets accomplished.

- *Reductio ad absurdum* (There, I helped. Now are you happy?). "Reducing to absurdity" deflates others by making their wish, complaint, or idea sound foolish. That's hurtful in itself, plus it's only a short step from *your view is ridiculous* to *YOU are ridiculous.*

- *Insults* (Such a jerk). Long after an argument is over, insults linger in the mind like emotional napalm, part glue and part gasoline, sticking and burning. Frequent insults are abusive, a grinding assault on the other person's sense of worth.

- *Character attacks* (You can't talk without getting hysterical). There's a world of difference between saying, *What you did was bad* and <u>*You*</u> *are bad.* When one person takes shots at the overall character of another, the target of the attack feels that his or her good parts are completely discounted, and is likely to fire back in kind.

- *Side issues* (Your mother spoiled you rotten, but I don't have to take your crap). These are distractions that shift the focus away from the real issue.

- *Demands* (Leave my family out of this!). Every communication contains two messages: the explicit content and an implicit statement about the relationship between the speaker and listener. We all have deep needs to feel both autonomous and connected in our relationships. When the implicit message threatens either need, that becomes the overriding issue. For example, any demand says implicitly *I get to boss you around* and limit your autonomy. Most people fight back against attempts at dominance, which turns up the heat and diverts attention from the explicit topic.

- *Threats* (Or I've about had it!). Both the explicit meaning of a threat, that something bad could happen, and the implicit one, that *I get to intimidate you* are alarming. Threats crowd out other issues and foster threats in return, like: *Fine! Just see what your relationship with the kids is like if you do!*

How to Help a Conversation Go Well

The key to a good conversation is each person's *purpose.* For example, is it your intention to speak your truth clearly, find out what is really bugging your partner, discover what you need to do differently, and solve problems? Or is it to avoid responsibility, dump your feelings, look good, or win? In your heart, where do you truly want to be coming from?

When each person's intentions are positive, they find ways to connect and mend, rather than distance and wound. A good conversation may start messy or heated, with a flurry of diverging volleys, but then one or both partners starts to settle down, and they converge on mutual understanding and practical solutions. Let's replay the dialogue above, but this time with each partner keeping a civil tongue:

- **Start by connecting.**

  HE: (*Walks through the front door. Sees the mess, feels like grumbling, but thinks better of it. Takes a big breath. Picks up his daughter and jiggles her in his arms while she giggles and makes him laugh. Smiles at wife.*) How'd it go? (*They chat for a few minutes. He says something nice about what she did that day. There's a pause, and he takes the plunge.*) I don't want to hassle you, but could we talk about the clutter?

  Leading with connection sends the reassuring, implicit message that *we are together, you matter to me.* Whenever you can, start by *joining* with your partner, rather than detaching or distancing, through warmth, touch, showing interest or concern, or saying what you agree with from the outset. And see if you can keep that sense of connection going.

- **Speak with accuracy and restraint.**

  SHE: (*warily, but with a touch of humor*) You're doing pretty well, this is the first time you've complained about that this week.

You can usually take your time to think before you speak and avoid exaggerated or inflammatory language like, *You've abandoned your children.* Explain how intensely you feel or how important something is to you by scaling it, as in: *On the 10-point scale of being mad, this is just a 3.* Imagining that the conversation is videotaped could help you avoid saying something that would make you wince later.

- **Take responsibility for your experience.**

    HE: (*knows the subject is charged, so he takes the time to say clearly how he feels*) I know Caitlin's a little mess machine and you're doing the best you can. It's just that I feel stressed at work and the commute's getting worse, so when I walk through the door and the first thing I see is clutter, it really bothers me. Plus we've already talked about you picking up before I get home. When it's still a mess, I feel you're not listening to me.

    When you talk about your own experience, using mainly "I statements," your partner understands you better and doesn't feel attacked. No one can dispute your experience (though he or she may not like it!), and it does not need to be justified or defended.

    In general, *try to practice the 80–20 rule*: focus 80 percent on what *you* can do to make things go better and no more than 20 percent on what your partner needs to fix. You have great control over the former, but little influence over the latter. Realistically, if you want the relationship to change, you'll have to do some changing yourself.

- **Stay on topic.**

    SHE: (*starts to get defensive and shift the topic to how Caitlin was especially active that day but catches herself*) OK. Let's talk about this. But I want to start thinking about starting Caitlin in preschool. Can we talk about that later tonight? She's getting so restless at home. I put one toy away and meanwhile she's taken out two others.

    Try to finish one issue before moving on to another. Sometimes it helps to set a time limit: *Let's do ten minutes on how I need to get the house straighter by the time you get here, and then ten minutes on how you need to come home on time.*

- **Focus on what is accurate or useful in what the other person is saying.**

    HE: (*thinks she's trying to justify herself by talking about Caitlin and starts to veer off topic to rebut that point, but he knows that would just get them fighting, so he stops himself*) You're right, Caitlin is getting real active. I know that makes it harder to straighten up, so let's talk about preschool later. But you have to admit, when you're firm with her, she behaves better.

When you can, begin your response with what you like or agree with about what your partner has said. Emphasizing common ground conveys respect and moves you toward positive solutions.

- ***Keep your dignity.***

    SHE: (*Liked the first part of what he said, but then he slipped in that last part about being more firm. Feels her heart start to pound. Speaks with intensity but maintains self-control.*) Look, I really don't like hearing about how I ought to be firmer with Caitlin. You try spending day after day with a two-year-old. You just can't be firm every second. You don't do it—no criticism, just fact—so you have *no idea* what it's like. Please don't be so free with your advice. I am actually quite firm with Caitlin, and you know people say she's well behaved.

    You could recall someone who embodies an attitude of self-respect and uprightness in the face of provocation and imagine speaking in the same manner. Try to talk in a way that makes you feel proud of yourself.

- ***Address concrete specifics.***

    HE: (*resists the temptation to refight old quarrels, and refocuses the conversation*) OK, OK. I know you're pretty firm, though I wish you were ten percent firmer. But that's not the issue. Here's my basic point. I don't really care about the rest of the house. I'd just like to be able to walk through the front door into a living room that is peaceful and orderly. And I thought we'd agreed you'd straighten up before I got home.

    Nothing can be done about a vague complaint or a global assault on someone's character. But you *can* solve well-defined problems. For example, clarify how much of a change you want, as the father did above with his "ten percent" comment.

- ***Concede points when you can.***

    SHE: (*Still calming down from the "you're not firm enough" side issue. Considers arguing with whether she needs to be "ten percent firmer," but thinks better of it.*) You're right, I did say I'd keep things cleaner. I didn't realize you only care about the living room. That's doable. But I have to tell you, I want more respect about how I do discipline Caitlin, and how hard it is to ride herd on her all day.

If it's more important to you to discover what is true and what will work than it is to be right or to win a power struggle, you can be good-humored about conceding a point. Plus, that's the fastest way to get your partner to stop bugging you about it. The true winner of an argument is the one who learns or grows the most.

- ***Make requests, not demands, and agreements, not threats.***

  HE: (*wants to fire back but has learned that the impulse to do so is actually a big, flashing warning to BUY SOME TIME until he has calmed down*) Hmmm. Let me think about that for a minute. (*Discreetly takes a few big breaths. Thinks about whether he's gone overboard. Remembers that people do say that Caitlin is well-behaved for a two-year-old. Remembers the time he had Caitlin for most of a Saturday and how he had to loosen up on the rules. Looks at his wife and feels compassion for her, hassled on one side by her daughter and on the other by him.*) OK. Would this work: Picked-up living room, so-so rest of house, and we try your firmness level for a while?

  SHE: (*Still irritated, but softened by his tone and partial giving in. Considers whether she can actually keep the living room straight up to the time he gets home, and makes a counterproposal.*) Well, I like where you're going. But what if you're late and Caitlin leaves out some new stuff, and you yell at me about it?

  HE: (*Sees her basic point and doesn't get distracted by the exaggeration about yelling. Nods.*)

  SHE: I can keep it clean between 6:00 and 6:30. If you get home later, bets are off. OK?

  HE: Sounds like a plan. I'm tired of arguing, anyway!

If You or He Is Upset

It's hard to be civil when the need is greatest: when you or your partner is upset. But you can help yourself in many ways. You might like to take a quick look back at the methods for coping with upsetting experiences in chapters 2 and 3. The suggestions below build on that foundation to focus on your relationship, and each one is also something you can ask for from your partner.

Stepping back. When you step back from and observe your reactions—including your body sensations, wants, emotions, and thoughts—that is the beginning of *you* being in control, not them. Rather than being your reactions, you *have* them. Fundamentally, you can always detach from reactions instead of identifying with them. With practice, you will get better and better at it—and raising a family will give you plenty of that!

You can step back from his reactions, too. Remind yourself that you are separate, perhaps imagining a boundary between you like a picket fence, or if need be, a thick wall. Or visualize a shield around you, like one of those force fields in science fiction, that blocks anything negative; you have total control over this shield and only you decide what gets through. You could imagine that you are looking at him through the wrong end of a telescope, so he looks small and far away, or that you are turning the volume knob down on his voice. Let his words or feelings move through you like wind ruffling the leaves on a tree; when the breeze has passed, you can decide for yourself what is accurate or useful in what he has said. Perhaps lighten up the seriousness or intensity by visualizing him wearing a funny hat. In particular, look past the most provocative words to the softer feelings and wants that lie beneath, using the empathy skills discussed on page 218.

When it's your turn to talk, you know your partner's hot buttons, and you can usually make your point without punching them. Clarify from the outset that you are not blaming or criticizing him (unless you truly intend to). Be careful how the issue is being framed, which is often what irritates most, and put it back in the proper context if necessary. For instance, are you approaching him as a normally on-top-of-it dad who slipped up, or as a perennial klutz? You can anticipate his concerns: *I'm not suggesting we take Steve out of soccer. I'm just wondering if there is a way for him not to get so banged up when he plays.* Try to be aware of the presence of implicit negative messages, such as *I know more than you, you blew it,* or *I'm the boss here,* and conscious of the absence of positive ones: Remember that he, like you, has worries or doubts that need to be *actively* reassured with messages like *I've really appreciated how good you are with the baby* or *You've been much more consistent lately* or *I know you've been working hard to make more money.* We aren't suggesting you walk around on eggshells, simply that you exercise reasonable sensitivity.

Working with your body. The stress relief techniques in chapter 2 can help calm down your body, such as breathing from the diaphragm, tensing and then relaxing, or imagining the upset draining out like liquid through valves at the tips of your fingers and toes. If your body is so upset that there's no sense in even talking, come back to the issue later, maybe after you've taken a walk around the block.

Managing anger. Of all the emotions, anger is usually the most challenging for a couple. On the one hand, suppressing it feels bad, plus it denies the other person important information. On the other hand, anger makes partners back away from each other, crowds out other messages, and breeds anger in turn. As an experiment, you—and hopefully he, as well—could try not to speak in an angry way for a day or two, or even longer, and see what happens to the atmosphere in your home. You can still explain what's bothering you, but you'll find yourself pausing longer before you speak and talking in a more heartfelt way.

Working with the mind. Our experiences growing up can't help but color our relationships. For example, women who were verbally abused as children are likely to have old feelings of hurt and anger well up in an argument with their mate. You can use the questions in the box to help sort your reactions into those that are proportionate to what is actually happening here and now, and into those that are transferred into the current situation from childhood (for more examples of this method, see chapters 2 and 3). Then, when it gets intense, you will be more able to help yourself and your partner by saying something like: *Look, part of my reaction is my thing with getting yelled at as a kid, but still, I don't think you should use that tone of voice with me, especially about something as small as dirty dishes.*

This idea of sorting is useful in other ways as well. Try to zero in on the current issue in its own right, not linked to other situations that make it seem like everything is falling apart. For example, a mother told Jan this story: **On the way home one night, John forgot to buy a special jar of baby food, and I just exploded. He was apologetic and ready to zip out to the market, but all I could do was think about other times his mind was clearly elsewhere. What was really just a half-hour delay in getting a jar of baby food became a huge issue.**

You can also separate out the ways that your reactions have been shaded or amplified by your temperament. Let's say you have an anxious disposition, and today your husband says Tommy needs a bigger bike. You would notice how your temperament shifts your response toward excessive alarm. These are perfectly normal reactions. But for yourself and your spouse, try to keep in mind the true scale of the problem: *This is quite upsetting, even though I know it's just a fifty-to-one-hundred-dollar problem, and maybe less if we can pick up a used bike at a yard sale. I get so worried about money. But I guess we can figure this out.*

Additionally, you can sort out where your husband has a role in the topic of your conversation from where he does not, by saying something like: *Our overall situation is tough, but nobody's the bad guy. The only part that is about you in what I'm saying is that it would really help if you could pick up Sophie at day care.* You'll be anticipating the questions any listener might have: *What does this have to do with <u>me</u>? Is there something I need to do? Are you saying I screwed up?* Make it clear whether you want him to simply listen, to help you solve a problem outside the family (e.g., with work or a relative), or to change the way he's been acting.

How Childhood Affects Our Reactions to a Partner

Consider the questions below for yourself.
Then, if you like, you could apply them to him.

Your feelings as a child:

What did your parents do that hurt, angered, or otherwise upset you? How do these emotional reactions to your parents come up when your partner acts similarly?

Your wants as a child:

How did you feel about how your parents responded to your wants as a child? How do those reactions come into play today when your partner responds to your wants? In your childhood, what did you yearn for that you long for today from your partner?

Seeing your parents together:

How did your mother act toward your father, especially when things were tense? Do you react to your partner in any similar ways? How did your father act toward your mother? How do you react today if your partner treats you in similar ways?

Then, sort out the specific ways he's involved by distinguishing *faults* from *putting in correction* or *gracious gifts*. A fault exists when a person falls short of a reasonable moral standard, such as not keeping an agreement with a partner or getting too angry with a child. Putting in correction means becoming more skillful in the future without being at fault about the past: no blame, but there's a better way. For example, it is not a personal fault if your toddler will only eat if she is watching a video, but you could find ways to wean her from the tube and still get some food into her. A gracious gift is when you do something nice for its own sake, not to remedy a fault or lack of skill. Suppose your husband drives faster on the freeway than you are comfortable with. But let's also suppose that he's not reckless, and most other drivers are going as fast or faster. You could ask him to shave five miles an hour off his pace when you or the children are in the car as a favor that would make you feel less stressed, not because there is anything wrong about the way he drives.

We all hate being at fault, in the wrong, to blame, the bad guy. Since (hopefully) each partner cares more about things going better in the future than making the other person feel bad about the past, why not cut to the chase and go for what each of you wants without complicating things by trying to make the other person agree that he or she was, in fact, a jerk? For an example of how to do this, let's go back to Sophie and day care: *Look, I'm not saying you should feel horribly guilty when you're late getting Sophie* (making it clear there's no fault). *But you've said it yourself that you want to improve at wrapping things up in time to get out of the office by 5:30* (asking him to put in a correction). *And one way you could be real nice to me is by picking up Sophie* (requesting that he offer a gracious gift).

If your husband thinks *you* are at fault, and you do not, try to be active within your own mind, a free agent who can decide for herself what is true or not, what's his stuff and what's your own, how your own personal code applies to the situation, and what you are going to do differently—if anything at all—in the future. If you get defensive, treating his communication like an unwanted message, he will just try harder to deliver it. Paradoxically, the fastest way to get someone's grievance to move on is to let it move in. The way to do that is to:

- Really hear the complaint.
- Take maximum reasonable personal responsibility for it.
- Express the maximum reasonable remorse or apology.
- Commit to appropriate changes from this point on.

Staying in bounds. If need be, try to agree on explicit ground rules for talking together, such as no name-calling, screaming, or threats. You could agree in advance to take a break if one or both of you needs to calm down; the person who calls time out should propose a specific time to speak again.

During a quarrel, follow the ground rules yourself, and if your partner does not, ask him to; if you can, speak from your heart about how you feel when he talks that way. If he continues to break the ground rules, you could call time out, and if necessary, walk away. Fundamentally, all you can control is how *you* speak, and your civility will create the best chance that he will communicate in a positive way.

A change of setting can foster civility, like going for a walk together or sitting in a coffee shop. A well-considered note or a message on voice mail can get your thoughts in order and express them through a buffer that may make it easier for your mate to truly hear you. It might help to propose tape-recording a conversation, both to learn from later and because it puts people on their best behavior.

Having another person present while you discuss a touchy subject can be calming: perhaps a minister, trusted friend, or therapist—but not your kids. A professional is especially called for if there is emotional abuse, drug or alcohol problems, frequent contempt or criticism, or intense fights in front of the children.

If there is actual or threatened violence—the ultimate breach of civility—you should immediately tell a physician, minister, therapist, or the police, or call a woman's shelter; shelters, including emergency housing for children, are usually listed in the Yellow Pages. Domestic abuse is, sadly, not uncommon: about one woman in ten will be seriously assaulted at least once by her husband, and the odds of this increase—sadder still—if there are children in the home. It might feel shameful to admit that there is actual or threatened violence in your marriage, but literally millions of other women have been in a similar situation. You're not alone, it's not your fault, and the most important thing of all is for you to tell someone who cares about you. Then, it's usually wisest to start with support for you, and later on, perhaps involve your partner (rather than the first step being couple's therapy).

In less serious situations, consider agreeing on a "no-fight rule" for several weeks. Civil disagreements are all right, but if they escalate at all, you would both stop and regroup. This is an admittedly artificial and short-term arrangement, like a cast on a broken arm. It allows the stress chemistry in your bodies to settle down while you build up a recent history of at least neutral interactions. If you add in some positive experiences of being together, you've got a powerful, one-two punch. In our experience, if a couple can just get three good days in a row—and even better, build on that for ten or twenty—they can turn a corner toward a much happier relationship.

Empathy

Empathy is the foundation of the experience of "we" rather than just "I" or "you." If you sense that your partner really gets how it is for you, you feel less stressed, plus closer and more trusting, and more inclined to give empathy to him. We are all able to be empathic, if we choose; it's an innate human capacity: even infants are moved by the distress of other babies.

Receiving Empathy

Let's start with the understanding we think you should be getting—and therefore have a right to ask for.

Your husband should give you empathy for both the good and the bad, how life is in general, how it feels to be a mother, and how he affects you. Often, it's the little things that you really want to share: how it felt when your baby—finally!—went to sleep, the humor in a toddler's repeated efforts to hold mashed potatoes in a spoon that's upside down, the frustration of trying to schedule an immediate appointment with the pediatrician for your daughter's umpteenth ear infection. Or it could be something big, like the fact that your own father may need more care, or that you are sick and tired of picking up after everybody, including your husband.

He should offer empathy for how you feel worn out, for any health problems you have, for how you might be depleted. You're not saying you want to lay the

---

How to Be Civil

Lead with the positive.

Make a connection.

Speak with accuracy and restraint.

Take personal responsibility. Follow the 80–20 rule: Focus 80 percent on yourself and 20 percent on your partner.

Stay on topic.

Don't interrupt.

Focus on what is true and useful.

Keep your dignity.

Address concrete specifics.

Concede points when you can.

Make requests, not demands.

Make agreements, not threats.

Research on Mothers

Studies have generally found that:

- Mothers are more emotionally affected by parenthood than fathers.

- Child rearing and housework are mainly done by mothers.

- Inequities in the total workload make mothers upset, angry, and even depressed.

- A mother is likely to feel sometimes pulled in opposing directions by her partner and her children.

- Child care hassles rattle mothers more than fathers, and working mothers experience more stress and overload from juggling both roles than their husbands do. A mother is probably more affected by the pressures in her husband's job than he is by the pressures in hers.

- Women typically experience a sharper drop in marital satisfaction after children than men do. Marital problems wear more on women, who usually place a higher value on relationships and are more economically vulnerable to the impact of divorce.

- A woman is more likely than her husband to be dissatisfied by her marriage, and twice as likely to seek a divorce.

burdens down. But you'd like them to be understood, especially by the person who helped put you in this position.

He should understand that you entered a new kind of life when your baby was born. For instance, you're no longer a free agent, but nested now in a web of connections and obligations that tugs at your every move. As one mom said: *I was feeling down and my husband asked, "Would you be happier if you had some new goals and went after them?" I smiled and said, "You're a man." "Huh?" he said. I explained, "Try going after a goal with a child holding on to you!"* You think about how you will affect other people, and you'd probably like more of that consideration from him.

He should give you empathy for how you're feeling pulled in different directions. For missing your job while also wanting to stay home. For loving time with your kids while hating housework. For feeling incredible compassion for your son who's in a tantrum combined with an incredible desire for him to please shut up. For the darker thoughts and feelings that come with parenthood, like the desire to shake a baby who won't stop crying—and wanting to hit yourself for having such a wish. He should understand that you have ups and downs for *reasons,* that you're not out of control or weird, that millions of other mothers have similar experiences. He can see it in your friends, in the news, and in the research on mothers (see the box opposite).

It's in your partner's interest to know how it is for you. It gives him useful information about your inner world, what's important to you, and the reasons behind your feelings and actions. It's also in his children's interest that he understand you better, so you two can work well together, and so his kids can have a mom who feels well nourished in her marriage.

He'll be especially able to empathize if you:

- Focus on yourself instead of events or him.
- Share your experience without justifying or defending it.
- Speak from your heart.
- Emphasize the softer, deeper, sometimes "young" feelings of fear, sadness, hurt, or shame that usually underlie feelings of resentment, disapproval, or anger.
- Speak in the form of, *When you do* _____ , *I feel* _____ , rather than being accusatory or saying, *You made me feel* _____ .
- Make clear the essence of what you are saying.

This way of speaking is responsible, open, and dignified. It feels rewarding regardless of his response. Hopefully, he will be understanding, but if he is not, you could openly ask for empathy. It is as legitimate to ask for understanding as it is to ask for a hand with your child. His empathy is real, even if you have to ask for it. And you can ask him to give you more empathy without you always having to ask!

It's also possible that he is already more empathic than you think. Since men tend to view *receiving* empathy as a sign of potential weakness, they often *give* it indirectly—using action, advice, or joking—as an expression of consideration and respect. For example, a year into parenthood, Rick was grousing to a friend about his life being turned upside down. Larry had just sent his own son off to college, and he said reassuringly, **Don't worry, it's just a phase. It'll be over soon.** Then he smiled and added in his Texas twang, **In about eighteen years.** Try to sense your husband's tacit empathy for you (and be empathic yourself about any issues he has with giving empathy). Additionally, you can ask him to express his empathy in a style that reaches you better. Humor is fine, but you may prefer a tone that is warm and forthcoming, one that envelops you in a caring embrace. You might like more words, more details about his understanding of you, more self-disclosure that shows he gets it from the inside out. And whether his empathy is implicit or clearly stated, take a moment to let the experience sink in.

Giving Empathy

Now let's look at *giving* empathy, because that's something you can each do for your relationship. Also, the more skillful you are at giving empathy, the more you'll know deep down what you can ask for when you'd like your partner to be more empathic with you. In sum, when someone is being empathic, he or she is *paying attention, inquiring,* and *double-checking*.

Paying attention. We can all tell if someone is fully present, rather than thinking about something else—such as his or her rebuttal! You and your partner can help yourselves be attentive in these ways:

- *Consciously choose to give your attention.* Attention is a gift. See if you can let your partner have your mind, in a sense, for a time. You can take it back whenever you like.

- *Focus on your partner's inner experience,* the feelings, wants, images and body sensations more than surface details or words.

- *Listen with your body.* Try sensing into your partner's experience from your heart and gut, not just your head.

- *Only listen.* Try not to look for holes in your partner's statements, offer advice, or explain why there's really no reason to get so bothered. The listener's role is simply to understand, without agreeing or disagreeing, letting the other person's communication flow through without resistance, like a breeze through a willow tree.

- *Listen proactively.* Inside your own head, actively sift through your partner's words, looking for the deeper truth. You could ask yourself questions— *What was it that felt so hurtful?*—or imagine how it would be if you walked in those other shoes.

Inquiring. Empathy is a process of discovery in which you try to gain an ever-deepening sense of the inner life of another person (for some possible questions, please see the box). Through inner reflection and outward inquiry, the empathic partner:

Empathy Questions

Here are questions your partner can ask to deepen his understanding of you, or you can use with him.

Can you say more about _____?

What do you mean when you say _____?

Can you give me an example of _____?

How was it for you that _____?

How did you react when he told you about _____?

Could you say it in a different way so I can understand it?

How mad were you? (Or worried, hurt, alarmed, sad, etc.)

What was the most upsetting part? (The most irritating? The most worrisome?)

What do you wish would have happened instead?

What do you feel underneath all that?

Did you also feel hurt (or embarrassed, ashamed, helpless, etc.)?

What does _____ remind you of?

How does the history of _____ affect how you feel about _____?

Deep down, what is really bothering you about _____?

- *Tries to get a sense of the softer feelings* of sadness, hurt, fear, or shame that lie behind a controlled, tough, or angry façade.
- *Considers the underlying, positive wants* the other person is trying to fulfill—such as desires for closeness, safety, autonomy, or being valued—though the way he or she is going about them may be a problem for you.
- *Thinks how the other person's childhood might be a factor today,* and listens for the younger wants and feelings.
- *Imagines the inner being* behind the other's eyes.
- *Listens for the different parts of the other person's experience* so that each can be understood in its own right. For example, if a mother is fuming about

her older sister interfering with the fortieth wedding anniversary party she is organizing for their parents, one part of her reactions might be feeling overloaded by all the details, another could be resistance to a bossy big sister, and a third part might be a long-standing prickliness about criticism from anybody who is linked to a childhood with perfectionistic parents. Her partner could try to imagine how each of those parts feels for her, or how they tug at her emotions in different ways.

Double-checking. A listener needs to let a speaker know, "Message received." Otherwise, the other person will have to express him or herself more intensely to get through, or give up and feel unheard. You can show you got the message by saying back, as best you can, both the explicit content and the implicit feelings, wants, and context. If you do this before launching into a reply, your partner is more likely to feel heard even if you have a different point of view.

Empathy for a Father

One of the best ways to encourage your husband to give you empathy is to express it yourself. Here we draw on Rick's experience as a dad and our conversations with fathers to suggest how it may be for him to be a parent; this is a composite, a generalization, of a father that will not fit the partner of any woman in every way.

Now I'm a dad. As profoundly as you, he loves the child you have made together. He has many of the same feelings you do, like happiness when the baby first curls her tiny fingers around one of his own, delight at the first step, and worry over crying that won't stop. And sometimes his sense of things may differ: he might feel less concerned about a knee bloodied by a tumble or more embarrassed if your son freezes onstage at the preschool holiday party.

Since he probably spends less time with children than you, it is natural for him to be less sure of his skills. Feeling awkward or inept is uncomfortable for many men and makes it hard to ask for help. If you poke fun or criticize him if he does, it gets even harder.

Plunged back into the sights and sounds and smells of childhood, long-forgotten feelings and yearnings from his own early years may be reawakened. That could trouble anyone, but especially a man who is leery of murky or childlike emotions.

Tugged in different directions. He shows his love for his children and you in part by stepping up his efforts as a provider. Yet that tends to draw him into working longer hours when you wish he'd put more energy into your children and home. Unfortunately, his workplace almost certainly couldn't care less about the needs of his family no matter what the personnel manual says; even though the Family and Medical Leave Act entitles him to twelve weeks off without pay if he works for a large company, ninety percent of the employees surveyed in such companies in one study said he should not take a single day. He's stuck between a rock and a hard place. He's probably more engaged in child rearing and housework than his own father was. Nonetheless, if you are like most mothers, you'd still like more involvement and help, and he feels uneasy and resentful that he is not coming up to the standard of what you want in a partner.

The changing, unclear societal expectations about what it is to be a father make it harder to find his footing. There are no cultural models of a man's man who fully shares in parenthood with his wife. Nor is there much respect for the role fathers play in the lives of their children. For example, he has probably had this experience or a similar one: walking down the street with you and the baby in a stroller, strangers come up and coo over the baby and you, but mainly ignore him.

Married to a mother. He is awed at your ability to make a baby and deeply grateful that you have enabled him to have a child. He probably appreciates your sacrifices more than he has been able to say.

He's also worried by their effects on you, by any fatigue, depression, or other health problems that have developed since you became a mother. He wants you to feel better because he cares about you, you'll have a better mood with the children, and you might be nicer to him. But when he offers well-meaning suggestions, like you getting more exercise or using more child care, there's a fair chance you get irritated, wanting empathy rather than problem solving, thinking his idea is impractical, or feeling he's trying to make you give less to your kids. After a few rounds of this, maybe he stops trying.

When it's your turn to offer suggestions, this time about his parenting, he probably feels uncomfortable, even annoyed, at being instructed by anyone, especially a woman, especially his wife. As one father told Rick, ***Most men wouldn't want their wife to be their boss.*** Maybe he's asked you what he could do and been told he should already know. Maybe he's tried to dive in and help and then been told it's all wrong. He picks up your underlying attitude about his parenting skills, and the way many mothers talk to each other about their partners is remarkably disdainful. He may experience you squeezing him out of the parent role while complaining that he's not involved enough.

Where did my wife go? He loves his child incredibly, but as a moment-to-moment matter your daughter or son may not have the same centrality in his life that she or he has for you, not being flesh of his flesh, bone of his bone. His relationship with you is still a priority in itself, not merely as a framework for raising children. He (usually) didn't marry a mother; where did his wife go?

He feels keenly the loss of the attention, energy, affection, cherishing, and love you have shifted from him to your child. The natural egocentrism of the mommy-baby unit can make him feel like little more than a means to its ends. One father said: *I go out in the world like a caveman who brings home the meat. I drop it at her feet, she says "thanks" and goes back to our daughter. It's like I'm not in the room.* Your husband may have had the lurching moment of truth that Rick describes for himself: *One day when Forrest was about a year old, he and Jan were laughing and cuddling on the couch. She smiled at me and I felt her love, but it just hit me. She loved him more than me. He was the sun who lit up her day. I had a jumble of feelings: sadness and loss for myself, bittersweet happiness for Forrest, a sense that this was how it was meant to be, resignation, and acceptance.* There's an Oedipal competition all right between father and child for the mother, much as Freud thought, but for many years at least, Dad is usually the loser. (This shift in a mother's caring away from her partner is made painfully concrete by the disinterest many have in sex—a subject for the next chapter.)

Does my wife understand me? The deepest question of all in any important relationship is, "Do you really understand me?" Unless each of you can answer "yes," that question will keep troubling the waters of your marriage. He needs to know that you understand him just as much as you need to know that he understands you.

You cannot make your husband understand you, but you can try to understand *him*: that much is in your own power. You could ask him about the description of a father just above. Or you could simply observe him for a while without any assumptions, wondering how it feels to be him deep down inside.

Since you give understanding to your children all day long, you might have "empathy fatigue." So it may take a conscious decision to bring understanding to your husband. But if you do, he will notice your interest and appreciate it and be more empathic with you as well. And when the two of you have a better idea of the feelings and wants of each other, you will be more able to solve problems together.

Translating Mom-Speak and Dad-Speak

To paraphrase a comment Oscar Wilde once made about the British and American peoples, a mother and father are one couple divided by a common language. Consider this typical exchange:

SHE: (*wanting to share her concerns about their three-year-old son and explore their options*) I was thinking about Ryan and preschool and after care, and wondering about his teacher, she seems irritable or something, and Ryan gets upset when I drop him off, maybe we need to think about how many hours he's there, and perhaps reducing them for a while and I could cut back at work, or talking with his teacher, or maybe thinking about another school. But it could be just a phase and he has to get used to it. You know what I mean?

HE: (*confused about what the topic is and what actions he is supposed to take, and alarmed at the prospect of her income dropping*) He's fine. Every kid fusses about school. He'll be OK. And we need your income because [*he lists reasons like a lawyer making a case*]. Honey, you worry too much. (*He pauses and thinks the matter is finished: she asked him a question and he answered it. Time to move on.*) How'd it go at work today?

SHE: (*Irritated that he closed the discussion, as if giving his opinion settled things. Hurt that he blew off her detailed observations with vague generalizations about "every kid fusses." Feeling pushed back by him when she wanted to feel closer. Flustered that she has to match his argumentative tone to justify her concerns.*) Wait a minute. You're not listening. I've read about this in some of those books you never look at. [*Gives three warning signs of a child not adapting well to preschool.*]

HE: (*Getting irritated himself at her pressing him. Defensive about not reading parenting books. Resistant to getting drawn into a conversation he doesn't really want to have right now. Sees no point in worrying about Ryan's reactions because the issue is moot: they cannot afford a more expensive school or a cut in his wife's pay, so why argue about it? Does not understand that his wife also doesn't want to argue, but to connect.*) Look, I feel like you're trying to talk me into something I don't want. Even if I did, we couldn't afford it. Besides, we've talked about this before. Can't we talk about something else? I've GOT to change clothes. (*walks out of room*)

SHE: (*Major annoyance. Thinks he is acting like a jerk by being bossy and cutting her off. Feels stymied in her concerns about Ryan. Follows him into the bedroom, her voice rising.*) We can't "talk about something else" because he's our SON and we don't settle things around here by you saying the way it's going to be and stalking out of the room like King Henry the Eighth!

BOTH: (*Now they are each yelling, fighting in earnest . . .*)

Common Gender Differences

Although it seemed like they were talking together, this mother and father were actually having two different conversations. She thought they were going to explore how they felt about their son's distress, and he thought they were making a policy decision. Her priority was joining and his was independence. She was speaking in a way that made sense to her as a woman, and he in a way that made sense to him as a man.*

Women tend to focus on connection in their relationships, while men are more attentive to status and dominance. As a result, a mother might think her husband will welcome her knowledge because he wants to come together with her in raising their children. Yet he could interpret her parenting tips as condescending or controlling.

In conversation, women emphasize the process of being together, concrete consequences for specific people, and feelings, while men emphasize tasks and outcomes, impersonal perspectives, and information. Consider how a mother might start talking about family finances: *The baby's mostly off the breast—though I worry whether she's getting enough to eat—plus it's not good for her when I get cranky because I'm cooped up at home, and of course money is tight, which puts you in a bad mood, but I don't want you getting home any later, so maybe we should make a change. We don't have to right away, because she'll be in kindergarten in just a few years, what do you think?*

In her opening statement, this mother is really trying to take her husband into account and give him all the information he needs to join with her in making a good decision. But he feels somewhat lost in a swirl of topics, back stories, emotions, implicit criticisms, and future possibilities. That feeling prompts him to do the opposite of what she wants: to step back and regain a sense of control by getting analytical and taking charge.

His approach to the subject probably would have been quite different: *I went through the bills and the numbers are clear. We need you to get a job right away.* For him, this is only the opening statement in a negotiation, and he's waiting for her response. But she feels he has already made up his mind without hearing from her. She's hurt that her intimate partner is talking to her like she's the bookkeeper. His matter-of-fact bluntness is to him a way to respect her time and get to the bottom line. But she's just getting warmed up! In a sense, it's like sex: she wants more foreplay and time lingering together. If he plays devil's advocate, expresses his views rat-tat-tat, or points out the grain of truth in his mother's criticisms of his wife's parenting, he's acting appropriately, according to the standards of his gender. But to her, it's jarring, like a lover who is too rough. By the standards of *her* gender, he's

---

*Of course, individuals vary in the degree to which their communication style is "masculine" or "feminine." Even when there's a major difference between his way of speaking and hers, it's worth remembering that the similarities in communicating will always be much greater than the differences.

speaking in a way she'd only use with someone she disliked. She feels dismayed and disoriented, thinking, *But I thought you were on my side!*

Appreciating the Other Style

Each gender style is valid, like it's valid to be Italian or Swedish. And the differences are not black and white. Women value autonomy; they just don't think it's threatened by joining with their partner. Men value connection; they just don't think it's threatened by acting independently.

We can all learn from the opposite sex. You might appreciate how your partner has a sense of connection with you that does not need much reassurance, and how he can be sympathetic and kind in his own way. He could appreciate how you can juggle multiple topics at once; how you really do get many things done in your conversations, including maintaining important relationships; how you have such a deep confidence in your autonomy that you don't need to defend it with preemptive strikes; and how you can be incisive and decisive in your own way.

Skill with the other gender's style lets you shift gears effectively, depending on what's needed. For example, the masculine style often has advantages at work, and the feminine style with children. Some conversations with your partner are mainly about connecting while others are about solving a problem, and it helps to be clear about what kind of interaction you're having. Even when it's problem solving, starting with connection-talk helps you feel good about each other and make better decisions.

> Kind words can be short and easy to speak, but their echoes are truly endless.
>
> —*Mother Teresa*

Bridging the Gender Divide

HOW DO YOU WISH YOUR HUSBAND WOULD SPEAK WITH YOU?
YOU CAN ASK HIM TO:

- Nod, smile, make eye contact, say "yeah" frequently, etc., to let you know he's *with* you; encourage you to say more; focus on the conversation going well more than any practical outcome
- Touch you (usually nonsexually) as a way to say *we're connected*
- Let himself be moved emotionally; express an empathic understanding; offer relevant self-disclosure
- Accept your feelings instead of trying to talk you out of them; hear you out instead of trying to solve the problem

- Understand that your (often greater) expertise about the children is not a threat but an asset for him and the family; be confident enough in his own parenting to ask for suggestions or help

- Realize that you need to ask him questions about his schedule, whereabouts, or plans in order to coordinate with him, not to be bossy; recognize that you are not trying to control him

- See that your desire for ideas and support does not mean you are unskilled or insecure, but that you want to be in this together and you respect his need to be informed

- Be willing to talk about problems instead of thinking they might reveal an embarrassing flaw

- Recognize that you need to be able to talk about your children or marriage with close friends

- Ask questions about your thoughts and feelings; ask three or more questions in a row (not "How am I doing?")

- Above all, communicate that he cares about you and wants to stay connected

HE MIGHT APPRECIATE IT IF YOU WERE TO:

- Pay attention to his sensitivity to issues of power, dominance, and status; be careful about orders, put-downs, or ultimatums

- "Knock before entering" by asking him if this is a good time to talk (he should name another one if it isn't)

- Explain the principles, values, or goals that guide your thinking; be direct about what you want

- Consider sometimes listening as one man would to another, with less of the chiming in and personal statements you might use with another woman

- Understand that he may not feel his passing thoughts are worth sharing, so his quiet after you speak does not necessarily mean he's not listening; understand that he may regard personal questions as potentially intrusive, so his lack of inquiry into your world could be respectful rather than uncaring

- Realize that his detached verbal style does not mean he wants to distance himself from or abandon you

- Recognize that his debate-style challenges are to him fair play in an on-going interaction, not a personal attack: more like a strong move to the basket than walking off the court
- Be judicious in what you say about him or your family to others
- Above all, communicate respect for his autonomy; make it clear that you are simply trying to work together as equal partners in the best interests of your children

Speaking Your Mind

There are surely times to bite your tongue. Let's say you've had a chance to go out to a movie while your husband minds the kids. When you get home, the house is a mess and no one's been fed. A complaint swells inside you. But you remember who got the break and who didn't, that you hate it when a criticism is the first thing out of his mouth, and that you can always make your point later. So you take a big breath, smile, and say something nice instead.

But repeatedly holding back your true feelings will lead to a general atmosphere of emotional distance (as well as wear on your health). Family is about closeness if it's about anything. When parents talk to each other mainly from their heads or about impersonal matters, that sends a message that it's not desirable or safe to connect in a deeper way. Children notice and become more cautious themselves. You feel stifled, weighted down with what you're holding back. Your partner misses out on important information about how you really think and feel, losing chances to learn and grow. And you have to be able to openly address any issues in your partner—such as a drinking problem or depression—that affect him, you, or the kids.

Again and again, we've seen that the single most beneficial step a couple can take after children is to make deep, open communication a regular and fundamental part of their relationship. By building civility, empathy, and skill with the "second language" of the other gender, you can make it safe enough to be more transparent, vulnerable, accessible, and authentic.

This way of communicating is explicit and unmistakable. You are in your experience as you express it. For example, if you were to tell your mate, *I felt disrespected when you criticized me in front of the kids,* you would feel your hurt and anger as you spoke, and he'd hear them in your voice and sense them in your body. In this instance, you are speaking your truth freely, focused on your own experience and viewpoint, not on getting him to agree or change. You are not watching to see how he reacts. You are *unilaterally* communicating what you need to say to feel complete. There is a lovely sense of freedom and dignity, of being real, of taking care of yourself.

As great as this feels, it's not easy for most of us to speak in this way. Growing up as a woman or being a mother may make you think that your first concern should be the feelings of others, that you shouldn't rock the boat, that you should never get angry or make anyone feel uncomfortable: *If you can't say something nice, don't say anything at all.*

Simply understanding why it makes you nervous to speak your mind fully helps remove any of those soft muzzles over your true voice. Tell yourself that you have a right to your experience and to express it. You do not need to justify your feelings; no one can argue with your description of your own state of mind. Nor are you stuck with what you say; in fact, communicating your experience or viewpoint can lead these to flow into becoming something else. And your partner will probably be more open himself if you put your own cards on the table.

Positive Support

When you and your husband are worn out by raising a family, it's harder to give each other positive energy. But that's when you need acknowledgment and reassurance the most, since researchers have found that receiving emotional support from one's partner is a powerful way to reduce the stress of parenting and increase personal well-being.

Acknowledgment

Now that you're a parent, you *deserve* recognition, appreciation, and praise more than ever. You're having to learn new things all the time, restrain the universal urge to rant and rave, and dig deep for love while working day and night. You also *need* acknowledgment from your mate more than ever: others can be critical, the culture puts out a Supermom myth that no one can live up to, and you worry about doing a good enough job. Unfortunately, you usually *get less*: he's too busy to notice, or too worn out or grouchy to say anything, or he's waiting for a kind word himself.

So it's natural if you'd like to feel more acknowledged by him. One way is to notice his appreciation when it's not stated outright, but sits behind his words or his eyes. Another is to ask for it directly. Some of the most powerful moments in a relationship come when one person is brave enough to ask questions like: *In what ways do you think I am a good mother? A good person? What do you respect about me? What do you see as my strengths? Why do you like me?* You can also ask for more information after he says something, as in: *What did you think was good about the [way I handled that tantrum, thing I said at the teacher's conference, etc.]? Could you be more specific about what you thought I did that worked?*

Yet asking could be hard: perhaps you were taught to be humble, or you worry that he might laugh or have nothing to say. To overcome these self-doubts, remind yourself of all that you do, and consider how it is good for your kids to see him being appreciative. He will probably be large-hearted when you ask him sincerely. If he is not, you will have learned about an issue you need to deal with as a couple. Either way, something good will have happened.

Sometimes we sit down at the banquet table of life, in front of an acknowledgment we have richly earned, and then take tiny bites, leaving most of it on the plate. Instead, try to treat it as an honest expression of his view of the facts. An acknowledgment is a gift, and it would be rude not to receive it. Even if you think you don't deserve it, he does—and he's probably right.

Turnabout can't hurt either: giving him acknowledgment both recognizes his efforts and virtues, and it encourages him to return the favor to you. You could reflect on why you fell in love with him in the first place, on his positive qualities, on the kind soul deep within him, looking out from behind his eyes. When you acknowledge him, you are not ignoring his foibles, but simply recognizing some of the good tiles in the mosaic of the person he is. Unless you have stumbled into a relationship with a complete loser, the positive tiles greatly outnumber the negative ones. Do your statements about him have roughly the same ratio of positive to negative? You might think back over the last few days: About how many times did you praise or thank him compared to the times you were critical? Besides what you said out loud, how often did you have acknowledging thoughts rather than caustic ones?

If the balance of your words or thoughts is not consistent with the total mosaic of who he is, he will feel unseen and misjudged, and you will feel worse about your relationship than you need to. On the other hand, think of a time when you acknowledged him: How did he respond? How did you feel? You might quietly do an experiment for a week of saying one true thing each day that acknowledges him—in addition to what you would normally do—and see what happens.

Of course, you are a mosaic yourself, with many more positive characteristics than negative ones. You can certainly ask him to talk about you in a way that is consistent with the total package of who you are, rather than concentrating on the tiles he wishes were different.

Reassurance

If raising a family doesn't make you worry about one thing or another—whether it's a child that's ill, how to pay the bills, or where your toddler put your car keys—you'd better check your pulse. Strong partners offer reassurance to each other; besides giving it yourself, you can ask for it directly, in one or more of these forms:

- *Solidarity* that he is on your side, that you are in this together.

- *Encouragement,* whose root meaning is to give heart. He can remind you of your strengths, of the capabilities you've marshaled before and will call on again. He can look in your eyes and tell you, in his own words, what he knew on the day he asked you to marry: *You are a strong and capable person. You have guts and character, and I believe in you.*

- *Hope* that Mother Nature is on your side, that your children will eventually learn to sleep through the night, wipe their own bottoms, and be nice to each other.

- *Realistic perspectives* about the facts and the risks involved in whatever you are concerned about. He could feel that there is less to worry about, or more ways to solve the problem, than you might have thought. Of course, this kind of reassurance goes down better *after* he has heard you out, and when it is offered respectfully, without patronizing or dismissing you.

Making Repairs

Like anything that is precious and fragile, a good relationship needs regular maintenance. Within an interaction, couples with a strong relationship make little repairs on the fly, clarifying intentions, correcting misunderstandings, revising their choice of words, dropping in grace notes to soothe a ruffled feather, lightening the mood by cracking a joke, or softening a criticism with a self-deprecating admission. And over the long haul, they act on any sense that there's something festering under the carpet, seeking out and repairing unresolved grievances or misunderstandings.

After years of working with couples, we are convinced that you can almost always find ways to mend what's frayed in any relationship, *if* both partners try hard enough. You have powerful tools and skills that you can use in your functional partnership as coparents and in your intimate friendship as lovers and mates, and when you do, both aspects of your marriage *will* get better.

Partners in Parenthood

*I*F A MOTHER AND FATHER do not come together about how to raise their kids, there's more stress on the person who handles the bulk of the day-to-day parenting—typically the mother. Also, unresolved disagreements about sharing the load wear most on the person who is doing the majority of the work—again, typically the mother. Besides being personally depleting, these nagging conflicts about raising a family eat away at the bonds that hold a marriage together. But they're really not that hard to solve. It just takes skillful communication, clear principles, and a little negotiation. Let's see how.

Parenting from the Same Page

One mother told Rick: *I think Angelina, our four-year-old, should watch only an hour of TV per day. My husband mumbles, "OK, honey," but when I leave the house I come back to see her glued to the tube. It's not just TV. I say no sweets, he says just a couple. I say no spanking, he thinks a swat is OK. I say bed by eight, but that means I've got to do it. I read books about parenting and he reads the sports section of the paper. I'm afraid we are confusing our daughter plus driving each other crazy.*

It's hard to get on the same page, since parents often have different values in child rearing, and issues of who gets to be right or in charge muddy the water. Yet children get confused when their parents have different approaches, and they're more likely to play one parent against the other: *But Dad said I could!* And it is disheartening when your partner approaches the most important undertaking of your life in a way that seems wrongheaded or cavalier.

Minor differences in parenting style are all right. Besides helping children prepare for a variety of teachers and (eventually) bosses, complementary approaches can build on each other, like Mom being more of a tender owie-kisser and Dad an exuberant horsieback-ride-giver, so kids get the best of both worlds. But major differences in parenting values or actions are a problem. To solve it, the first step is to pin down exactly what they are, so we suggest you take a moment to fill out the questionnaire in the box on page 234.

Taking Steps Yourself

While it may seem unfair to be the one who makes the first move, trying to be a better partner yourself will evoke positive behavior from your husband, reduce his reasons for being irked with you, and if nothing else, let you stand on principle if he is dragging his feet. And there will be a better result when you and he take steps *together,* as we discuss in the next section. Here's a buffet of options, focused on the common situations of a somewhat disengaged father or one whose parenting style differs in some ways from his wife's; if these are not issues in your marriage, you could skip ahead to page 247.

Have confidence in his fundamental ability to be a parent. Hundreds of studies have shown that a father is just as able to parent with love and skill as a mother. For example, when babies cry, the typical father gets just as upset inside as his wife does, and just as relieved when the baby settles.

Encourage him. Try to be encouraging (though not patronizing) if he is learning a new skill. Suppose he feels awkward holding a little baby: reassure him that he's doing fine, and perhaps disclose ways you, too, have felt a little klutzy.

Acknowledge him. Admit it when his way worked even though it was different from yours, or when you learned something from him. Emphasize what you appreciate about his parenting rather than what you wish were different. See the strengths in his approach and understand the values it is based on.

Let him learn. Let him be the one who handles a tantrum from start to finish or tries to get a child to eat some carrots. Occasionally direct the kids to him for things you normally provide so he gains more experience with those parts of child rearing. If you can, arrange for him to spend extended times alone with your children, such as an entire evening from dinner to bed, or better yet, a full day or two while you go on a business trip or (best of all) take a mini-vacation.

Are We Parenting from the Same Page?

Indicate the degree to which you and your partner agree on the topics below, using this scale:

1 = We mainly disagree.   2 = We somewhat disagree.
3 = We somewhat agree.   4 = We mainly agree.

Values—The importance of . . .

_____ Being sensitive and responsive to your children

_____ Respecting their wants

_____ Preventing their discomfort or unhappiness

_____ Accepting and encouraging their self-expression

_____ Personally interacting with your children

_____ Physical affection toward them

Actions

_____ Where your children sleep

_____ Bedtimes

_____ How they are put to bed

_____ How you deal with them if they wake up at night

_____ How long to breast-feed

_____ Their religious upbringing

_____ How many sweets or snacks they are allowed to eat

_____ Expectations for their behavior at mealtimes

_____ How much TV or video they are allowed to watch

_____ What sort of TV shows, videos, or movies they see

_____ How many toys to buy them

_____ Use of swats or spanking for discipline

_____ Yelling at the kids when they misbehave

_____ Other consequences for misbehavior

_____ What to do when a child has a tantrum

_____ How to intervene when siblings quarrel with each other

_____ What a parent should do if he or she has made a mistake with a child

Add up your total score. Here is a rough estimate of the degree to which you and your husband have similar approaches (if you skipped some questions, just adjust downward the ranges given on the next page).

81–92	Together, you are raising your children in a very consistent way.
66–80	You agree more than you disagree, but there could be some significant differences.
51–65	There are major differences in how you approach child rearing.
Below 50	Your husband and you are parenting from different books.

When there's a meeting with the pediatrician or a teacher, do what you can to have your husband come, such as saying that the person wants to talk with both parents. When you're there, try to have roughly half of the conversation be with your husband. For example, if the professional asks a question, you can remain silent, or smile at him and ask, "What do you think?"

Let him experience the consequences of his actions, so he can see for himself why you do things differently. For example, if he wants to play roughhouse with the kids just before bed, tell him he can settle them down for sleep.

Try not intervening in situations where you normally step in (unless something truly abusive is occurring), and see what happens instead. Things may turn out better than you feared, or perhaps your husband will see from his own experience that he needs another approach.

Understand the whole picture before you jump in. Be aware of how your emotions, beliefs, or previous experiences can make a situation look worse than it really is. A father once told Jan: *Our five-year-old son, Pete, whines and gets upset real easily. If we roughhouse, he gets mad over nothing, and then my wife, Joanie, comes in and yells at me. We were playing basketball in the backyard one day, and I was letting him win and he was happy. Then he missed a shot, and I got the ball for my turn. But he wanted the ball. I explained it was my turn but he started to cry. Joanie heard him and ran outside, glared at me, and said really nastily, "Can't you ever play without making him cry??!" But I didn't do anything! First she tells me I don't do enough with him and then she's mad at me when I do. She's always watching, ready to pounce for the least thing.* Again, try to get the full story before you react.

Don't micromanage. Try not to be controlling, dogmatic, or self-righteous about small matters. That way, you'll be more credible when you discuss the big ones, and your partner will probably feel less defensive. Many disputes about parenting are inherently minor: if he puts an orange top and purple pants on your preschooler, maybe you should just smile to yourself and let it go. Every time you argue with him about how he parents has an emotional cost for each of you, plus it discourages his involvement; sometimes the issue is worth the price, but often it's not.

Get a reality check on the actual seriousness of your differences by being clear about the facts: how much TV does he actually let the kids watch, how many times a night does he speak in a scolding tone, how often does he let your child stay up past her bedtime? Find out whether he is acting within the normal range of child rearing or is over the line by finding out what other families do, reading books, taking a parent education class, asking your pediatrician, or getting a consultation with a child development specialist.

Be respectful. When you do offer suggestions, be respectful and specific. Give a positive idea of what he *could* do rather than what he *should not* do, like saying *It's been working for me to change Emma's diaper with that little music box going* instead of *This time, try not to make her cry.* If you can, filter out any implicit criticisms or commands in what you say.

If he offers a suggestion or criticism to you, try to be a model of how you'd like him to react when he's on the receiving end. Make sure you understand his idea. Next, *join* with him as much as you can: offer empathy, acknowledge the problem he's identified, agree with the positive aims behind his idea, and say how it could in fact be useful. Then share your concerns, if you have any. Finally, offer a specific suggestion about what happens from here, ranging from maintaining your approach to agreeing to his idea, or some kind of compromise in between.

Taking Steps Together

Parents often work out their differences informally: maybe you mention something over dinner, there's a testy exchange, one of you makes a point that's too sensible to disagree with, and you come together. But other times, you'd benefit from a process that's a little more structured. Hopefully, your husband will read this section, but if not, you can bring up its points with him.

Talking about values. A good place to start is to set aside time to talk about the values that guide your parenting. You can use the questions in the box opposite or come up with your own. This should be an empathic exploration of how each of you feels rather than an attempt to change anyone's mind. Be as supportive as you can and emphasize where you already have common ground. Really try to understand how your partner came to feel the way he does, and encourage him to do the

> Before I got married I had six theories about bringing up children; now I have six children, and no theories.
>
> —Lord Rochester

Questions About Parenting Values

Ask your partner these questions and consider them yourself. Some come at the same topic from different directions; feel free to change or eliminate questions as you like. If you are confused by an answer from your partner because it seems at odds with his actions, you can ask him to clarify, but avoid arguing. Take your time; these questions are not always easy to answer, and it will normally take several conversations to explore them thoroughly.

How you approach being a parent:

What does it mean to you to be a parent?

If parenthood were pie divided into four slices—direct child rearing, housework, coordinating with each other, and providing for the family—how big is each slice for you?

How does your personality affect your parenting?

How has becoming a parent changed you as a person?

How you want to raise a child:

What do you think are the most important things to give a child the age of our own?

From your own life experiences, what do you feel are important personal characteristics you'd like to see our child develop? What are the top three or four? Is there a number one?

There are three central aspects to parenting: nurturing, disciplining, and supporting learning and achievement. Is there one that's most important to you? If a parent can be high, medium, or low on each aspect, how do you think you should be?

What do you wish your mom had done differently? Your dad? How has that affected the kind of parent you want to be?

How did your parents work out their differences in parenting styles? How has that experience affected the ways that you approach working out differences with me?

Your values in action:

Do any of your values related to raising a family pull in different directions?

How do you feel you have been able to act consistently with your values as a parent? How do you feel you have not?

How do you feel you have become more skillful as a parent? How would you like to become more skillful in the future?

same. For example, what experiences have (hypothetically) made him feel it's important to "toughen up" his children?

It's all right to say how you want the two of you to act as parents. Women who say what they feel and want are generally more satisfied in their marriages than women who don't. But you may have to push through some resistance—yours or his—to say your piece. If so, get some support from other mothers for the validity of your needs and your right to express them and remind yourself that you're just advocating for the sake of your kids.

Of course, when you discuss your differences, try to avoid an accusatory, blaming, or disdainful attitude. Unless your partner is outrageous, he is parenting like millions of other people. Most differences in parenting style call for compromise or skill building rather than indignation.

Being supportive of each other. See if you can get agreement on the general goal of supporting each other as parents. For starters, keep each other up-to-date by sharing information like *I think Charlie's getting a cold* or *Patrice has to bring something to share to kindergarten.* And try to back the authority of the other parent in front of the children whenever possible, handling disagreements behind closed doors, with voices that do not fill the house.

Children take their cues for how to treat their parents from seeing how they treat each other, and insulting, hostile, threatening, or raging speech gives children the message that it's all right to speak that way themselves. You both could consider how a child's gender might affect his or her reactions. For example, a boy hearing his father routinely berate his mom may think that is how men are allowed or even ought to act with women. A girl observing her father act in that way may come to believe that such treatment is normal, and perhaps even unconsciously seek out a man who will treat her similarly when she becomes a woman herself.

You can encourage the children to accept parental authority by going along with it in each other. If Mom calls the family to dinner, Dad should not dawdle. If Dad says it's time to get in the car for a family vacation, that's not the best moment for Mom to make a quick call to a neighbor.

Finally, try not to polarize roles so that one parent is the disciplinarian while the other gets to be more nurturing or playful. This cuts both ways. A mother may feel she has to do mainly humdrum, plain vanilla activities with children in order to get through the daily marathon while her partner gets to come in with a flashy sprint of high-energy play that kids love. On the other hand, a father is usually leery of being pegged as the source of big punishments—*Just wait until your father gets home!*—especially if that's a role his own dad played. You can talk about this is-

What Promotes Optimal Child Development

- Good food and health care, a safe environment, and a supportive community
- Many loving and affectionate interactions each day between parent and child
- Sensitive and rapid responsiveness to a child's wants—whether to fulfill them, offer an alternative, or compassionately deny them
- A generally positive emotional atmosphere in the home
- Discussion and modeling by parents of character and moral values
- Encouragement and prodding to develop age-appropriate skills, and ultimately achieve in life up to the child's potential
- Clear expectations for age-appropriate behavior
- Consistent rewards for good behavior and penalties for poor behavior
- Minimal or no spanking
- No harsh, erratic, or abusive parenting practices
- Parents who work together as a strong team

sue and sometimes deliberately shift who does what. There is no rule that says you can't be the one in the middle of the pillow fight while he finishes up the dishes!

Using a tie-breaker. A book, professional, or class is a neutral guide that can break a deadlock between parents. For example, if there's a conflict about how to punish your child, the two of you could read a book in the *Positive Discipline* series, mark any parts you don't feel good about, and then use the rest of the book as an agreed-upon "manual" for that aspect of child rearing. If a big issue comes up— like you want to try a family bed while he feels the baby should sleep down the hall—the two of you could discuss it with your pediatrician. Many parent resource centers or local therapists offer classes, and taking one together would give you a common experience and an opportunity to hear ideas from other moms and dads.

Informally, you could have another couple over and ask how they handle issues like time-outs or tantrums. This can be reassuring: behind what appears to be the perfect family is usually a messy reality that looks a lot like your own. Even if you don't get any new techniques, there's the calming sense of perspective that you are grappling with a normal-range problem and if you hang in there, things will work out like they have for countless other parents. But avoid getting drawn into a fight, whether it's yours—or theirs!

Parenting is still more art than science, but in the last thirty years, much excellent research has established some of the facts of optimal child rearing; the box summarizes those studies. Disputes can be resolved or at least clarified by finding out what science has discovered about that aspect of raising kids. But keep in mind that many disagreements are fundamentally about values and cannot be resolved by facts alone, that each child is an individual who may differ from the average tendency of the groups that are the basis of most studies, and that any parenting expert who sounds completely sure of himself or herself is suspect.

Negotiating your differences. Strong couples negotiate all the time, whether it's how to answer a child's questions about God or what to watch on TV tonight. It doesn't mean you don't love each other if you sometimes find yourselves striking a bargain like shoppers at a flea market. Getting skillful at negotiation can only serve your marriage—plus help you with your child, whether she's two or twenty. Good books have been written about negotiating in general (e.g., *Getting to Yes* by Roger Fisher and William Ury) or for parents in particular (e.g., *Why Parents Disagree and What You Can Do About It* by Roberta Israeloff and Ron Taffel, Ph.D). In our view these are the six essential steps:

1. Know what you want.
2. Establish a favorable foundation.
3. Communicate clearly.
4. Respect feelings.
5. Work out the details.
6. Make a commitment.

1. Know what you want. Negotiating is all about wants. To get what you want, you need to know what it is. As we saw in chapter 2 (pp. 42–44), our wants are layered, like a parfait, with less important and fleeting desires on top and vital and enduring ones underneath. The deeper you go, the more you will get to what you *really* want. And the more that you and your husband can talk about what you each really want, the more teamwork and friendship you'll have in your marriage.

Therefore, try to probe beneath the surface of your wishes or complaints—such as being peeved that he routinely comes home late from work—to find the deeper stakes, which in this case might include wanting to feel you matter enough to him that he would care about how his lateness affects you, or that you can trust him to keep his agreements. Try to sort the wants from your childhood into a pile that's separate from those that come from a more adult place within your mind. For example, suppose that people frequently kept you waiting a lot as a kid, you hated the boredom and powerlessness of it, and the strong desire to not let that happen again is getting mixed in with your need as a grown woman for him to get home on time to help you during one of the most stressful times of the day, the mad dash before dinner.

When you acknowledge and accept the child wants, you'll usually feel a softening inside and a nurturing kindness toward yourself. You'll also see ways that the situation you faced as a child was different from the one you're in today. That simple understanding has an amazing power to lower the emotional charge on your wants. When it's time to talk about your desires, try telling him the parts that come from your childhood so he can have a better understanding of what's linked in your mind to seemingly small issues, like being fifteen minutes late. Your openness will probably evoke more compassion and support from him—and if it doesn't, you can ask for them.

Take a close look at any thoughts that argue against your wants, such as *Oh, it's just not practical for him to get home on time every night.* If the thought has merit, it could lead you to adjust your wishes, like telling your partner that you can live with him coming home late one night in five, or that you just want him to give you a call when he knows he's going to be late. But many thoughts are not good friends to us, trying to talk us out of wants that are in fact legitimate, reasonable, and positive. Try to challenge those thoughts like this: *Is there really some rule that says I can't ask for that? Would the world come to an end if I got what I wanted? Does he make the same assumptions when it comes to his own wants?* Your partner may not give you what you want, but that does not mean it was bad to want it in the first place, or bad to express it. For example, it's reasonable to want your husband to be more supportive when you are struggling with a preschooler's tantrums. It is valid to want him to use a different tone of voice while disciplining a child. It is completely OK to want him to do something within his own head like clearing his mind of work clutter during the drive home so he can be mentally present and ready for kid-action when he walks through the door.

2. Establish a favorable foundation. Create a context of mutual rapport, empathy, and good wishes. Choose a good moment and place and be prepared to take the time you need, rather than tossing off comments as you rush on by.

Frame the issue as a "we" problem rather than an "I" or "you" problem. You are in the same boat together, each affected by the other's actions or suffering.

Try to treat each other as teammates rather than opponents. If that doesn't feel natural, you could do an experiment in which you act *as if* you were teammates, and see what happens.

3. Communicate clearly. Try to say what you want explicitly and without apology, rather than hinting or saying nothing while hoping he'll somehow just know. Of course, this can be hard for several reasons. For one, you may think that what you want should be obvious by now. But, it often isn't—since he probably is not holding as much information about the kids in his mind as you are, and he has his own preoccupations as well—and even if it is, it can't hurt to go on record with it one more time. Second, you may want him to figure it out on his own, as a sign that he understands and cares about you: *I anticipate his needs without him asking, so why can't he return the favor?* But there's a good chance that that the issue for him is not a deep matter of whether he cares about you but simply a practical question of finding out what he's supposed to *do,* since many men show their caring mainly through action. You can pursue more direct and effective ways to feel understood and cared about, like finding times for good conversation, or any of the other suggestions in the next chapter.

A third reason is contained in this comment from a mother at one of Rick's talks: ***It really, really irritates me for him to say, "What do you want me to do?" Then I have to be the mom with him and say, "Well, you could do this or that."*** Understandable as these feelings are—since you've probably been telling your kids what to do all day—try to step out of the mom frame and into the colleague frame with your husband. Certainly you shouldn't have to spell out every detail like a contract. Yet if you do not tell him what you want, how can you expect him to fulfill his part?

Finally, it is common to have had experiences as a child that make it feel scary to come out with what you want. Using the tools in chapters 2 and 6, try to be aware of those inhibitions. Inside your own mind, challenge the expectations from childhood that are probably not valid today, and give yourself encouragement to push forward and let your true voice ring free. (A structured exercise that could support you in expressing your wants is shown in the box opposite.)

Once you start talking, try to explain your point of view in terms that will make sense to him, given his values and concerns. Avoid distractions such as other issues or arguing about what happened in the past. Anticipate his doubts: *I know you want to be able to feed Emma yourself, and I'm willing to pump milk so you can, therefore I don't think we need to wean her right now.* You can make it easy to try the approach you're suggesting by framing it as an experiment, putting a time limit on

Sharing Wants with Your Partner

In this exercise, one partner asks the other one a simple question over and over: ***What do you want from me?*** Then you switch roles, and the one who was asking the question now starts answering it, over and over. Start by agreeing that you will respect what the other person says and not use it against him or her later. Try to create a context that feels safe.

As a questioner, all you need to do is ask the question genuinely and listen empathically to the answer. Please do not comment or criticize, although you can ask your partner to clarify something you don't understand. After he has answered, say *I got it* or something similar, and ask the question again.

As a speaker, look inside each time you hear the question and see what else you want from your partner. It is fine to express wishes that seem whimsical, silly, embarrassing, or taboo; you are only sharing your experience in the moment, not committing to a position. You are trying to dump the whole bag on the table, including wants that are general (e.g., that you act more loving) and specific (e.g., that you put the cap on the toothpaste). It is all right to express wants that come from the younger parts of yourself, including those that are more about your own parents than your partner. Try to push through any holding back and say what you really long for, whatever it is.

Set aside half an hour or more to do this exercise. Try to get through at least a dozen rounds of questions per person. If you can, let yourselves go into a deep place of honesty and intimacy with each other. Afterward, talk about the exercise, but do not argue about it.

If you'd like, alter the form slightly by having the questioner respond to each answer by saying either *Yes, I can do that* or *Let's talk more about it.* You can also use this format with related questions, such as: *What would you like for our family? What do you need from me to trust me? What are you afraid of? What is bothering you? How could I be a better husband/wife?*

how long you'll give it a go, and perhaps linking it to certain conditions: *Could we just try for a week insisting that Serena eat some vegetables before dessert and see what happens? And if she goes on a hunger strike, we can do something else.*

It's especially useful to translate general wants into concrete specifics, using examples of how things will be if you get what you want. This brings issues down out of the clouds of abstractions like "spoiling children" to solid ground where you can actually *do* something. It lets your partner know exactly what you'd like him to do, and it enables you to tell if it gets done. For example, instead of saying, *You're too permissive,* try: *I think you let the kids have too many sweets. I'm willing for the kids to have dessert at dinner but not a candy bar in the afternoon, too. OK?* Overall, focus on positive behaviors by saying what you want more of rather than less.

Of course, it's also all right to be clear about where you are unclear: *I think we ought to try a new baby-sitter but I'm not one hundred percent convinced; what do you think?* Or: *I feel like we need to push harder on toilet training, but I'm not sure how to do it; do you have any ideas?*

To be sure, you need to find out what he wants, so you have to ask or give him the space to say. If it is not obvious, try to get at the wish or complaint embedded in his communication. Don't shy away from differences. Sometimes a couple will avoid conflicts by ignoring their issues, but the result is a relationship that is just not anchored in truth; the issues will come out one day, anyway, or some unrelated challenge—an unexpected pregnancy, a lay-off at work—could blow the relationship away like a tumbleweed with no roots. Ask questions even if you fear the answers: *What is really bothering you? What's the most important part of this to you? What would make things better? What would it look like if we did it your way?* It is OK to discover that your partner wants something from you that you do not want to give; it is all right if he does not love every single thing about you or approve of everything you do; you cannot please him—or any person—all of the time.

Prevent misunderstandings before they happen by double-checking. Ask him what he thinks you want. Or say what you think he wants.

4. Respect feelings. Communicating wants often brings up emotions, some of which can go all the way back to childhood. If these feelings are not acknowledged, they will clamor more loudly, like a child raising her voice to be heard. If you are nervous or irritated underneath, try to say so explicitly, because your partner is probably sensing your disquiet and may react to it instead of to the topic you want to focus on. For example: *I'm a little nervous about bringing this up, but I don't think our child care is working out.* Or: *I'm getting frustrated that Amy is still crying most times you wash her hair.* Explain why your wants are important to you, how they are linked to deeply felt values, and try to find out the same about him. If emotions are clouding your discussion, you may need to shift gears to talking about them for a bit, and then get back to negotiating.

5. Work out the details. Adopt a mind-set in which you are driving toward positive solutions instead of wrangling about negative problems. Study the times when all goes well as a model of what you each can do to make things work. Consider, at least to yourself, any payoff you are receiving from the current situation—such as getting to feel morally superior or like a virtuous victim—then consider the costs, and decide what you really want. You and your partner could ask yourselves, *What would it be like to no longer have this problem?*

Push to narrow your differences: *It's not that I'm a Nazi or you're a hippie, it's that I think Latrell is old enough to put away his clothes and you don't.* Or even closer together: *Can't we just insist that he put his coat on the hook when he gets home instead of dropping it on the floor?* Since people in conflict usually overestimate their differences, chances are that you're closer together than you think. It's a lot easier to bridge a smaller gap.

Sometimes in the throes of a negotiation (or argument), you start to realize that you might be able to live with some difference in parenting style. Ask yourself some questions: *Is it that big a deal? Is it really harming my kids? Is it worth straining my marriage or stressing myself out?* Seemingly opposing practices might in fact be complementary, such as how being highly nurturing to a child promotes independence, rather than dependence, by giving her the sense of a safe base from which she can explore. Maybe it's all right for one parent to put a higher priority on something than the other parent does—like being more zealous about saying "please" and "thank you"—as long as you don't undermine each other: *It's OK that I don't care about this as much as you do, but I won't get in your way, and I'll support you when I can.* Different approaches can often coexist; it's not the end of the world if the kids know that one parent is a softer touch for a cookie.

Another way to live with differences in parenting is to agree that each partner has veto power if he or she feels strongly about an issue, such as risks to a child's safety. Of course, no one should abuse the veto, and you can take back that power if it gets out of hand.

If important conflicts remain, be willing to make a deal. Consider offering a compromise, or budging on one of your priorities if he gives in on one of his. For example, you could agree for your values to rule in one area while his prevail in another: *I'll loosen up about what the kids wear if you promise to be stricter about bedtimes.* Or find out what parts of the total job he might prefer, and see if it works for you to other ones.

Try to anticipate potential problems and then presolve them. It does not put a hex on your plans to imagine how they might go awry.

Finally, it could make a lot of sense to help him to give you what you want. For example, maybe he could use a little coaching on a particular skill or an occasional reminder. But sometimes this can be hard: You might feel too worn out, or sick and tired of prodding him. Or perhaps a young part within you feels disappointed in the care she received as a child and yearns for a partner who knows without saying what she needs. Yet you only help yourself when you ask yourself: *What could I do that would enable him to give me what I'm asking for?*

6. Make a commitment. When there is a clear understanding of what you and your partner are going to do, check your gut feeling. Do you and he really think this is going to happen? Or are you kidding yourselves? If your plan feels solid, treat it as a personal commitment and ask him to do the same. You are each giving your word, and that is not a thing to be taken lightly. Then acknowledge the process you have gone through. It's not easy to work out issues in parenting, yet you've each stuck with it.

Finally, try to avoid snatching defeat from the jaws of victory. You've probably seen some of the common methods: Not noticing it when your partner has come over to your side, continuing to fire after he has put up the white flag, remaining irritated that you had to talk about it in the first place, or shifting with hardly a breath to another issue.

Talking about misunderstandings or broken agreements. Fulfilling commitments is the basis of trust in any relationship. Nonetheless, no person manages to keep all of his or her agreements. Maintaining trust requires communicating when an agreement is broken. If you did not do what you said you would do, try to bring up the matter yourself. Say if this was a one-time event that does not reflect your true intentions. Or explain that you think the plan is unworkable and should be revised.

If it is your partner who departs from the plan, talk about it openly, since silence on your part can be taken as tacit approval. Plus, you need to know what is going on. Perhaps there was an ambiguity in the original arrangement, or maybe you misunderstood something and he actually did what he agreed to. Or it could in fact have been a broken agreement. If so, perhaps it was just a temporary lapse and he's back on track. But you may discover that you need to do some more negotiating.

Even though they can be uncomfortable to discuss, if you do not talk about misunderstandings and broken agreements, they will happen again. In particular, if your partner is often flaky or unreliable, if he does not seem willing to make the most fundamental commitment of all—*I agree to keep my agreements*—you've *got* to talk about it. You are entitled to bring a moral seriousness to the discussion, to confront broken agreements for what they are, breaches of trust that erode the foundation of any relationship. If he says something like, *You can't pin me down so much, things change,* a possible reply is: *If you had a colleague at work who said one thing but did another as often as you do at home, how would you feel and what would you do? You would probably feel let down and frustrated, and you would tell the person that there needed to be changes in the way he or she was acting. It's the same here.*

If talking together doesn't work, consider involving a professional such as a therapist or minister. Besides letting your partner know you're serious, the thought of airing dirty laundry in front of another person could be enough to prompt a change in behavior. More than once, Rick has made a first appointment with a mother for couple's counseling only to receive a second call a few days later canceling the session because, *To get out of going to therapy, he started acting differently.* Whatever works!

Sharing the Load

The amount of mental and physical work required to raise a family is staggering, whether it's painting your baby's bedroom or—eighteen years later—helping her pack for college. Without supportive communities, the work of raising children mainly lands on Mom and Dad alone, pushing them into Condition Yellow even when they have a strong partnership. If either does less than his or her share, the other one is shoved toward Condition Red: more to do, less time to sleep or eat right, more guilt over not keeping every ball in the air, more dismay and resentment and anger. Compounding things, the parent who is dropping one end of the log may have the audacity to wonder, "Why don't we ever talk/go to the movies/make love anymore?"

Many couples share with equality the work of making a family, handling condition yellow with tenacity, skill, and grace. But that's the exception, and the rule tilts mainly against women, as the following list shows.

- *Tasks.* The average mother works altogether fifteen to twenty hours more per week than the father of her children, whether or not she is drawing a paycheck. It's not hard to get there: an hour in the morning, an hour at night, a few hours on each weekend day . . . it adds up pretty fast. Even when a mother makes as much or more money than her husband, typically she still does more housework and child care. And he'd be hard pressed to say he's pulling more weight on the job: studies have shown that women usually clock more minutes on-task at work than men do.

- *Emotion work.* This part of making a family may not look like much on the outside, but it is often the most draining. It includes settling squabbles between siblings, worrying about a fever that won't break, or comforting a child who's being picked on at preschool. Women do most of the emotion work in families, much as they do in relationships in general. For instance, when both parents are in the room, it is the mother who is most likely to be emotionally available to their child, rather than off in another world going over the bills, reading the paper, or watching TV.

- *Stresses.* Since tending to young children is more stressful than most jobs, if Mom stays home while Dad goes off to work her day is usually more stressful than his. When both parents are home, even if each of them spends about the same amount of time doing tasks, the mother typically does the high-stress ones while the father does more peaceful projects he can schedule at will and carry to completion. And when there is nothing left for her to do, a mother often feels stressfully vigilant and on call at a moment's notice, while her husband is more likely to do his tasks and then relax.

- *Responsibilities.* Children live in your heart and weigh on your mind. The consequences of your decisions can be monumental: literally, the health and welfare of an innocent child. For all the advances in the workplace for women over the past thirty years, little has changed at the "board of directors" level in most families: it is still usually Mom, not Dad, who does most of the planning, worrying, and problem solving about the children. It's lonely at the top of the typical family.

These inequities impact the children: Studies have shown that fathers who are less involved tend to have kids who are less responsible, less able to solve problems, less confident, and have lower self-esteem. Inequities also eat away at a marriage, reducing the satisfaction of each spouse. And they deplete a mother, increasing her stress, giving her less time to recharge her batteries, and lowering her mood; for instance, lack of help from the father exposes a working mother to more stress than any other factor. As one mother told Jan: *I did all the planning and organizing for Sammy's birthday, thinking that Bob would help out during the party itself. But no, he stood around the whole time talking with his buddies while I raced around doing everything, except for when he cut the cake and then looked at me like he deserved some kind of reward! I want someone who doesn't need me to stamp my feet to get some help, who takes initiative with the kids and the house, whose mind is not elsewhere all the time. Somebody who does things because he* wants *to do his share, not just to get me off his back. I need to feel like I have an-other half.*

Lapses in sharing the load aren't good for a father, either. Avoiding the nitty-gritty tasks of tending to young children—like getting them dressed—usually makes a father feel less connected, competent, or satisfied with parenthood.

It is fine to do different things, such as Mom puts in a load of laundry while Dad gives a bath. But significant unfairness poisons the well of a family. The *why* of sharing the load fairly is clear. The real question is *how*.

Clear Facts

The place to begin is to establish what the facts are. You and your partner may al-ready agree on how the load is shared, but commonly a father feels he is doing more than his wife thinks he does, which sparks recurring quarrels; for example, one study asked dual-earner couples how they handled child rearing tasks, and 43 percent of the men answered "fifty–fifty"—but only 19 percent of their wives agreed.

Therefore, if there is any question about what is actually happening, we suggest that each of you (or you alone, if necessary) track, for at least a few days and ide-ally for a week, who does what and for how much time. Each day, just jot down how you spent your time. One way to do this easily is on daily copies of a simple form you can create in which the rows are fifteen-minute intervals and the columns are different kinds of activities, such as interacting with a child or doing housework (or both at the same time!); you can create the form by hand or use a spreadsheet. Additionally, you could each make note of the stresses you experi-enced that day as well as the sense of responsibility you felt for planning, worry-ing, and problem solving.

Alternately, each of you could simply list what you did with the kids or house-hold that day. If even that would be overwhelming—since the typical mom does several hundred such tasks daily—make a list for an hour or for a specific part of the day, such as the morning or evening.

At night, compare notes, and see if you can agree on the basic facts of that day without nit-picking whether something took five minutes or ten. At the end of the period, try to agree on what the facts are, plus or minus ten percent. If you can't, consider involving a third party, such as a therapist.

If your partner suddenly becomes an angel once the spotlight is on, you can comment on that. You could also suggest continuing to track time for a few more weeks, which would have one of three outcomes, all of which are good: (1) you

If evolution works, how come mothers have only two hands?

—*Ed Dussault*

might discover that you've had a better partner than you thought; (2) his true colors would be revealed over time if he could not sustain the miraculous transformation; or (3) what started as an exercise in looking good could become a habit.

But in the usual case, people remain more or less true to form, and the results on paper are eye-opening. Rick once worked with a couple in which the mom felt overworked, but the dad thought she was exaggerating because she was mad he was putting so much time into his hobby of music. They tracked their time for a week and saw in black and white that he averaged one hour of sleep and two hours of personal time more than she *each day.* He couldn't ignore that difference or justify it, so he started spending more time with their child.

Clear Principles

Even with clear facts, parents can disagree about what they *mean.* Cultural factors influence our expectations about the proper sharing of roles after children arrive. In some regions of the country, or within certain groups, it is common to find support for a view of family life in which the woman does most of the child care and housework, even if she's employed, and she may defer to her husband in other matters as well.

Psychological factors also determine how we share the load. A father's active involvement with child care depends in part on his enjoyment of parenting, his beliefs about the importance of fathers to children, and his feeling that masculine men can be skillful with little kids. The amounts and kinds of housework he does are shaped by his ideas about the fundamental equality of the sexes. Your psychology influences him, as well, through your expectations and willingness to assert yourself. But speaking your mind can be hard if you:

- Believe in traditional gender roles
- Think that making money counts for more than child care or housework, or feel one down in the relationship because he makes more money than you
- Fear he might leave you or take his anger out on the children
- Feel guilty about pursuing your own career and try to compensate by going overboard on child care and housework
- Are embarrassed about asking for help, perhaps thinking it makes you look needy, or that you should have already handled everything on your own
- Think he'll do it all wrong, or feel territorial about your role

The real test of a society is how well it socializes its males to care for their young.

—Margaret Mead

Biology plays a part as well. Men vary in their innate interest in child rearing, much like women do, but to a greater degree. For some perspective, consider that males do next to nothing for their young in ninety-five percent of the mammal species, including the primates that are our close relatives. "Mating effort"—sowing seeds far and wide—is in most species a more effective reproductive strategy for males than "parental investment," the strategy usually used by females for passing on their genes.

In this light, what is remarkable about human fathers is that they do anything at all. Our species seems to have evolved a mixed strategy in which both inclinations—mating effort and parental investment—interact with each other, and the relative weight of each varies from man to man. We make these points about biology not to let fathers off the hook, but to highlight the poignant reality that is the backdrop of many domestic disputes. That way, you can take your partner's natural inclinations less personally—wherever they are in the range of men—and have compassion and respect for the ways he's trying to work with them. The balance of power in a father between mating effort and parental investment is greatly affected by social and psychological factors. He can help himself by spending time with other dads who are deeply involved with their children, participating in groups that support engaged fatherhood—such as religious organizations, Indian Guides, or Cub Scouts—or reflecting on his ethical duty to his children and their mother. He could read about fatherhood, perhaps a book such as *Father Courage: What Happens When Men Put Family First* by Suzanne Braun Levine. He could apply the same ideals of learning and competence that he lives by at work to his parenting. He might reflect on his relationship with his father, both what he gained from his dad and how he would like to parent in a different way (perhaps using the exercise in the box on p. 253).

In gentle ways, you can support his involvement by helping him see what a difference he makes to his children. You can point out models of masculine and competent fathers—especially him! Or do little things to help parenting be enjoyable for him, like having him come see your son with his hair shampooed up like a rooster's cock's comb.

In the end, though, no matter what the cultural, psychological, or biological forces may be in our lives, we still have to make choices based on principle. You are entitled to make a case for certain values, to say what you think your children need, and to name what you feel is fair or unfair. Here are examples of principled responses to various objections we've heard fathers make to carrying more of the total load; please adapt them to your own needs and voice:

- "I'm not as good at it as you are. Plus the kids go to you anyway." *Like anything, you just need to practice a little. The kids will get used to you doing certain things, and I'll direct them to you more. Plus you could initiate and not wait for the kids to come to me. Additionally, even if I'm the one who always washes Angel's hair, you could still help more by reading to Michael or cleaning up the kitchen.*

- "You always interfere, and I've quit trying." *I don't <u>always</u> interfere, but I do sometimes. I'm trying to help, anyway, not interfere, but I can understand that you feel crowded, so I'll promise to back off.*

- "You just want someone to do things for you." *Nope, I want you to do things <u>with</u> me. It's not just about getting stuff done. When you do your part, it makes me feel connected to you, like I'm not alone and we're in this together. I made a baby <u>with</u> you and I would love for us to share that experience in a happy way together.*

- "I do more than my dad did." *That's great, and I appreciate it. But there is still more to do if we're going to be fair about it.*

- "My job is so stressful that I need to rest at home." *Remember how you nearly fainted with relief when I finally got home after you were alone with the kids that one time for a few hours? Now imagine doing that for many hours instead of a few, and for a thousand days instead of one. If we're talking about getting a break based on the stress level of our typical day, in fairness I deserve rest at least as much as you.*

- "Making a living counts for more than raising children." *I believe that it's the other way around. Child rearing counts for more since it so directly impacts our precious children. And it's usually harder, day after day. I am not setting child rearing above making a living. But it is at least equal.*

- "I make all the money, so you should handle the housework and kids." *I <u>do</u> handle the housework and kids while you are making money. I'm talking about what you do when you're not commuting or at work. You wanted children and now we've got them. You can see that it's best for them when we are both involved in the morning, at night, or over the weekend. Speaking personally, it does not feel fair for me to keep on going while you watch TV or go out with your friends. How would you feel about someone at work who did that sort of thing while you kept getting things done? Would you feel resentful? Would you be eager for them to do their share?*

- "I make *more* money than you." *I appreciate all the money you bring into our family. But that does not change what is good for our children and our relationship when we are both at home in the mornings, evenings, and week-ends.* (And follow with the points just above.)

- "It's because you're working that the kids need so much and there's so much housework." *I think that's hitting below the belt. If I didn't work, our kids would still need you to help out in the evenings and weekends. We need my salary, and even if we didn't, I have as much right to work as you. Besides, we could just as well turn the point against you: The kids wouldn't need so much if you, their father, stayed home. In fairness, the hard choices between career and time with children should fall just as much on a father as a mother. We both work, we both need to parent, and we both need to do housework.*

- "That's woman's work." *There is no law that says so. You did dishes before you met me, and it wasn't women's work then. I don't think you take it easy while I wash clothes or give the kids a bath out of high moral principle, but simply because that's your personal preference. You're just as capable as I am of putting a child to sleep or feeding a toddler.*

- "Quit telling me what to do." *I don't want to tell you what to do. Usually I try not to. And if I ever do, it's because you won't make a reasonable agreement with me about who does what—or you make one but don't stick with it. I'm*

A Man's Reflections on His Own Father

In addition to thinking about the questions below, you might like to discuss them with your wife. You could also write your answers as a letter to your father that you will probably never send.

When you were a boy, what was your father's role in the family?

How was your father there for you? How was he not?

Did he spend so much time at work that you felt his job was more important to him than you?

How might he have affected how your mother acted towards you or your brothers or sisters? Did he help her be a good mother? Or did he make her job harder?

What are the ways that you are glad you are acting like him? Are there any ways you are acting like him that you wish you were not?

How do you think your own children will feel about you when they are reflecting on their dad like you are today?

the messenger of what our kids or home needs, so please don't be angry at me for just bringing the message. If you saw what needed doing in the first place, I wouldn't have to bring a message at all. Besides, why is it fair for you to tell me what to do about the car or computer or mutual fund or whatever but I can't tell you anything about what to put in a lunchbox?

- "Get off my back, or else." *I'd be glad to talk about this when you're calmer. But I'm going to ask: What's the "or else"? Are you really going to hit me or walk out on your kids because I'm tired of picking your socks off the floor? Because I'd appreciate it if you'd get home sooner? Your kids need you to be more involved, I need it, and our marriage does, too.*

Clear Agreements

Once you come together on basic principles, agreements about actions are pretty straightforward, especially when you use the negotiation skills you've already learned. Here are some practical solutions that have helped many families, including those in which the parents are already sharing the load fairly and the real issue is only how to work together even better.

Apply organizational principles. A family is an organization, and many of the same approaches used in other organizations will work in your home as well. First, you could create a base schedule that guides your week, knowing that you'll almost never stick to it perfectly. For example, if you're staying home while your husband works, he could agree to get home by 6:30 most nights and you'd agree to have already fed the kids so you two can have dinner together.

In your base schedule, build in breaks that are fair for each of you. One dad said to Rick: *My wife gets Wednesday night "off" while I take care of the kids. I'll get up early on a weekend morning and go for a hike with a buddy, getting back by 12 or so. I think about that hike all week, like she thinks about what she'll do Wednesday night. It's a lifesaver.*

But be sure to take your break when it comes! Many mothers feel like they have to overcome an invisible gravitational field to lift out of their orbit around their children. Remember that you deserve and need this time to yourself, and that your children will benefit from a reinvigorated mother when you get back. You might also arrange to take some of your time off *with* your kids as long as your husband assumes the major responsibility for caring for them. For example, Rick's idea of a dream vacation is a trip to the mountains with a buddy and no kids, while Jan's is a week in the sun somewhere with her children nearby while Rick watches them.

Second, we suggest you distinguish between *responsibility,* which you both share for the family's overall well-being, and individual *accountability* for specific tasks. Then create a basic understanding of what you are each accountable for: Who does what when? You could write it down, and if you have to, post it. Just walk through your day mentally and think about what would help things go well. Could you get the kids dressed while he showers, and then he feeds them while you shower? Would he rather clean up after dinner or put the kids to bed? Should you pick up take-out food on Tuesday nights? The details are usually not that hard: most of it is just being good roommates, and there are many tips for a smoothly running household in women's magazines or various books.

Coordinate with each other. Check in before making plans like committing to a golf date for the weekend. Rick and Jan got a big lesson in this just a few days after their first child was born, and Jan describes what happened: ***Our good friend, Bob, was coming to visit, and Rick mentioned they were going sailing Saturday. I was dead tired already and asked in disbelief, "You're going to leave me home alone for a day with a baby while you play around?" Rick was startled. In the past, he'd go off with a friend, and it was no big deal. But now what he did really affected the baby and me, and he had to take us into account. He took a long, slow breath and it was like a lightbulb went on. Then he said, "You're right. Now I need to ask."***

Keep things in perspective. It's the overall performance that matters. Nobody's perfect, and overreacting to small lapses can undermine a general spirit of cooperation. See if you can let your husband do housework his way; for example, unless dishes are getting broken each night, don't hassle him about how he loads the dishwasher. As a general rule, let the person who is doing the task be in charge of how it gets done.

Try to be flexible and creative for the greater good, which includes him feeling positive about being fully involved in child care and housework and you feeling less stressed. If he suggests paper plates for most weeknights, maybe that's not so crazy. Perhaps you both can live with a semimessy kitchen until Saturday morning, when you spend an hour together cleaning it up, drinking some coffee, and talking.

Children are passionately unpredictable in their nature, so it's a good idea to cut each other some slack. For example, a mother told this story: ***We were going somewhere, and I was getting Marion ready while Frank was on the phone. He came in and snapped at me because we were running late. He hates that, and he is Mr. Punctuality at work. But a child doesn't always follow a schedule. He should know that, because if he's the one trying to get her to cooperate, we never leave on*** *time!* Or better yet, step in and help out instead of judging the other parent's performance.

It's all right for you to take the lead. Unless you and your husband truly share all aspects of parenting—an unusual yet potentially wonderful arrangement described by Diane Ehrensaft, Ph.D., in her book *Parenting Together: Men and Women Sharing the Care of Their Children*—it is natural for you to have a leadership role sometimes when it comes to the kids. He is probably entering a flow of activities that you've been managing, and he is just being a good team player when he asks you, the quarterback, what the play is. We suggest that you tell him at the time how he can help. Later on, if you like, you can talk about similar situations in the future and figure out what he could do in them without you having to say anything.

Look for ways to involve him with the children. If he is hanging back, invite him to share in the fun moments, not just the chores. He could think about the interests he'd like to share with his kids, like a love of the outdoors, or the values he wants to help them develop. For instance, perhaps reading certain stories to them would be a way to talk about similar experiences he has had or what he thinks is really important in life.

He might say that he'll get more involved when the kids are older and it feels more "natural." This may well be true, and meanwhile he could do more housework while you do more tending to the baby. On the other hand, your child's life is still going on, and your husband may need to get comfortable with settling a baby to sleep ahead of schedule. There is no good reason why a guy who can do what he does at work all day can't manage a young child.

You may also have to deal with him pulling back from the kids because he's upset with you. Men are more likely than women to let their relationship with their children be affected by their feelings about their spouse. Doing the right thing by his kids is ultimately up to him, but you can help in several ways. Tell him how much the kids need him no matter what he thinks right now about you. And if you need to, you could play hardball, asking questions like *Do you think a man should walk away from a responsibility just because he feels ticked off at a coworker?* or *When your kids are older, what will they wish you had done?*

Work out housework issues. One mother said, *He comes home from work and expects the house to look immaculate. I just don't care as much as he does, and even if I did, I would have to follow behind the kids every minute.* On the other hand, a father commented, *She thinks it's her house, that she has some kind of God-given wisdom about housekeeping because she's a woman. She freaks out if the dishes are not immediately done after dinner. She literally cannot sit still at the table and relax and talk if there's a dirty glass in the sink.* A few suggestions: Agree to lower your standards while kids are little. Keep one room as an orderly sanctuary. In age-appropriate ways, relentlessly prod kids to pick up after themselves.

Tackle high-stress situations together. For instance, analyze the morning madness. It all starts the night before, so perhaps he could promise to quit extending your daughter's bedtime with extra stories even though she loves them. Later that night, you could lay out her clothes while he sets up for breakfast. Maybe wake up fifteen minutes earlier to have a moment for yourself and a chance to get ready for the day. He could get your child into the car while you put on your makeup. And off you go.

In particular, pay special attention to working well together on any issues with your child, such as a challenging temperament. Try to talk about the different meanings that the situation may have for each of you; for instance, a mother often feels that a child's difficulty must somehow be her fault. He could read books on child development or on the particular issue. Make a clear plan together that will effectively address your child's needs; if you can't on your own, get a consultant or tiebreaker.

Balance the total stress load more or less evenly. Take into account the nature of each parent's job, the age and temperament of the children, and any other circumstances that pile on stress. Notice if one parent lets the other one handle the stressful jobs, or if one parent automatically jumps in first. Usually it's the mom who walks through the door and immediately dives in to settling a squabble or doing a load of laundry while Dad goes off to change his clothes or sort through the mail. Maybe she should take a page out of his book and relax a bit first. And maybe he could agree to take more initiative with the kids and the household.

If he slides into fun jobs with the kids like reading stories while you fold laundry or figure out the checkbook, that could be a break for you from mommy mode, but it could also mean that you're getting stuck with more than your share of the housework, which is often boring, unpleasant, and even depressing. To deal with this, try divvying up strictly household tasks, including paperwork, coordinating with others (like planning a birthday party), maintenance (who stays home to wait for the plumber?), and yard work. You could make a list of the major tasks in one column: scary! Then add two other columns, one for each of you, and mark who gets which job. Factor in that some jobs take longer or are worse than others (toilets . . .), consider alternating jobs (if it's an odd day, he does the dishes), and create something that's reasonably fair. If there's an impasse, you can flip a coin.

Perhaps you could afford an occasional housekeeper; it's cheaper than a couple's counselor—or divorce lawyer. Worst case, you could go on strike and not do a particular job until there's some resolution; this would mean letting go of any compulsion you feel about it, but remember that *he* doesn't feel compelled, and that household tasks are not life-and-death matters.

Address the impact of work on your family. It's very challenging if you both work full-time and get home around 6:00 or later to a mad flurry of activities ending in a collapse in bed. (Unfortunately, the effects of the two-career family are commonly framed to blame women; that's not at all our point since, in principle, a man could as readily scale back his career.) Alternately, you might work part-time or not at all while he puts in sixty or seventy hours each week, including business travel. A demanding job may be one way he fulfills his sense of responsibility as a provider, but some men use their work to hide from their family. Even with the best of motives, his big job is like an elephant in the living room, limiting the space that's left for family. In that situation, children frequently grow up with a subtle sense of fatherlessness. The dad misses out on a special time that will never be repeated, trading it for career moves that often could be postponed a few years. The mom becomes a de facto single parent. And it is hard to work around the elephant to maintain a deeply intimate marriage.

Sometimes absolutely nothing can be done about the jobs you or he have. The best you can do then is to try to reduce your other stresses (e.g., lower your standards for housework, don't take on another puppy), increase your resources (like getting a neighborhood kid to do some yard work), and improve your psychological coping (see the tools discussed in chapters 2 and 3).

Usually, though, you *can* do something about your circumstances, especially if you persist. Let's use the example of him working long hours while you stay home. The first step is to create a positive atmosphere for tackling the issue, approaching it as a "we-problem" with no bad guy. For instance, you could express your respect for how hard he works to provide for his family and your understanding that his career is very important to him. Second, challenge the assumptions that box you in. You could consider going back to (perhaps part-time) work ahead of schedule to ease the economic demand on him. He could do some soul-searching about:

- How this time with children is fleeting and unique, and worth making a special effort to spend with them
- How his children, wife, or marriage would benefit if he were home more; how he would benefit himself

- The beliefs that make him feel embarrassed about saying he needs to leave at 6:00 to get home to his kids, or the ways he may be getting caught up in a business warrior culture that prides itself on insane hours

- The extra work he might be doing for personal rewards distinct from what his family actually needs; personal fulfillment is a valid aim, but it's not selfless sacrifice

- How a small reduction in his time at work—say ten percent—would probably have little effect on his career but would double or triple his time with his kids, the epitome of a highly leveraged investment.

Third, make a long-term plan that is consistent with your deepest values as well as financially realistic. Perhaps your overall quality of life would improve if you moved to a less expensive place or spent less money on discretionary items so you could spend more *time* with each other. The questions in the box can help clarify the values that shape these choices.

Unnecessary fears drive many financial decisions, and the antidote is clarity about money and the specific facts of your current expenses and future needs. It's not that hard. Books and websites can guide you through the details; please see the resources below for suggestions. On your own in an hour or less, you could probably come up with a family budget that is accurate within ten percent. Estimating your needs down the road is more complicated, so it's wise to use a good book or a financial planner, especially if you and your husband disagree about priorities or methods. But with less effort than it took to equip your baby's bedroom, you can come up with a rational plan that makes your jobs serve you and your family, rather than the other way around.

A rich child often sits in a poor mother's lap.

—*Danish proverb*

Resources for Financial and Planning

Smart Couples Finish Rich by David Bach
9 Steps to Financial Freedom by Suze Orman
Your Money or Your Life by Joe Dominguez and Vicki Robin
How to Raise Your Family on Less Than Two Incomes by Denise Topolnicki
www.aoa.gov/retirement/default.htm
learningforlife.fsu.edu/fp101/
financialplan.about.com/money/financialplan/mbody.htm

Your Values for Life and Money

Please consider these questions:

- *Imagine looking back on your life at age eighty or so: What will you be most glad about, and what will not have mattered much? From that perspective, how will you wish that you had approached money and career?*

- *Imagine that you have just a few years to live: What would your priorities be? Are there ways to be truer to those priorities if you were to live for fifty more years?*

- *How do you want your life to make a difference?*

- *What's your preferred pace of living? How important is leisure compared to accomplishment, status, or expensive toys?*

- *How much do you value time with your children, especially while they are young, compared to furthering your career or making money? How willing are you to defer saving for a few years when your children are little? At this time, how rapidly do you want to pay down any debts?*

- *What's your bottom-line limit on the number of hours each week you want your spouse or yourself to give to work (including commuting and business travel)?*

- *At this time, what standard of living are you determined to have, from weekly spending on lunches out to big-ticket items like major vacations or remodeling your home? What standard of living do you want to have in a few years?*

Staying Intimate Friends After Becoming Parents

Raising children together can nurture a relationship in many ways. Doing activities as a family—playing a game, going to the park, making popcorn—creates a circle of love that includes your mate as well as your children. When things get hard, as they do for every couple, having children can motivate partners to dig down and do the work necessary to maintain a strong relationship. Nonetheless, children innocently yet inevitably bring consequences that tend to nudge their mom and dad apart—like fatigue and depletion, conflicts over child rearing, or little time to be together as mates.

That's why we have to tend to our marriage in a new kind of way after kids come along. Otherwise, it's easy for a little more distance to come between you each day, a little more irritation or disdain. Love is hard-won—and so precious. Staying intimate friends with your partner helps you feel cherished and secure. It lifts your mood, brings you companionship, affection, and romance, and even bolsters your resistance to illness. And it naturally evokes more consideration, compassion, and help from your husband, and makes it infinitely easier to stay out of nasty quarrels.

A strong and enduring love between parents casts a light and a warmth that envelops their children as well. Even when very young, children can sense the quality of feeling between their mother and father. Visible friendship, love, and passion between parents make children feel secure. And they give kids hope, when they're older, for their own dreams of lasting intimacy with a beloved mate.

With just a little effort and attention, a loving intimacy can be preserved, or reestablished, between you and your husband. Much as the buildup of little, negative things can slowly tear the fabric of a relationship, the growing accumulation of little, positive things can reknit it together. In this chapter, we'll discuss overcoming barriers to closeness, finding time for your relationship, having good conversations, healing old hurts, and rekindling romance and a comfortable sexuality.

People approach their relationship from different places. Hopefully, you and your partner have preserved a reservoir of love and passion for each other and just need to carve out more time to talk or spark up your sex life. But maybe you have grown a bit distant: even if you work well as a team, your hearts are not as connected as they once were. And for some couples, it's sad to say that their relationship is in real trouble. We'll present a range of suggestions in this chapter for this range of needs; if things are generally good between you and your partner, please don't be alarmed by the comments or options offered to couples that are in a more difficult situation.

Of course, improving your intimate relationship has the greatest chance of success when there's a foundation of civility, empathy, and teamwork, since it's normal to be reluctant to get close—especially physically—to someone you feel routinely let down or hurt by, or angry at.* If there's currently a good deal of arguing, we suggest both partners make a personal commitment not to fight for at least a week or two—and hopefully longer. When it starts to get heated, take a break to cool off, talk about it after you've eaten or slept, or bring in a third party to help you stay calm. If you can manage even just a couple of weeks without angry conflicts, it's remarkable how much better it will feel between you. Down the road, when your relationship is stronger, you'll be able to have the normal quarrels of any couple. But now's the time for each of you to choose words carefully and be on his or her best behavior.

The more strained the relationship, the more effort that's needed to turn it around—but that's also when it's hardest to bite your tongue, or be understanding, friendly, or affectionate. How do you motivate yourself to move toward each other when you want to pull back, give when you're aching to receive, respond to the other person's grievances when you feel so wronged?

It's not easy. At different times in our own relationships, we've faced very tough issues, so we know how hard it can be. But several perspectives can help you stay motivated to work on your marriage:

---

*As chapter 6 said, if there is threatened or actual physical abuse in your relationship, please contact a therapist or women's shelter immediately. You should not attempt to use this chapter with your partner until there is no possibility of violence between you.

- Remember the love you once had. There was a time when you were very fond of each other: if it could happen then, it can happen again.

- Understand the reasons why you and your husband have distanced from each other (these are discussed in the next section). Insight into them lessens their power over you, and makes it much easier to put fondness and goodheartedness into your relationship.

- Have faith that if you make a serious and sustained effort yourself, the relationship will almost certainly get better. Imagine a scale running from zero to one hundred: zero is no effort for the relationship, and one hundred is the absolute maximum that anyone could possibly do. In our experience, when either partner (ideally, both) consistently operates in the thirties or forties on that scale for several weeks in a row, the relationship always gets better. By two or three months, there's a *dramatic improvement*. And if they can get up into the eighties or nineties for a good deal of this time, the change in their marriage is extraordinary. Most of us have made this much effort numerous times: pushing hard at work for a few months, a tough semester in college, training for a marathon—or for long stretches while raising children. We do this with hardly a thought, yet when it comes to a marriage, suddenly it seems like an odd idea to work this hard. But why not? The stakes are greater and the chance of success just as good. Marriage is like anything else: it gets a lot better when you work at it.

- If your relationship has really deteriorated, you can sometimes motivate yourself to work on it by remembering that divorce is painful and difficult. Yes, there are times when things have gotten to such a state of rancor that separating is the least-bad alternative. But having read the research and seen many divorces—or, in Ricki's case, lived through one—there is no doubt in our minds that all children suffer in a divorce, and many are injured psychologically as well. The initial breakup is stressful for both parents and children, and even when things settle down, there's usually a wound in the family that lasts for years; it can include more room to diverge in parenting practices, financial disruption, grappling with new partners or stepparents, or hassles scheduling holidays. You'll probably see your children less, and when you have them, solo parenting is no picnic— one reason why single mothers tend to have worse physical and mental health than married ones. Children—and their moms and dads—do survive divorce, but the costs are such that we think it's both principled and self-interested for parents to do *everything* they can to prevent it.

As we said earlier, while it would be best if your husband went through this chapter with you, we couldn't be sure that would happen, so it's directed largely at you. That focus on what *you* could do, understandably, can make you feel like you have to do all the work. We feel strongly that a father should make a serious effort to nurture his partner and their relationship, and if anything, he should be the one to put more into the marriage since she is probably more depleted than he is. But meanwhile, there are two kinds of things you can do that do not depend on him: you can keep telling him what you need in your relationship, and you can try to be a better partner yourself.

Neither of these means that you are letting him off the hook, "enabling him," or putting the burden of the relationship entirely on your own shoulders. You are just doing what you *can* to build the intimate friendship that will nurture you—and the effort alone will make you feel strong in yourself, active instead of passive, dignified and honorable. Your efforts will likely evoke similar steps from him over time, and if they don't, you will know in your heart—and someday, you will be able to say to your children—that you did everything you could to help your relationship get better.

If things have gotten bad in a marriage, there's often a kind of no-win standoff in which he says, *I'll change if she changes,* while she says, *I'll change if he does.* The only way to break that deadlock is for someone to focus on his or her own efforts to make the relationship better; the 80–20 principle (p. 207) applies to intimate friendship as much as to teamwork. Ideally, both partners would do so. But if he doesn't, what's your best option? Even though it's hard and it's not fair, the most direct way for you to have a better relationship is to take action on your own—for weeks, and perhaps months—to improve it.

Understanding and Overcoming Blocks to Intimacy

As much as you know in your head that you should make these efforts, your heart could be pulling in a different direction. To be sure, sometimes the reasons are healthy. For example, it may be all too clear that a partner is impaired by drugs or alcohol, violent, or mentally ill—in which case a mother should always seek professional help. And under any circumstances, we each need to maintain a sense of being an autonomous individual—even when we feel most connected. There's also a variation in natural interest in closeness; some of us would like to be around people all day, while others prefer and need much more time alone.

Then, besides the positive reasons for not getting *too* close, there are the ones that aren't so good. See if any of these eight problems that can block intimacy apply to you or your partner; if one does, take a look at its solutions. (To avoid a numbing repetition of both personal pronouns, we focus specifically on a mother or a father in most of these problems, though every one of them could apply to either gender.)

1. *It seems like there is no time to be together.*

   Solutions: See pages 270 to 273 for practical ways to create time for the two of you. You might also consider whether busyness has become an excuse for avoiding closeness. For example, one father admitted to Rick: *I wasn't really aware of it until recently, but for a long time now, I've been quite happy to work late. It was tense when I got home, and I knew Hallie would be on me for one thing or another, so I found myself leaving the office later and later.* And a mother said: *Serena, our two-year-old, still needs me to lie down with her for her to go to sleep. Doug says I have to let her learn to sleep on her own, but she cries and is so upset, so I keep doing it. But I usually fall asleep too, so we're never together at night for talking or having fun together, which frustrates him to no end. The truth is, I just don't feel very interested in him right now, especially when it seems like all he wants to talk about is this business he's starting. He always notices my mind drifting off, which hurts him and often starts an argument. So I don't mind falling asleep at all. It's easier this way: he can't pester me, and we don't get into a fight about me not listening to the details of some deal he's trying to pull off.*

   If you have been using (perhaps unconsciously) your circumstances as a means to the end of distancing, please know that almost every parent has done this in one way or another, including us. Then, decide if you want to continue doing so. If you don't, you could acknowledge what's been happening to a friend or your partner as a way to get it out in the open and have more conscious control. With your partner, try to talk through and resolve the issues that make you feel like distancing. For instance, in the examples above, the father could give his wife more support so that she would feel less drained and irritable, and he could ask her not to hassle him the first moment he walks through the door; the mother could ask her pediatrician for ways to help Serena fall asleep on her own, and suggest to Doug that they talk about some of her interests as well as his.

2. *You are emotionally drained from tending to children.*

   Solutions: At the practical level, see if it's possible to get more help from others, including your husband—especially respites in the middle of long stretches of solitary child care. Psychologically speaking, look inside to see if the boundaries between you and your children are too porous; it's one thing to be deeply empathic, and another to feel so merged that their needs or pain become your own. Try to do more of the things that give you a stronger sense of self, like an avocation you enjoy, exercise, or meditation. When you're together with your child, pay attention to the intensity of your feelings, and try to relax and release them if they start to seem overwhelming. Also consider if you have a greater sense of responsibility for your family than is necessary or nurturing to you; if so, you could talk about it with a friend and ask for more help. Remember the many things besides yourself—so it's not all on your shoulders—that are promoting the welfare of your family, from a child's natural development (Mother Nature is on your side!) to the support of your partner and friends.

3. *Your husband is stressed out by and preoccupied with work.*

    Solutions: When you're the one who is concerned about something, he should empathize with you (see chapter 7, starting on page 214). But now, the most direct way to feel more connected is to start with empathy yourself, by talking about the difficulties he's facing, his concerns, and any underlying issues in his mind (e.g., competitiveness with colleagues, fear of looking bad). Then, the two of you might be able to come up with ways he could think about or approach his job that would make it less stressful or worrisome—from psychological methods (like recalling his past successes) to more concrete ones, such as asking for administrative support in getting out quarterly reports. Finally, try to make agreements about the "mindspace" work occupies when he's with you or his children. Maybe he needs ten minutes to shift gears when he first gets home, rather than having kids shoved into his arms when he walks through the door, and then he can be fully available for his family. He could probably agree not to take business calls at night. And he should accept the general principle that it's important for his kids and his marriage that he be emotionally present when he is home.

4. *You think he should not ask for much from you while the kids are little, and then you'll have energy for him again.*

    Solutions: While it's realistic for parents to expect less from each other in the way of intimate friendship while raising young children, it's a mistake to think you can put your partner in the deep freeze for a few years, and then pop him in the microwave and expect everything to be warm and tasty between you again. During peak demand times—such as the first months after childbirth, while an infant is colicky, or when either of you is sick or flat-out exhausted—it's understandable if you need a sabbatical from physical or even emotional connection, but otherwise, there's no way around a simple fact: we have to keep investing in an intimate friendship if we want to continue to have one. Your partner's needs for closeness are probably not as fulfilled through contact with the children as yours are if he spends less time with them then you do. He is a human being with feelings, and there's a good chance he misses you in some ways.

We've heard moms contemptuously describe the yearnings of their partners for more attention and affection as weak, needy, or childish. But it's as wrong to view them like that as it would be for your partner to characterize your own desires for closeness in the same way. Whether they're his or yours, we're talking about normal needs here—plus it usually takes surprisingly little to keep a partner reasonably happy. Find out what he has in mind—both what he'd really like and the minimum that could sustain him during this chapter in the making of your family. It probably won't take that much from you to do little things for your relationship within that range. And, of course, you can ask for the same sort of thing from him.

5. *He's withholding attention, warmth, or affection because of his issues with you.*

Solutions: The fastest way to encourage someone to treat you better is to address his issues and treat him civilly yourself. Find out what his grievances are, sort out the reasonable wheat from the unreasonable chaff, and then do what you can about his legitimate needs. Then, if he keeps holding back, you're on a solid footing to talk with him about it.

6. *You are wary of getting hurt or disappointed.*

Solutions: On page 277, we discuss how you and your partner can work through lingering upsets in which you felt let down or mistreated. In particular, try to make realistic agreements that will prevent that kind of painful event from ever happening again.

Inside your own mind, you could double-check that you are not overestimating the likelihood of your partner acting in a hurtful way; the intensity of your reactions if he does; or your inability to cope with the reactions you might have. Try to become increasingly aware of any ways that thoughts, feelings, or wants from your childhood are intensifying your reactions.

Reach out to other sources of nurturance for you—like friends, spiritual practice, sports, or art—and take in what they give you, making it a part of yourself so that your emotional reserves are more filled up and it's less disappointing if your husband feels distant. And when he does connect with you, let it sink in, feeling the love that is actually there for you, letting yourself feel more trusting and comfortable with closeness; if the moments of lovingness between you these days are few and far between, that is all the more reason to drink deep when you can.

7. *He feels overwhelmed or frightened by closeness.*

Solutions: Talk about your sense that he wants to be emotionally close, but it seems uncomfortable for him. It may seem he doesn't care much about relationships, but in fact, the opposite is probably true: because he cares *so much,* because he is so affected by an intimate partner, he feels the need to put up buffers—like how a person whose pupils are dilated needs sunglasses. Otherwise, he feels intruded upon, swamped, or exhausted. (This is often the case with someone who was introverted as a child or who had invasive or controlling parents.)

He could look at his tendency to seek an optimal distance, tacking back and forth between closeness and disconnection; the closer he gets, the more he wants to distance—to the point that he wants to move closer again. He can become more aware of the methods he uses to keep you at arm's length, like getting lost in the computer at night. He can also look at any ways his mind has found to simultaneously reach out and distance, like bickering or quarreling: the perfect method for staying both safely separate and just connected enough.

Based on this self-awareness, when you're together, he should try to keep relaxing his body, allowing your words and presence to flow through him, all the while noticing that he is still his own person, still intact, still in charge of his own mind. He can remind himself that your experience is over *there* while his is over here, and that he can make any decisions later, when he's had time alone to reflect. He can let you know when he needs you to dial down the emotional intensity and give him some breathing room, in order for him to really hear your words and feelings. All of this should help him to feel safe enough to stay more connected.

On your part, try to respond to his signals to take a step back and not take his withdrawals so personally. When you respect his need for distance, he will be more able to renew his capacity for coming closer. You can also reassure him that he needn't fear he will be overwhelmed or controlled: maybe it was that way when he was a kid, but you're just not like that, and it's not going to happen today. You and he can talk about the distance or closeness you each prefer, and then come to understandings in which you both stretch to meet the other person's needs. In particular, the two of you can take steps to get out of vicious cycles in which his distancing leads to your pursuing, which makes him distance further, and so on: your acceptance of his need for space will interrupt the cycle, and on his side, he can give you more regular experiences of connection, making you feel more fulfilled and secure, and thus less insistent or possessive—which in turn will help him feel more comfortable with closeness.

8. *It feels like overcoming sheer inertia to be loving.*

Solutions: Although it takes just a little warmth to make a connection—a touch, smile, quick hug, compliment, or simple *I love you* immediately brings both of you closer—it can feel so hard to make that first move. Soon walking past each other in the hall can seem like two ships passing in the night, disconnected, yet trailing thoughts in the wake like *I wish she'd smile* or *Why is it so hard for him to be a little affectionate?* On a typical day, how frequently does your mate express fondness to you—or you to him? In many couples, the answer would be zero for each person. To be sure, there is a range in how much people want to express fondness or hear it; some of us are gushier than others. Nonetheless, if either partner is acting loving less than a handful of times each day, it's reasonable to have some concern about the relationship.

Certainly, there are moments when you feel so angry, wronged, or unsafe that it would be utterly false to do something to connect; the light is red: full stop. But mostly, your feelings probably move around on a spectrum ranging from orange (you're irritated but could still find some warmth for him if you tried) through yellow (neutral, task-oriented busyness) to green (a positive attitude toward him). Anywhere along that spectrum, a person really could find a genuine fondness inside and then express it. But it takes an act of will.

We use our will many times a day, whenever our inclination is to do one thing but we ask ourselves to do another: crawl out of a warm bed to walk a crying baby, listen politely to Uncle Fred tell the same story again, or tidy up when it would be nice to collapse on the sofa. Nonetheless, it's uncommon to bring one's will to a matter of the heart—but it is so helpful. Early on in a relationship, love bubbles up unbidden, and it's natural to think that wellspring will overflow forever. Yet with the passage of time, and the usual accumulation of irritations and hurts, it's normal for love to sink underground. Therefore, over the course of a typical marriage—and especially when the relationship is troubled—the only way love will be openly expressed is if someone reaches into that well, finds some fondness, and shares it.

No doubt, this can feel hard, if not impossible, to do. But each partner probably uses his or her will every day to do even harder things. And after being willfully warm a few times, there's a good chance that love will start flowing more freely between you.

Sometimes the love is close to the surface, while at other times, a person has to stretch way down for it. Either way, it is real, not fake, and expressing it does nothing except benefit yourselves and your children. You honor your commitment to your family by caring enough to make an effort to offer simple gestures of fondness to your partner: loving at will is actually twice loving.

Finding Time for Your Relationship

Josie—raising two sons, age four and eight—frowned when Rick asked about her marriage: *We're treading water. You're busier than ever, the days blur by, and then you look up and there's your husband, and you realize that it's been weeks, literally weeks, since you've done anything pleasant together. When we do get some time, it's great and there's a little glow in our relationship that lasts a couple days. We keep saying we have to do that more often. But it's really hard.*

Yes, time apart can contain warm thoughts of each other, and grinding out tasks side by side may give you a nice sense of camaraderie (and we each need time alone as well, for our own well-being). But that is just not enough to recharge anyone's relationship over the long haul, particularly while it's being challenged by each partner's stress and weariness, and by conflicts related to raising a family. You need time together that feeds your relationship. The question is *how*—amidst the kids, the bills, the dishes—and here are some suggestions.

Make it important. When you make a personal commitment to set aside more time for your relationship, you will always find some ways to do so. But without that resolve, the world, the kids, the job will grab your time and suck it up and there'll be little or nothing left for your marriage. For a motivating dose of reality, you could track (casually or carefully) the minutes each week that are actually spent talking fondly, being affectionate, or having fun together. Try to discuss these facts—with nobody being the one at fault—and say how each of you would like things to be.

Do tasks together. Understandably, parents often divide their tasks in order to conquer them: Dad's in the kitchen doing dishes while Mom's giving Junior a bath. But then there's zero opportunity for closeness. Instead, try to do more tasks jointly; for example, when you're both cleaning up after dinner or bathing a child, it's easier and more fun. Additionally, look for chances to connect even while you're getting things done, like comfortably touching shoulders at the sink, sharing glances of amusement at a child's play with a stuffed animal, rubbing a partner's foot as he or she reads a story, having a friendly conversation in the car while running errands, holding hands as you walk your child into day care, and so on.

Create family fun. You can also do more family activities that are fun and connecting for Mom and Dad, not just the kids, such as roughhousing together, making music, playing hide-and-seek or other games, doing arts and crafts, making cookies, or planting flowers.

Make time for pillow talk. Arranging to go to bed at the same time gives you more private moments for talking and snuggling, but that's hard for many parents. For example, sleep is at such a premium for a nursing mother that she often goes to bed before the father does. And Rick has listened to couples quarreling bitterly about one partner—often the father, but not always—insisting on staying up later to read or watch TV, since *That's the only time I get to myself.* Yet the difference in bedtimes is usually small enough—an hour or so at most—that it's easy to bridge with a gracious compromise. You could split the difference: if he's the night owl, he might come to bed a half hour sooner while you stay up for half an hour. Maybe he could get the kids going in the morning, giving you more time to sleep so you can go to bed later with him. Or he might come to bed with you, talk and cuddle for a while, and then go back out to the living room.

> We're too busy being parents to be friends.
>
> —A mother

Establish daily routines. Try to build time for just the two of you into the normal rhythm of your day. Tell the kids to leave you alone—perhaps after setting them up with an activity—and make the rule stick; soon enough, almost any child past two will come to respect it. Some couples have a glass of wine or cup of tea together when they're both home in the evening. You could arrange for the kids to eat early so you can have a peaceful dinner with each other. Firm bedtimes will give you time to yourselves in the evening. Or pay an older child to play with your younger ones for a few hours over the weekend while you hang out together in another part of your home; a friendly ten-year-old is a preschooler's dream playmate.

Schedule regular date nights. By the time most infants are six months old (and for some, it's sooner), they can handle their parents going off for an hour or so in the evening. At this point, try to schedule a "date night" for at least once a month, and maybe even weekly. The first time or two, let yourself be as careful or nervous as you like: call home every fifteen minutes, carry a pager, leave the movie early because you can't stand being away from your baby, whatever—we've been there. But soon it will feel very natural, and the kids will see it as simply part of the weekly routine, even if they howl for a few minutes after your car pulls out of the driveway. No question about it, get really good care: sometimes a child care provider would like to make a little extra money, or a relative will help out, or you could ask around for a mature and trustworthy teenager. Some couples swap baby-sitting with each other, so you get your date night this week and they have theirs the next one. Baby-sitting co-ops are a more elaborate version of this basic idea; you could ask around to see if there is a good one in your area—or start one yourself.

Refresh your relationship. But now that you're spending time together, sometimes it's been so long that you're not quite sure what to do or how to be! As one mom put it: ***We went out for the first time after Luis was born, ordered dinner, and then just kind of stared at each other. Finally, we both started laughing, it was so silly and awkward. We had been so busy for months with the new baby that we had sort of forgotten how to be together as just us. It felt strange, shy.*** For ideas—plus rekindling fond memories—you could talk about what you liked doing together when you first started dating, or at any time prekids. It's also worth thinking about new activities that would bring fresh interest and energy to your relationship. How about taking turns picking something novel to do each month? Or watching a documentary on public TV, going to a concert or play, or reading to each other in bed? You could take a class together, from aerobics to zen. Or try some athletic or outdoor activity you would both enjoy, such as doubles tennis or riding bikes.

In general, try to share the load of orchestrating these activities. It often falls to the mother to make all the arrangements—extra work for someone who typically is already juggling more tasks than her partner. Maybe your husband can set up the baby-sitter, even if he has to ask you for her name and phone number. He can make the restaurant reservation, recommend the movie, or dream up something special.

Let good moments last. As much as you both want things to be good between you, it's striking how hard it can be to let the nice moments last. Every one of the barriers to intimacy discussed in the previous section can get in the way. For example, it might seem like a part of you absolutely doesn't want to give way to strong feelings of liking or love. Perhaps you fear that would imply you're letting him off the hook for the ways you think he's been a jerk or a goof-off. Maybe you're afraid to melt, afraid to let yearnings for love and support stir within you, unwilling to chance being hurt one more time. This part of the self—though completely understandable, based on real events—makes you overlook opportunities to build a nice interaction, or it nudges you to do something that spoils the moment and puts you at odds with each other again.

Instead, try to remember all the reasons—from the long overdue healing of your heart to the benefits for the kids—for letting warm feelings linger between you. Take the moment for what it is: it doesn't negate the past or delegitimize anyone's grievances, nor does it mean you've agreed to anything from now on. Try to locate in him that which calls forth warmth and fondness in you. When he offers something positive, build on it rather than letting it hit the ground with a thud.

Protecting these moments makes a sanctuary for your love, giving it room to live—and grow.

Spend the night away. Sooner or later, you'll probably take the plunge and spend one or more nights away, just the two of you. It's usually rejuvenating to a relationship, but the concern is always how a child will handle it; please see the box on page 274 for suggestions on taking good care of your kids while you're away for the night.

Asking Three Questions a Day

Many couples would say that talking together was once the best part of their relationship. One mother told Rick: *He always made me laugh. When we started dating, sometimes we'd talk on the phone for three hours. It was just stuff: office weirdness, where to go skiing, some hassle we'd had. But I could hear him breathing, he felt so close to me. I really miss that. We still talk, but never for very long, and it's usually very practical: the kids, the house, info, problems. I'd say we still have a strong marriage, and I'm grateful for that. Yet it's strange: I miss him even though I see him every day.*

Yet now, real conversation—that goes beyond *How'd it go with the kids today?* or *I called the guy about the insurance*—gets pushed to the side by child care, housework, and the pressures of making a living: Who's got time to talk anymore?! So when we do, it's usually much more about exchanging information, driving toward decisions, or quarreling, than it is about an open-ended exploration of the inner world—that once so charmed and nurtured us—of our partner. It's a pity, since conversation is a crucial way to stay connected, especially for a woman, and especially one who's spent most of her day in the company of children.

That's why we recommend asking each other at least three questions a day. Questions about each other, not the bills, the dry cleaning, or the company picnic. Questions that do not carry implicit criticism or advice. Questions that contain real interest, that reach out, like: *What do you think about that? How did it make you feel? What would you really like?* Questions that make you feel more connected when you're done than when you started. Some of these questions, naturally, come on the run, but we also suggest trying to spend at least twenty minutes a day with your partner having an extended talk; it could be in the kitchen while you make dinner together, on the couch after getting home from work, or in bed once the children are asleep. (You might like to look back at the listening skills in chapter 6, p. 218.)

Yes, each of you has to have time to yourself; for example, after kids come along, a mom often craves, as one put it, *Just a few minutes each day, alone, no*

Taking Good Care of Children While You Are Away

Designed for preschoolers and multiday trips, these suggestions can be adapted for younger children and briefer times away.

- *Solid planning* will make the time go better for your child and help you feel more comfortable leaving. As a rule of thumb, adjusted for your own family, we recommend no more than one night away if the child is less than three years old, and no more than three nights if he's less than five; we're cautious because we've seen the lingering impact (occasionally, years later) on some children whose parents went on multiday trips when they were little. While you're gone, you'll want excellent care, provided by someone who can handle sensitive moments with a young child, like putting him to bed. Arrange for some kind of check-in and backup, just in case, like a neighbor looking in on the baby-sitter each day, or a relative who could take the kids in a pinch. As far as the child is concerned, it's generally best to stick with familiar routines. On top of these, you could add some neat activities—like a special time with Grandma, or going for a dip in a new backyard wading pool—that would keep him having fun. If you are nursing, plan ahead for your needs, not just your child's. Besides leaving breast milk frozen at home for him, bring along a pump to avoid any discomfort.

- *Introduce the idea to your child* that you'll be going away, and explain why, saying something like: *Your daddy and I enjoy spending time together, and it's good for us when we do. We're really going to miss you, but it's OK for us to do this.* A few days before your departure, show the child a calendar with the days of your trip marked out, and gently emphasize all the time you are spending with him beforehand and afterward.

- *Be empathic* with any protests, anticipatory grieving, attempts to bargain (*I be good if you stay, Mommy!!*), threats (*I die if you go!!*), etc. It's normal for you to feel wistful, torn, or regretful, but there's no reason to feel guilty: you need this time to yourselves, you have a right to it, and it can only help your child in the long run. It's fine to mention the goodies he'll experience while you're gone—like a trip to the zoo, extra dessert, or lots of time with his favorite aunt—but do not try to talk him out of his feelings. If it's called for after hearing him out, gently but firmly restate the fact that you will be going. Try to share this "emotion task" with your partner; it gets dumped on Mom more often than not, setting the child up to blame her for the separation.

- *Set up a regular time each day to call* your child if you'll be gone more than one night, thinking ahead to what will be least upsetting. Mornings and early evening often work best; if it's too close to bedtime, a phone call from Mom or Dad can trigger a meltdown.

- *Have a card and present for him to open each day* that do not depend on whether he was "good." His caregiver should also mark off the day with him on the calendar, showing him how soon you'll be home.

- *Bring something special back for him.* But don't be surprised if you get the cold shoulder: it's natural for a young child to be angry or reproachful after a separation. After a day or two, things should settle down, though there may be a week or more of extra clinging or sensitivity to separations.

questions to answer, no one pulling on me, no one I have to respond to. Peace. Quiet. That's all I ask. It's also important to be able to feel a sense of connection without talking. In our experience, though, parents are more likely to make sure they get time to themselves than they are to make a space in their busy lives for happily chatting together. And when they're sitting together without talking, they're more likely to be off in their own private worlds. We're not suggesting that your home become some sort of hit-and-run therapy group—just that you try to spend at least two percent or so of your waking hours (i.e., twenty minutes) taking an interest in each other.

Many times, you'll be asking about reactions to everyday matters. Additionally, partners in lasting relationships usually know a lot about the more fundamental pleasures, interests, struggles, and concerns of each other; if you don't already, then there's plenty more to ask about. It's also important to understand the hopes and dreams of each other, with questions like these: *When you were a kid, what did you want to be when you grew up? Are you generally satisfied with your life, or do you feel something important is missing? If you suddenly had three extra hours each day, what would you do with them?* You can appreciate what you have in common, including love for your children, values, spirituality, sense of humor, taste in music, or a passion for chocolate chip cookies. You could acknowledge your shared challenges, like a very stubborn toddler, aging parents, a nutty landlord, or an alcoholic neighbor. Or talk about the future, such as what it might be like to have the kids in grade school (high school?!) or where to go on vacation next summer.

No matter the topic, though, try to stay out of an argument when you're in "asking three questions" mode. Studies have found (no surprise) that humor oils the machinery of a marriage, so look for chances to laugh at yourself, the kids, or—gently—each other. In particular, these conversations may not be the best time to get into "our relationship." For women, broaching that subject usually comes from an effort to connect, but for many men, it seems to contain a built-in criticism; if the discussion brings you closer, fine, but if not, see if you can save it for another occasion.

Since men are less likely than women to value conversation for its own sake or to turn to it as a way to feel connected, in the majority of relationships, if the man were to ask the woman three questions in a row about *herself*, it would be a pleasant surprise. Rick describes a lightbulb moment on this point: *I'd be clipping along—scheduling appointments, reading a story to Forrest, taking out the garbage, whatever—feeling good about getting things done, and then Jan would try to draw me into talking with her, for its own sake, which seemed at odds with the long to-do list in my head. Finally, somewhere I read the phrase "relationship*

Men fall in love with what they see, women with what they hear.

—*Oscar Wilde*

tasks," and I realized that talking and giving her that feeling of being connected was part of what it was to be a husband. Redefining my role that way made chatting with her part of what I was **supposed** *to be doing, rather than a distraction from it.* You might suggest to him that talking with you is one aspect, and a very important one, of his "job description" as a father and husband.

Of course, taking a greater interest in one's mate is not just a guy thing. Many a dad complains, rightfully, that his partner is so absorbed with being a mom that she no longer asks about his experience of raising a family, or his work, dreams, and worries—or if she does, it's perfunctory, with eyes that soon glaze over. In this regard, what do you feel—in your heart, freely, not because of any role imposed upon you from the outside—is included in *your* "job description" as a wife or life partner?

For either parent, we think there's a place for graciousness, for bringing your attention to something that may not be your preference in the moment. A place for shifting gears inside your mind and letting yourself be drawn into a topic—and more important—into a sense of relationship with your partner. After some minutes pass, you notice that it feels satisfying to talk and to listen, and when the conversation comes to a natural pause and you shift to something else, you're glad you took the time to be together.

Often, when you're talking the connection between you will be like a light touch, more a reminder of the depth that's latent in your relationship than a direct experience of it. If you like, though, you can reach for an even greater sense of intimacy. Either one of you—and ideally, both—can cultivate a quality of being fully present, your body and mind given over to this moment together, not distracted by your own ideas or agendas. When this happens, your throat and eyes soften and your heart opens, and the feeling in the conversation changes, as if you were lifted by a warm humming swell of caring and closeness. Words might recede or fall away—honest words bringing you to a wordless intimacy.

Simply making an effort to be present will develop these faculties within you. As well, try to pay attention to the mental chatter that takes you out of the moment; you'll learn things about yourself—like when you typically check out—that will help you take fewer rides on those trains of thought. General practices of mindfulness—art, music, meditation, and so on—will also make it easier to let your mind be full of your partner. Additionally, in order to let yourself to be very close without feeling overwhelmed, controlled, or frightened, you must—paradoxically—preserve a core sense of self, remaining so fundamentally your own person that it is safe to let yourself fall deeply into relationship with another; if that's hard, please see the discussion of the eighth barrier to intimacy, page 269.

Healing Bruises to Your Relationship

In any important relationship, occasional misunderstandings, disappointments, and resentments are the rule, not the exception. Many of these fade with time and good experiences together. But some may linger, darkening the mood of a relationship, leading partners to shrink it to a size that feels safe, and adding dynamite to quarrels over little things (see the box below for common issues). By healing old wounds, you and your partner will feel more trusting and loving. You'll like each other more, your relationship will be stronger when the next challenge comes, and there won't be any explosives gathering dust in a corner of the living room.

Common Relationship Issues Between Parents

Many couples face one or more of these issues related to having a family:

- They had serious disagreements about having children in the first place.
- They had to deal with upsetting and expensive fertility procedures in order to conceive their child.
- She felt he distanced during her pregnancy, or he wasn't understanding when she had a miscarriage; or during childbirth, he wasn't emotionally present or supportive.
- They had widely different ideas about how to raise their children.
- She felt he hasn't pulled his weight as a father.
- He felt she indulged herself in the private pleasures of being a mother and hasn't pulled her weight in bringing money into the family.
- She felt pressured by him to go to work when she wanted to stay home, or to stay home when she wanted to go to work.
- He felt stung by her micromanagement of his parenting, her obvious view of him as a kind of clueless Fred Flintstone.
- She's sick and tired of him criticizing the housework, especially when he does so little himself.
- She stopped being interested in him sexually.
- He felt abandoned by her, emotionally and romantically, once children arrived.
- Someone said or did something terrible during a fight.
- Someone had an affair.

Out with the Old

Over the years, we've found certain questions to be helpful in healing hurts and getting a relationship back on track. Besides considering them privately, you can discuss them with each other, either informally or by setting aside specific times. When you do talk, try to keep in mind the methods covered in the two previous chapters, including civility, empathy, and sharing your own experience without blame or defensiveness. It could work best if one person at a time talks about a question completely (or several questions in a row), before the other person does—or you may prefer to go back and forth within a question in a less structured way. You can also explore the questions in any order that suits you. Take your time with them: they cover a lot of ground, and some may be so loaded that you have to approach them gently. If you can talk productively on your own, great. But if not, try to have a third person present, like a minister, trusted friend or relative, or therapist.

Here are the questions, which each partner could answer:

1. What were your original hopes and dreams for your relationship before children? What did you want to give? What did you hope you would receive?

2. What did you imagine life with children would be like? What did you anticipate would be the effects of children on your relationship?

3. What have been the *actual* effects of children on your relationship? Such as on your energy level, finances, time, romance, sexuality, intimacy, or conflicts?

4. What has made things go badly between you? (No blame, just the facts; don't refight those quarrels. . . .) To be honest, how have you brought out qualities in your mate that bother you? (Like how one person's stonewalling of criticism makes the other person more insistent.)

5. How have you suffered in your relationship? And—painful question— how have you made your partner suffer? Related to each other, how have you each felt anger? Hurt? Shame? Loss? Fear? Sadness? What could you have more compassion for, both in yourself and in your partner?

6. How might you have misunderstood some of your partner's motives or feelings? How might you have interpreted his or her actions in an unnecessarily negative way? How might your childhood have affected,

intensified, or distorted your reactions to your partner? Your life experiences prior to marriage? Your growing sensitization to certain issues?

7. What have you tried to do to make your relationship better? What has worked well when you stuck with it?

8. What has kept you from sticking with the things that work for your relationship—both external circumstances and internal thoughts, attitudes, or feelings? For example, how have other parts of your daily life gotten to be a higher priority than caring for your relationship? What has felt scary to you about being vulnerable, or giving your partner a fresh chance? What might be the hidden rewards to you of the problems in your relationship—like proving that he's done you wrong, or making you feel justified (and not a bad person) in seeking a divorce?

9. What feels correct and wise to take more responsibility for in your relationship? To apologize for? To ask forgiveness for?

10. Stated cleanly, without blame or rancor, what would you like to request from your partner? What would you like him to take more responsibility for? Apologize for? Do differently in the future?

11. What could you do differently to make your relationship better— both outward behaviors and internal actions within your own mind? How could you help each other stay on track? How could you help yourself?

As a speaker, try to focus on communicating for yourself, not on any response you might want from your partner. Be clear on your purpose: to express whatever you need to in order to clear this upset, to get it out of your nervous system and out of your relationship—that's your priority, ahead of being right, winning the point, or paying him back. Explain how and why his behavior affected you, but take reasonable responsibility for your reactions: they occurred within your mind, not his, and they were shaped in part by your personal history. As you share your experience, try to sense that it's leaving your body and no longer troubling your mind. Let in your partner's compassion, his regrets and remorse, and his commitment to act differently in the future. See if you can let go of the upset, and move on.

When you're the listener, remember that you have an opportunity here to get this upset out of your relationship. Help your partner set everything out in the open, especially whatever is hard to say. Try to get down to the bottom of his upset; you want to pull the tip of the root so that it doesn't grow back. Say back what you understand—particularly the deeper feelings, wants, or bruises—so your partner knows you got it. Try to acknowledge as much validity as possible in his views. Take as much responsibility as you authentically can for your part of the upset. State your regrets or remorse for everything you can. Say what you would have done differently in the past if you had only known better, and what you will do differently from this point forward. See if you can let go of the upset, and move on.

In with the New

It is extremely important to keep any agreements you made with each other in these conversations. When you've been let down in the past, and then warily extend the open hand of trust one more time, there's a particularly bitter slump of disappointment if it happens again. Also, you could talk about any discomfort you feel with the growing closeness between you. It is common for couples to create a quarrel when they start feeling connected again: you could discuss some of the ways this might happen, and how you could prevent it.

Further, as you look to the future, how will you cultivate more love for each other? Healing upsets is like pulling weeds. But it's not growing flowers. A couple can get to a place where neither person is really mad at the other one, but there is a numbness or exhaustion in the relationship. Maybe you wonder: *Will I ever really love him again? Will I even like him again? Will he be loving with me?* Sometimes the heart has become so stony that it seems nothing green will ever grow there again. But when just a little effort is sustained, we've seen a kind of miracle happen many times: pockets of fondness and caring beginning to emerge, fragile at first, then spreading and getting sturdier, love taking hold, softening a once-hardened heart.

It feels mainly like love happens *to* us, but we can also consciously plant its seeds within ourselves, protect them, and help them grow. If you think about yourself—and these points apply just as much to him—the seeds of a lasting love include:

- A general attitude of being compassionate and kind toward everyone, including your partner
- A sense of the being behind his eyes, seen through the latticework—perhaps a little overgrown these days—of his personality
- Allowing warmth, liking, and love to come forward within you; not putting a lid on these to prove a point or pay him back

- Actions that are friendly, caring, interested, loving—even when they are not your inclination in the moment—which evoke those real feelings within you

- Doing things together that naturally lead to warm feelings, like recalling good times together

- Seeing him as your children do; honoring him as your coparent, joined in the difficult, amazing undertaking of raising a family

Sex After Children

Ah, sex. After children come along, it becomes an issue for many couples. There is little time or opportunity, and often not much interest in one or both partners. But based on a foundation of teamwork, emotional safety, friendship, and nonsexual affection, romance and lovemaking can help keep a marriage healthy, or help reknit one that's unraveling.

First, some clarifications. We don't mean sex when it's uncomfortable during pregnancy or for some months after childbirth. We don't mean sex on demand, sex that might lead to an unwanted pregnancy, or sex with someone you really don't like very much right now. But when the dust settles six to twelve months after a baby is born, we suggest making an effort to preserve a romantic and erotic dimension in your marriage, living together as lovers as well as friends and coparents.

If you and your partner are both happy with your sex life, that's great. But difficulties related to sex are not uncommon, as you can see in these blunt comments from one woman on a survey Rick handed out at a mothers' club: *We've got one child, eight months old. I work full-time, commute forty-five minutes to work each way, have two dogs to walk daily and handle one hundred percent of the housework. My husband works for a high-tech company, with lots of pressure, a long commute and a long workday, and he also has to get up at 5 a.m. to check e-mails. He'd like to make love once a week, but I'd choose about once every two months, so we do it about once a month. Every night, we are both exhausted. When he complains that I'm not interested, I try to reassure him that I'm just tired. Weirdly enough, if I walk the dogs for an extra-long period, he thinks I must be having an affair! Tell me, is there any mom with little kids out there with the energy for two men??*

Like many couples, you might be dealing with one of the following issues:

- One partner—typically the man, but not always—is more interested in sex than the other one.

- Neither of you cares much about sex, but something is missing in your relationship.
- Practical problems are getting in the way of your love life, like no good times, kids crying right when you get started, it's awkward to shift from mommy or daddy mode to lover mode, etc.

The first two of these are about *wants,* while the last one is about *arrangements.* Let's start with the more fundamental issue—sexual desire—and then tackle the normal difficulties that complicate a romantic, erotic relationship after children.

But I Don't Want To

At this point, it is possible that somewhere in your mind a voice is saying something like: *That's all well and good. But what if I just don't want to?*

Of course, you absolutely don't have to. In many marriages, that works out all right. But in some cases, if the father is more interested in sex than the mother, there's a fair chance that sex may remain an issue in the relationship.

Besides leaving things as they are, you and your mate have four options if there's a disparity in desire:

- You accept your differences.
- The one who wants more becomes satisfied with less.
- The one who wants less kindles the desire for more.
- You both make gracious accommodations.

Many couples weave their way through a combination of these, emphasizing one more than another at different times. We've tried each one and can vouch for them. But above all, whatever you do has to feel like it's your own decision, not forced upon you in any way—and this is *especially* true if you've experienced sexual abuse or assault, or grew up in an oversexualized atmosphere. Sex is highly charged, and partners can be very persuasive—or even threatening or intimidating—to get what they want. It's all right for him to make his case or express his feelings. Then he has to back off enough for you to pick freely. Let's look closely at what you might be choosing.

Helpful husbands are an aphrodisiac for their wives.

—A mother

Will Change Diapers for Sex: Accepting Your Differences

Ironically, coming together about sex starts with acknowledging the ways in which you are apart. Sex is one of those aspects of life in which there is enormous natural variation in desire and preferred practices. One source of this variety is, obviously, gender: in most couples—and especially those with children—the man has a greater sex drive. (If it's not like that in your relationship, please see the box on page 287; you can apply much of the rest of this chapter by simply switching the genders.) The difference in natural interest is often a source of friction, as you can see in this imaginary, plainspoken dialogue, a condensed version of what we've heard from many mothers and fathers:

She says: For starters, you need to understand that my body was already over-touched long before you came near me, I'm tired most of the time, and the last thing I'm looking forward to when I finally get to bed is an aerobic activity. It's not personal if I'd rather go to sleep. The truth is, I don't feel sexual a lot of the time—and I'm not just neutral about it: at those times, deep in my brain, I want to not be sexual. This is really how most mothers are. Ask a hundred women with little kids where they'd put sex on a list of ten pleasant ways to spend a half hour—including taking a long bath, reading a magazine, or chatting with a friend—and most of them would put it near the bottom. I know your list would be different, that sex would be at or near the top. That's normal for you. But my list is normal for me.

Once we get past that generic lack of initial interest, yes, I still enjoy sex with you. But it has to be based on something. Sure, I may fantasize at least once in my life about hot sex with a near-stranger, but in the real world, caring comes first. I need to feel that you care about me, the person, much more than you lust after the body I inhabit. Since many women have been treated like a sexual object, you can understand why I need your leading communication to be one of cherishing and respect. And it's got to be real, not a box you're trying to check off so you can get to what you want. I can't have sex in order to connect; I have to feel connected in order to have sex.

Foreplay starts in the morning, when you support me in the care of our children, pulling your weight, showing through your deeds that you value what I value. To be blunt, I need to feel that we're joined in raising a family in order to be very interested in joining my body with yours in bed. And foreplay continues throughout the day in how we talk with and treat each other. Don't take my head off when I call you at work and then expect me to be all passionate when you get home. There's a switch inside me (and most women, I bet) that's set firmly to "off" whenever it doesn't feel good and safe between us. I need to have made up with you before I can start making out.

And there'll be many times when you're doing everything right, and I still won't want sex. It could be the kids crying, which is a total turnoff. Maybe I'm worn out, or my body feels funny. Whatever it is, it's not about you. You really shouldn't take it personally. And when you do get mad at me about not having sex, I become even less interested.

He says: I'm a normal man, and I think sex is one of the major good things in life. My attraction to you hasn't changed just because we've had children. It still gives me a thrill to see you walk around the bedroom getting dressed. But none of that means I don't also see you as a whole person, or don't care about your mind or soul. I want to have sex with you because I love you. It's a physical expression of my love, one that's fun, sweet, and instantly connecting.

That's why it hurts so much when you act like I'm some sort of jerk if I come on to you sexually. When I was a boy, I had my share of painful moments of feeling embarrassed about my sexual desires, so I don't need any more of them.

Occasionally, I want to be seen and wanted as a lover, not just a breadwinner or someone who can give a child a bath. I can totally understand if you're too far along in a pregnancy or it's too soon after childbirth to have intercourse, but if that's not an issue, I hope we can make love regularly. That regularity reduces the hurt if you're not interested tonight, since there's a good chance we'll make love pretty soon.

I totally love our children. And I love it when we're all together. But I also want to have a relationship with you that's about just you and me. I married you because I love you, I cherish you, and I want to be with you. So when I try to draw you into relationship with me, whether it's just us talking or we're in bed and the door's locked, it is not in order to drive a wedge between you and your children. I don't want you to give them less, I just want you to carve out a little more space in your mind and in your day for me. It won't take much. How long does it really take to let me know you still like me, give me a kiss, or make love?

It's as if she's waltzing while he wants to tango. In some couples, there's a good-humored acceptance of these differences that makes it possible to work around them: they create a foundation of teamwork and intimacy that doesn't involve sex, he respects her need for a loving warm-up, she makes room in her heart for regular lovemaking—and they find ways to keep dancing together, mainly a gentle waltz, and occasionally a hot tango. But in other couples, there is a lack of acceptance of sexual differences for two kinds of reasons.

There's something wrong with you. First, one or both partners could think that their own way is what's natural and right, and that the other person needs fixing. We've done this ourselves, in our own relationships, and it's always led to conflict and pain. Instead, each parent should try to see the sexual nature of his or her partner in a neutral, open-minded way.

From your side of the bed, notice any lurking contempt for male sexuality—like *Men think mostly with their little head instead of their big one*—or any exaggeration of his behavior; as a mother said to Rick once: ***All he ever thinks about is rubbing up against me. It's disgusting.*** Try to find compassion for his feelings about asking and being routinely turned down, his frustration, his sense of being unwanted, his hurt that this need of his doesn't seem to matter much in the relationship.

From his side, he should understand that having children literally alters the sex chemistry of your body: it is normal for estrogen to be lower than usual for several months after childbirth (longer if you continue to nurse), and estrogen helps make women receptive to sexual advances; also, both stress and nursing* increase production of prolactin, a serious lust-buster. He can recognize that it makes complete biological sense for mothers to evolve internal brakes that stop them from conceiving one child right after the other.

Even without factoring in the effects of children, he can accept the fact that most women have naturally less sexual interest than most men, and that there is considerable evidence that the tidal wave of passion you felt early in your relationship was due in part to brain chemicals that inevitably recede after a few years, leaving behind a shallower sea of innate sexual desire. He can understand that the fruits of sex—pregnancy and twenty-plus years of motherhood—and therefore sex itself have been enormously more consequential for females than males throughout history, causing a woman to normally need more conditions to be met for making love than a man does: more stability and safety in the relationship, more vitality in her body, more confidence that he's going to love and support her in the years to come.

He should have compassion for you, torn between your wish to make him

---

*But the benefits of breast-feeding are so great that no one should wean her baby in order to improve the sexual aspects of her marriage.

happy and the plain truth that you'd rather not have sex right now, meanwhile feeling guilty about saying no—and irritated that you have to. He can see that it's not about him that you're tired after a long day with a job and kids, that it's a lot of work to shift gears from mommy mode to lover mode, and that much of the time, you just don't want to want sex. He has to respect your right to *not* want something he wants.

There's something wrong with me. The other main reason for a lack of acceptance is that one or both partners—more often, the mother—thinks there must be something wrong with herself, and tries to act like something she's not. It's understandable. Pop culture pours out images of women who feel sexy and are interested in sex—*So I guess I must be the odd duck.* There's a long history of women setting aside their own needs to satisfy those of others, and of wives expected to roll over and let their husbands have their way.

As you'll see further on, we think there's a legitimate option for gracious stretching by both partners when it comes to differences in sexual interest, for him to relax and let the erotic impulse soften and become a feeling of love without sex, and for her to encourage her mind to awaken erotic desire. But falsifying what's fundamentally true for yourself undermines the honesty, intimacy, and emotional safety that are the very foundation of a healthy, loving sex life. In fact, when you accept yourself, you create a kind of oasis inside, where you can freely cultivate your own natural sexuality, and over time, bring that into your relationship.

You might like to look back at the material on self-acceptance in chapter 3, starting on page 76. In particular, try to be aware of any ways you might be putting up a front about sex that's not the real you; if so, notice the reasons for doing it: perhaps guilt, or simply taking the path of least resistance. For reassurance that your level of libido is not unusual, talk with other mothers in similar situations (rather than comparing yourself to women who are younger, without children, or at an earlier stage in their relationships). Try to be at peace about your own nature. It is what it is, and being hard on yourself is both unfair and will not make it any different.

We need to understand each other. Perhaps you and your partner can talk frankly about your sexual natures at this time. One way would be to read the statements of the fictional mother and father above, and say what fits for each of you. You might even write a letter to each other that says what you understand about the other person and sex, what you'd like to have understood about you, and what you'd like to have happen in the future.

Less formally, both of you could simply talk about sex, your likes and dislikes, your similarities and differences. You might agree to a truce in which you accept your differences and put them on hold for a while, perhaps to get through an especially demanding time like the months following a mother's return to work. Alternatively, on a foundation of accepting each other, you could explore the options below.

When He's Less Interested in Sex than You Are

A man could have less desire for sex than his partner does for a variety of reasons. Some have nothing to do with being a father, such as naturally low libido that preceded children, physical shyness, concerns about performance, or a partner who has a naturally high interest in sex. Parenthood-related reasons include upsets with his partner about raising a family, not feeling attracted to her physically after her body has changed due to having children, seeing her as a motherly figure rather than an erotic partner, or being unwilling to approach her after being repeatedly rejected.

Some mothers are content with the situation because they have little interest in sex themselves, and a partner's disinterest takes the pressure off them. Others feel resigned, though the status quo is not their preference and they're troubled about the long-term implications for the marriage. But some women are hurt and frustrated.

If you wish your partner were more interested in sex, see if you can talk with him openly about it and find out the reasons for his disinterest. If he has no desire for sex at all (typically indicated by never or rarely masturbating), that often suggests depression, sexual dysfunction, or a medical problem. He should talk with a therapist or physician; your support will be a key element in things getting better in this aspect of your relationship. If he isn't interested in sex with you, it's prudent to make sure he's not having an affair or using a prostitute. Once you've eliminated these unlikely possibilities, find out if there is anything you could do differently, such as resolve an upset between you, reassure him in some way, give him longer foreplay (which men need as they grow older), adjust to his preferred times to make love, or perhaps try some new things in bed. But none of that means doing anything that feels emotionally wrong or degrading. And in the end, you can only do so much, and the ultimate source of the solution(s) to his sexual issues will have to be him.

Becoming Satisfied with Less

Much as a mother might take steps to encourage more sexual interest within herself (see next section), a father could just as well take action to lower his desire for sex.

Cultivate compassion and wisdom. Based on compassion, not guilt, he can let himself feel how his sexual interest may be a kind of burden on his wife and on their relationship. He might consider the chain reaction of effects on his children, his wife, and himself, and ask: are the rewards worth the price? Through wisdom, seeing the greatest good for the greatest number, there could be a natural relinquishing of desire.

Sublimate sex. Like people have done throughout history, he could sublimate sexual passion into other activities. He might take up an artistic pursuit. Or get into some sport, go fishing more often, climb more mountains. Or invest more emotionally in his own children.

Engage in spiritual practices. He could explore spiritual practices that channel erotic energy into higher states of consciousness. This may seem airy-fairy, but there are, in fact, well-established traditions that have cultivated these disciplines for thousands of years, such as tantra, kundalini yoga, and parts of Taoism, and he could read about these or take classes. Besides being an effective way to manage a difference in desire, these techniques can make lovemaking, when it happens, more fulfilling and ecstatic.

Find other ways to be connected or intense. Sexuality has many elements, some of which are not sexual per se, such as closeness, intensity, affection, feeling wanted or appreciated, and physical pleasure. He could satisfy these in other ways than sex, both within and outside your relationship. For instance, he and you could make a special effort to spend more time touching or in a state of loving closeness. He could deepen his friendships with other men, finding in their company some of the companionship he has sought through sex with you. He might explore activities that provide a different kind of intensity, like rock climbing, bicycle racing, or playing music—especially vital for a man who feels a strong pull toward the wild and has used sex in part as an outlet or safety valve.

Have sex with himself. He could take care of his needs through fantasy and masturbation (if that's not in conflict with his beliefs). Even under the best of circumstances, it is normal for a happily married man to masturbate. For most men, it takes nothing away from their relationship with their mates: it's a private act, instant stress relief, and then on with the day. Though it could well be uncomfortable for you to contemplate, his fantasizing about other women or pictures in a men's magazine almost never affects his feelings for you. Unless his masturbation directly impacts the marriage—eliminating or disturbing real sex, or drawing him into relations with real people—it's usually wisest to let it remain his own business.

Kindling a Desire for More

Many factors—some situational and others more fundamental—affect sexual desire. Starting on page 295, we'll look at practical ways to maintain a sexual relationship in the everyday circumstances of raising a family. But here, let's consider the foundations of a mother's sexuality. There are numerous ways to increase a person's authentic interest in sexual relations; you could try one (or more) of them below and see if it works for you. But to repeat a crucial point, these are simply options, and whether you explore them is a very personal choice that is entirely up to you.

Nurture your health. Any drop in physical health will usually reduce sex drive, which is one more reason to get a thorough assessment, and to take good care of your body (see chapters 4 and 5).

Look into your hormones. You could consult with a doctor, such as a gynecological endocrinologist, and assess the hormones that might be affecting your sexuality. Then there's the tough question: do you intervene or not? Taking hormones is a tricky business for any woman, but especially for a mother. Low doses of supplemental testosterone, estrogen, progesterone, or DHEA may bring back erotic interest, sometimes miraculously. But we've also seen these approaches backfire, producing side effects like irritability, aggressiveness, and insomnia, and disturbing a hormonal equilibrium that was already fragile in a depleted mother. If you and your doctor decide to try these approaches, it's wise to be cautious and go slowly.

Consider your medicines. Certain drugs, such as antidepressants or blood pressure medications, can lower libido altogether, not just make it hard to climax. You should discuss these possibilities, and the alternatives, with your doctor. Nonpharmacological interventions for depressed mood—such as therapy, social support, or exercise—usually help your sex life if they have any effect on it at all. Some antidepressants, such as Serzone or Wellbutrin, typically have fewer sexual side effects, and the natural antidepressants, Saint-John's-wort and 5-hydroxytryptophan (see pp. 174–75), usually do not affect sexuality. If you stick with the original medication, your doctor might suggest lowering the dose, or taking a "drug holiday" (e.g., skipping the antidepressant Friday and Saturday, and making love Sunday morning).

Get exercise. Exercise often seems to increase sexual interest. It also boosts energy in general and enables your body to shift more easily into the active parts of making love.

Try spiritual practices. Some spiritual practices can be used to raise sexual energy rather than lower it; these include certain kinds of yoga, or tantric techniques (see *The Art of Sexual Ecstasy* by Margot Anand).

Establish a loving intimacy. When there is anything awry in the relationship, sex for most women goes right out the window. If that's part of the problem, this chapter and the two before it contain many ways to develop a warmer, closer sense of connection.

Care for postpartum depression. Much like depression in general, postpartum depression (PPD) usually reduces or eliminates one's interest in sex. PPD calls for treatment as a whole, not focused on the symptom of low libido; with time and good care, an interest in sex should return if PPD is the main source of your lack of desire.

Try to lift your mood. A glum mood can rob you of any interest in sex, plus make it nearly impossible to get aroused or climax. If you've been feeling blue, "flat," or dispirited, or you've lost interest in activities that you once enjoyed, take a look at pages 60 to 71 in chapter 3, and perhaps call a therapist.

High levels of anxiety can have much the same effect as low mood. If that's a problem for you, see pages 71 to 76 in chapter 3, and think about contacting a therapist.

Consider your upbringing. In certain home environments or cultures, girls are taught that sex is dirty and embarrassing—and especially for women, who are not supposed to seek or enjoy it. Or there may have been early experiences of being punished or shamed for sexual activities (e.g., masturbation, kissing a boy, coming home late from a date). As a result, sexual desire may have become inhibited.

If you have an inkling that this might apply to you, you could use the techniques in chapters 2 and 3, read books written by women with similar upbringings, or talk about it with a close friend. But probably the most effective thing you can do for yourself is to see a therapist. If a person chooses not to be sexual, that is her absolute right, but the option itself may have been taken away from you. You have a right to reclaim it, and then decide yourself how you will express your sexuality, without anyone telling you what a nice girl is or isn't.

Find enjoyment in being excited. Sex is (in part) about excitement, but some girls grow up with little brakes inside on being energetic, intense, emotional, spontaneous, carried away, or loud. Occasionally turn up the dial to a higher setting in nonsexual situations and see how that feels. You might detect a fear of scolding or embarrassment, and if you do, you can work with and release that fear, using techniques that are by now probably familiar. The point is to make sure that the normal human capacity for excitement is wide open inside you, and then you can make your own choice about what you'll do with it.

Remember previous sexual experiences. If you're like many mothers, you might initially feel a resistance to sex, but after some minutes of sensitive and skillful foreplay, you often start to get interested. Remember that when your partner approaches you sexually, and see if doing so can help you feel more comfortable at the start of lovemaking.

The more you have, the more you may want. Many women report that the more often they have sex, the more they enjoy it. You could do an experiment in which you make love twice a week for a few weeks and see what effect that has on your libido.

Turn on your mind. Put your attention on romantic or sexual stimuli as a way to prime the pump of desire. For example, a client of Rick's, whose love life had become mundane after children, told him: ***Don't laugh, but I've been reading romance novels lately, and I'm telling you, they've got me more interested in sex. I know it's manipulative, I know it's dumb, but I couldn't care less: they're fun to read and I like the effects.*** There is a range of possibilities, starting with warm thoughts about your husband or an image of him looking particularly handsome. You could imagine teasing or dating him, or perhaps recall a time in your life when you felt especially flirtatious and sexy. Getting more explicit, other options include erotic stories or novels (a growing genre is written by women for women), sexually oriented Web sites, racy movies, men's magazines (many women find the pictures arousing), or adult films (a growing number are being made with women in mind). Or you could explore different fantasies in your imagination, maybe involving your partner, maybe not; the majority of women fantasize sexually at one time or another, and such fantasizing is associated with fewer sexual problems or dissatisfaction.

Experiment with being more active. When there's the opportunity for eros, ranging from a quick kiss to intercourse, you might experiment with acting more sexual than you would normally do. See what happens if you kiss harder, move more aggressively, allow your body to be more accessible to your partner, get louder, or reach for a more stimulating image in your mind. Notice any resistance, and see if you can tell what part of it feels like an essential part of your nature, and what part seems more related to how you learned to be while growing up, or to a censoring of your sexuality acquired in adulthood.

Get to know the lover within you. All of these suggestions are ways to nurture the sense of a sexual being inside, to make room for her and allow her to grow with loveliness and spunk. What is she like, this lover within you? If you were to imagine a conversation with her, what would she say, and how would she ask you to help her? When alone sometime, you might pretend to walk around your bedroom like her, and notice any differences from the ways you normally move. Perhaps she'd like to try on some of your clothes, maybe a sexy bit of lingerie you were given once and put away. Can you let her come out and play?

Give desire a try. But what do you do if you sincerely and actively want to *not* want sex? Let's start with the fact that you are far from alone. Even past the first year postpartum, many mothers in long-term, stable relationships have little or no innate desire for sex; we haven't seen a careful study on this subject, but our own experience would lead us not to be surprised if the number were as great as one woman in three, and it could be higher. And it's usually more than mere indifference: that switch is locked on OFF and some deep part of the self *wants* to keep it that way.

In some cases, the switch is set to off because of factors in a woman's personal history, like sexual abuse or assault, domestic violence, or shame from childhood. But more often it feels natural, even primal, and healthy. Evolution has given our species a variety of tendencies that are expressed more in some people than in others. Perhaps those mothers with low sexual interest are biologically inclined toward one effective and completely normal reproductive strategy: shift most of their libidinal energy to caring for their young, and avoid jeopardizing that care by allowing sexual interest to draw them into risky distractions.

Because we have met so many mothers who feel awkward or self-critical about their low sex drive, the point is worth belaboring: you're in good company, you are perfectly normal, and you do not have to change. On the other hand, you might consider the benefits to you, your relationship, and your family for seeing if it is *possible* to awaken more sexual interest.

If you do decide to try, the good news is that our wants are quite flexible. With a little effort, we usually can genuinely want one thing less, or truly want something else more. The mind is amazingly plastic, and most of us never make a sustained push to nudge it in one direction or another. We usually don't know what is really possible within the mind until we give it a try.

Making Accommodations for Each Other

Whether or not either of you takes steps to reduce any differences in sexual interest, you can still find ways to accommodate each other. It's usually easier than one might think. Disparities in desire often become so polarized that they look more extreme than they actually are.

We've seen many couples make accommodations for each other in the erotic arena. Honestly, we've done it ourselves. The couple comes to an understanding that works for each person, typically along these lines:

- Both maintain a foundation of teamwork and intimacy—as well as a sense of perspective about sex, so that it is neither a bigger nor smaller issue than it ought to be

- The father makes an effort to respect a mother's need to have surplus energy to even contemplate sex, loving preliminaries, and the right to say no without being hassled

- The mother makes an effort to feel comfortable with regular lovemaking

- Both share an expectation about how often they will, in fact, have sex

Regarding the big question—How Often Are We Going to Do It (which usually means someone has an orgasm, but not necessarily through intercourse)—there are several approaches:

- Never or rarely, for now: Appropriate at some point during pregnancy or the first months after childbirth; usually not healthy for a long-term relationship.

- Once a month: Often sensible during pregnancy or the first year or so after childbirth; will not satisfy most men—nor many women—over the long run.

- Two or three times a month: Probably the most common rate of sex for parents of young children.

- Once or twice a week: Typically the father's preferred frequency of sex (though many men wouldn't mind more); a stretch for many mothers, but if you can find your way to being comfortable with this amount, in most cases there will be a nice glow in your relationship, and sex will disappear as an issue.

- His week/her week: She agrees in advance to be sexually responsive during his week, unless something occurs such as a cold or her period, and he agrees to lay off during her week; not easy to do for a mother with a baby, but worth considering for mothers of older children or to break logjams around sex.

We have known some couples that made effective agreements about sex without ever getting explicit; if that approach works for you, great, but if not, then you will probably need to be more plainspoken. Even if it's awkward, it usually helps to be pretty specific about what you want from each other, both outward behaviors (*please do this, never do that*) and internal attitudes. Try to listen to each other without arguing. This information is pure gold: each of you is saying what you need in order to give your partner what he or she wants.

But even more than skillfully working out the details, it helps to be both gracious and willful when you try this option of making accommodations for each other. For example, there might be a loose analogy between having conversations and having sex. For many men, giving themselves over to an emotionally intimate conversation with their partner is not their most preferred way to spend half an hour, no matter how much they cherish her and are committed to the marriage. But a man can recognize that intimate conversation is good for his relationship and family, that there's probably personal growth available for him in pushing through his barriers to that form of closeness, and that he usually feels better and more loving afterward. So he brings both graciousness and his will to the encounter. He works with himself a little before sitting down, getting his mind into it: maybe he remembers past conversations that felt good, does a two-second review of the wise reasons for giving himself to this one, and shifts mentally from task mode to talk mode; in sum, he locates a genuine motivation inside for talking. In the beginning, he may not be very into the conversation and might have to make an effort to draw his mind back to it, but pretty soon he gets engaged and starts bringing his own interests into it. When they're done talking, he notices the nice feelings inside himself, and between them. He enjoys the aftereffects of the conversation in their relationship, and he's glad he took the time to do it.

Things can be pretty much the same for a mother and sex. There's a good chance it's not her first choice for the next half hour—and in fact, there's frequently a deeper, more visceral reluctance within her to engage in sex than a man has for emotionally intimate conversation. But she could remember the good reasons for making an accommodation, and bring graciousness and will to it. If there is a fair chance that sex is on the agenda for later in the day, she might think a bit about the things that draw her to lovemaking, like warm feelings for her partner or pleasantly erotic imagery. She could do what she can to keep the kids from running her ragged and to preserve some energy for lovemaking, including telling him that she needs more help. When they first start, she could make an effort to give herself to the encounter, and pretty soon her body and mind will probably become more naturally engaged. Afterward, she might notice the nice feelings between them, and be glad she took the time to do it.

In both sex and conversation, there is a middle place between being naturally excited and absolutely opposed. We would *never* suggest making love if it would be painful, unsafe, abusive, or degraded. But finding a genuine willingness within yourself to spend a small amount of time—almost always, less than an hour each week—engaged intimately in a way that usually ends up feeling good for you, helps your partner feel loved, and bonds you together, could be a nice way to nurture your intimate friendship.

Making Room for Two When Baby Makes Three

Now comes the logistical part. Sex was pretty simple before Junior came along: you were both interested, when and where were easy to figure out, and there were no interruptions. But now, making love seems to require a perfect configuration of children finally sleeping, no irritating interactions with kids (or each other) in the last few hours, somehow there's still some energy in your bones, the gods are smiling—and no one wakes up in the next room. These days, maintaining a spark of passion in your relationship, and igniting a fire when the time is right, takes more conscious attention than ever before.

Nonsexual affection. One of the members of a mothers' club made this interesting comment when Jan and Rick gave a talk there: *When we were first married, we touched each other all the time. At family events, people would even kid us about it. But now, I feel pretty touched-out from the kids, and it hardly occurs to me to touch him. Plus he'll think it means I want sex, and I don't, at least not then, and it would be awkward to say no, so that's another reason. And he mainly touches me when he wants sex. Which I don't like. But because about the only time we touch is when we're making love, touch has gotten equated with sex.* When she was done speaking, a dozen other women chimed in about similar situations, and we all came up with these suggestions:

- *Talk about touching.* Talk with each other about the sort of touching and affection you used to enjoy; just remembering how nice it felt will also get you moving in the right direction. Reflect on the ways affection was expressed in the home or culture in which you grew up, and how that might have put an unnecessary lid on what you're comfortable with today.

- *Ask for what you want.* Ask specifically for what you'd like, such as a kiss when you come home from work. You may think it's obvious, but your partner may have a totally different idea of what you want.

- *Let touching last.* Allow the times of touching to last longer; for example, instead of a quick pat on the back, let the hand linger. Notice any feelings that prompt you to withdraw a touch sooner than you really need to, like a discomfort with closeness or a fear that your touch will be misinterpreted.

- *Display affection in front of the kids.* Feel free to touch each other around the kids: a hand on the leg, a visible cuddle in bed. It's not appropriate for them to witness a major make-out session—let alone anything more sexual—but it's completely fine for them to see a warm and extended hug, even if they do try to worm between you and yell, "Gross!"

- *Reach out yourself.* Besides asking him to be more affectionate, you could start touching him more on your own: on the arm, little massages, back scratches—whatever he likes. Yes, it's more giving when you may feel pretty gived-out, but try it and see what happens. Usually, it will give you a nice feeling and he'll become more affectionate with you.

- *Experiment with affection.* Try a simple experiment, for five to twenty minutes each, in which you take turns being the giver and the receiver. As the giver, his job is to touch you in exactly the ways you like (in this experiment genitals are off-limits), and your job is to let him know when it feels good and when you'd like something different. Then you switch roles. Besides learning about the other person's preferences, you'll become aware of any ways that it's hard to tell each other exactly what you want—or to be told. After the exercise, talk with each other about what you experienced during it and what you learned.

- *Take sex off the table.* Paradoxically, one of the best things you can do for your sex life is to make it clear when sex is not an option. That way, you don't have to wonder what that hand on your hip means, maybe starting a downward slide of resisting his affection and launching a quarrel. You can enjoy the caress for what it is without fearing what it might become. Couples learn to send these signals gracefully, through hints, subtle shifts in the body, little jokes, or even straightforward statements like, *How about some hugs before we go to sleep?*

- *Put parts of your body off-limits.* Similarly, you need to be able to declare parts of your body off-limits at certain times. For example, some couples have nights when the erotic zones are not to be touched; besides giving each person—well, usually the mother—the sense that her boundaries are respected, it can build an erotic charge for the next time you make love. This ban may become semipermanent for many months, such as in the case of a nursing mother who does not want her breasts touched by anyone besides her baby. (On the other hand, some mothers notice that their breasts feel more "turned on" during the time they're nursing.)

- *Touch more in bed.* Time under the covers with each other is a great opportunity for affectionate touching. Now that you've got some clear boundaries, try to get rid of any pillows between you in bed, and maybe the pajamas as well. If you're using bedclothes as a kind of barrier, or a way to discourage his sexual interest, your words alone should be sufficient; if they're not, that's the real problem, which should be addressed through methods more direct than a nightshirt (see the two previous chapters). Lying skin to skin under the covers should feel safe and pleasant, not scary. A bathrobe at bedside—so you're ready for any 2 a.m. calls from a child down the hall—can let you relax and enjoy a naked undercovers night.

Romance. Remember the little romantic things you used to do for each other? Those gestures were a way to say *I cherish you apart from all the jobs you do for our family.* As a relationship continues, it is normal for romance to decline, becoming a more everyday love. But when romance disappears entirely, it can start to feel like the principal basis for your relationship is that you are yoked to a common plow.

Since caring for young children can be about as unromantic as it gets, give yourself a jump start by actively looking for things that help you feel romantic. It could be as simple as putting on lipstick, scented bath powder, or perfume, wearing nicer clothes, playing special music, setting out flowers, getting prettier underwear, or reading a romance novel.

Try to talk with your husband about what feels romantic to do or to receive. This applies to small gestures, such as a love note, roses, dressing up—or shaving! And to big events, like a special date. You could each describe your idea of a dream romantic experience, and invite your partner to do it with you as your guest. If your notion is the ballet in formal attire, he would agree in advance to escort you and be a good sport; the same applies to you if his plan is opening day at the local ballpark. If you're like most couples with kids, there's currently so little romance that a tiny effort will lead to a giant increase. You can wait for him to take the first step, but that might leave you feeling rather like the damsel in the tower; in addition to asking him to be more romantic, you could start making romantic gestures yourself.

Erotic affection. The territory between a quick kiss and sexual intercourse often shrinks to nothing after children, with parents acting like asexual, functional partners except when they make an appointment to be lovers. But when little moments of juicy contact are sprinkled into your relationship, it is easier to warm up to all-out sex, and interestingly, the partner who's more eager for lovemaking usually becomes less insistent about it since some of his or her needs are being satisfied in the ordinary course of your life together.

The key is to have an understanding about erotic touching—about when, where, and how—that works for both of you. For example, you probably don't like being fondled while stirring the spaghetti sauce, but there's a good chance he'd like spontaneous sexual attention. You just have to talk about it, respect the sexual natures you each have, and find a middle path. He needs to know that merely because you may not like being fondled out of the blue, it doesn't mean that you don't like him or lovemaking—when the time is right. You can understand that his impulse to give you a pat on the rear when you bend over to pick up a toy—probably jolting and even offensive when your mind is entirely in mother mode—is utterly normal for a man, a blending of lust *and* love.

Each of you can stretch a bit, whether it's him resisting the urge to give something a squeeze as he walks by in the hall or you going out of your way to give his ear a nibble as he heads out the door. Maybe you'd like passionate kisses every day that don't implicate you in going any further. Maybe he'd love a few minutes of genital fondling in bed at night; when you are having sex fairly regularly, most men are delighted and grateful to receive this pleasure and then drift off to sleep.

Going all the way. Here are some suggestions for the practical problems parents often need to get out of the way before they can go all the way.

- *The child's in the bedroom.* This is one of the prime physical obstacles to intimacy, especially when your children are babies. One mother described her solution for this problem to Ricki: ***It's the last thing you think would happen, but our kid has improved our sex life. She's made us be more creative. We put her down in the family bed, and then make love in the living room, her bedroom, even the bathroom—places we never would have thought of before.*** Other parents find ways to make love discreetly with a sleeping baby in their room, as we mentioned in chapter 4.

- *You might be interrupted.* Some disturbances can't be helped: if a sleeping baby wakes and starts crying, you just have to smile at each other in resignation and then tend to your child. But you can prevent other interruptions through a bit of planning, like letting a child stay up a little later to be sure he'll sleep soundly. Or get the kids out of the house altogether by arranging for a friend to watch them or hiring a baby-sitter to take them to the park (maybe "while we work on our taxes").

- *The kids might hear you.* It's fine for children to have a vague idea about the sexual aspect of their parents' relationship, but it's not appropriate to be in their face—or ears. Most of us can tone it down during lovemaking if we need to; whispered sex can be, in fact, very sexy. You can also use a pillow as a muffler, set the kids up with a read-along audiotape/storybook, or wait until a child who could sleep through a brass band is snoozing deeply.

- *You're too tired for sex.* A universal complaint among parents. Sometimes, you just go with it. But you could also go to bed early with a plan to make love in the morning—when libido is higher for most people—or postpone it to the weekend when you're more rested (if this seems all too pre-arranged, see "It's no longer spontaneous" below). Or try quickies: five to fifteen minutes of lovemaking, nothing fancy, and no pressure on anyone to climax.

- *There's never any time.* There's always *some* time: the real issue is usually fatigue or one of the other difficulties we're exploring here. And you can make time in the ways we discussed earlier, starting on page 270. For example, when the baby goes down, head for the bedroom. Don't turn to housework or returning calls. Take each other's clothes off, help each other get into it, and soon you'll be glad you did.

- *He can't maintain an erection.* Occasionally losing an erection is normal for all men, particularly as they age, but if it's happening often, he should speak with a doctor or therapist. The potential causes include physical complaints such as cardiovascular problems and psychological issues like anxiety about performing. With skillful care, this problem can be solved in most cases.

- *Your vagina seems "stretched out" after childbirth.* Usually, after a few months, the vaginal walls return to near their original shape and elasticity. If not, Kegel exercises often help, and if they don't, consult with your gynecologist.

- *Intercourse is painful for you.* Painful intercourse is normal up to a year after childbirth, and the lowered estrogen that comes with breast-feeding can leave vaginal walls dry and easily irritated. But it could also be due to a yeast infection (most common), broken tailbone that is slow to heal (rare), or a sexually transmitted disease. So be sure to mention this problem to your gynecologist. On your own, try longer foreplay to help stimulate vaginal lubrication, using a lubricant yourself, or slow and gentle insertion and movement of the penis. If those methods don't seem to be enough, talk with your gynecologist since there are many good options for treatment.

- *A medicine is making it hard to climax.* Please see the discussion of this issue on page 289.

Other issues are more a matter of the mind. If, deep down, there's little natural inclination toward sex, look at the section on desire, starting on page 289. But if it's more of a mental block, here are some suggestions:

- *Fertility procedures have complicated sex.* The medical interventions and sex-on-the-clock aspects of fertility procedures can rock a couple's sex life for years. Check with your doctor and perhaps do some testing to make sure there aren't any lasting effects of hormone therapy on estrogen, testosterone, or other hormones that regulate sexuality. With your partner, you could deliberately retrace the early steps of your romantic relationship, recreating the freshness and passion that are the best antidotes to any mechanical quality that has crept into your sex life.

- *You're mad at each other.* If it's a spat that day, try to talk it out before lovemaking. But if there continues to be an open sore in your marriage, you can use the methods we've described to deal with it inside yourself or between you and your husband. In particular, try to speak about any hurts in your sexual relationship, such as thoughtless comments about changes in your body or disdain about one spouse's (high or low) interest in sex. If you can't resolve these issues on your own, we suggest you consult with a therapist.

- *Something traumatic happened during pregnancy or childbirth.* Invasive procedures or insensitive professionals can leave scars on the mind that linger. The passage of time and just talking about it with your partner or a friend can really help. If that's not enough, contact a therapist since there are effective methods for dealing with psychological trauma.

- *Issues unrelated to being a mother are complicating your sex life.* For example, abuse during childhood, rape, or sexual humiliation can lead to intrusive images, feelings of panic or shame, intense dislike of one's body, an abhorrence of sex, or other complications of sexual relations; if this might apply to you, please see a therapist. Alternately, many women have difficulty having an orgasm; for help in that regard, please see the box on page 303.

- *You feel embarrassed about how you look.* If you feel your body is too heavy or not shaped the right way anymore, try to remember that if he wants to make love with you, it's because you are sexually attractive. Even more to the point, he's probably more excited about making love with *you,* the person inside, than he is about having sex with your body; the most thrilling moment for him is likely to be when you become passionate yourself. When that happens, he is not going to care about those stretch marks or any other detail about your body. If you share your concerns with him, there's a very good chance that his response will be reassuring.

- *It's been a while since you had sex.* You may feel nervous about making love again if it's been a while; sometimes a year or more can pass since the last time a couple with children had intercourse, especially if the woman was pregnant during that period. But you were able to have sex before, and you will surely succeed at it now. Go easy with it when you make love for the first time again, and tell each other what you need to feel comfortable.

- *Motherhood and sex don't seem to mix.* Our culture tends to draw a double yellow line between maternity and sexuality. When you look inside, can you find any beliefs like that? If you do, you can talk back to them (using the methods outlined in chapters 2 and 3), or examine and challenge them with a friend. Try to sense the ways your physical and emotional fertility as a mother are connected with your sexuality.

- *It's hard to shift gears.* Even with a moderate sex drive, most women have to make a conscious transition from mother mode to lover mode. If you think lovemaking might be on the agenda, maybe he could get the kids to bed while you take a nice bath or read a chapter from a steamy novel. Changing into a sensual camisole rather than a flannel nightgown might put you into a certain frame of mind when you're headed for bed. You could do some stretches or yoga—perhaps in the nude?!—to relax, loosen up, and get more into your body. Or take a shower together, dance for a few minutes, or give each other a brief massage.

  When you're tired or afraid the kids will wake up any minute, it's natural to skip the hors d'oeuvres and jump to the main course. Sometimes it's the entree or nothing, but try to linger with foreplay whenever you can, an important way to warm up and shift into being lovers. Lightly kissing each other's mouth and face for a few minutes, holding back from anything more intense, can be extremely exciting. You could also spread foreplay throughout the day, building a pleasant buzz between you.

- *It's no longer spontaneous.* Well, so what? Many pleasures, from dinner with a friend later tonight to a pleasant walk next Saturday, are increased through anticipation. Rather than fighting the way that sex necessarily becomes more scheduled after children, see if you can use that to make it even more exciting. If you're planning to make love Tuesday night, build up to it with sexy hints, teasing and pulling away (*Wait till Tuesday!*), writing little notes that suggest what you'd like to do, or simply playing with mental fantasies. Aiming for a certain time for sex can help motivate you to be nice to each other and stay out of wrangles. And if you can, try to be open to spontaneous sex at least occasionally, even if it's not really the perfect moment.

- *Sex is boring.* On top of the normal issues that usually make sex more prosaic as the years go by, becoming parents adds new ones, including diminished libido, less opportunity for anything creative, and a weariness that leads to plain vanilla sex. To rekindle some zest, you could start by thinking about or writing down a list of things you would like to try or change in your sex life, and be as specific as possible. Next, make a second list of the reasons it's hard to suggest these to your partner; when they're down on paper, you'll see that most if not all of them are nothing more than the familiar collection of general inhibitions on asking for what you want, or embarrassment or shame about sex. Understandable and normal as these thoughts are, you can let go of them like any other beliefs that dampen your well-being and the quality of your marriage.

    Then, unless you truly believe it would be risky in your relationship, try being very candid about what you like. Just talking about it can be a turn-on. Over time, if you can give each other at least some of what's being asked for, that could make lovemaking very satisfying again. You could also do a variation of the giver/receiver exercise on page 296, this time focused on pleasuring each other sexually; if you like, you could try this two ways (on different occasions), one in which you take each other to climax, and the other in which you get as close as possible and stay there without going over the edge.

    Perhaps read some books, alone or together, such as those listed at the end of this section (p. 304). Sex is many things, but one of them is that it's

If You Rarely Have an Orgasm

Around ten percent of women rarely or never orgasm, so you're not alone. It could be due to a medical problem, such as the ones discussed on page 289, or to psychological or interpersonal factors.

If you do not know how to have an orgasm on your own, we suggest using a mirror to look at your genitals and locate the clitoris, using this experience to get past any embarrassment and to appreciate the lovely, wondrous anatomy of a woman's sexual organs. Exploring masturbation* with your fingers or a vibrator is a good way to learn how to reach orgasm, knowledge you can bring into lovemaking with your partner (but don't get so used to the vibrator that you can't climax without it!).

If you can be orgasmic by yourself but not with your partner, there could be several reasons. For one, most women do not have orgasms through intercourse alone, but rather require direct stimulation of the clitoris. You may need to encourage your partner to give your clitoris more attention during lovemaking or let him know specifically what you like. Many men enjoy helping their partners climax. But if your partner doesn't seem motivated (e.g., lovemaking is over when he has had an orgasm) or skillful, try to talk with him about it. If that doesn't help, you could contact a sex therapist.

Another possibility is that it's hard for you to let go into orgasm, especially if someone, even a person you dearly love, is with you. Try to understand what the block is, such as childhood shame about sex, fear of losing control, reluctance to let someone have that power over you, or not wanting to give him the satisfaction of giving you an orgasm. Like any other psychological barrier, you can use the methods in chapters 2 and 3 to let it go. Building on your self-awareness, you can ask your partner for what you need in order to feel safer about letting go with him. Inside your own head, you can increase or decrease the sense of being-with-another by whether your eyes are open or closed, the amount of fantasizing you do, or the depth of emotional connection you let yourself feel; find the degree of being-with that still allows you to climax, and then gradually try to increase your sense of closeness while continuing to be able to come.

---

* *For Yourself* by Lonnie Barbach, Ph.D., is a sensitive guide to female sexuality and self-pleasuring.

a *skill* that anyone can get better at through a little study, attempting new things, and practice. Like many couples do, you might try looking at erotic pictures or videos, playing imaginatively (such as pretending it's the first time you made love), or experimenting with sex toys.

Some Resources About Sex

Our Bodies, Ourselves for the New Century by the Boston Women's
　　　Health Collective
For Yourself by Lonnie Barbach
Passionate Marriage by David Schnarch
Women Who Love Sex by Gina Ogden
The Mother's Guide to Sex by Anne Semans and Cathy Winks
The Art of Sexual Ecstasy by Margot Anand
Video instruction in various techniques; advertised in magazines such as *Harper's*
　　　and the *New York Times Book Review*
Seminars in sexuality, including tantra, an ancient system that integrates
　　　sexuality and spirituality; advertised in local magazines and newspapers

The most profound way to revitalize a sexual relationship is both the simplest and scariest: it is to open up more, *emotionally,* while engaged erotically with each other, from lingering looks to all-out lovemaking. Sex is so revealing that it is natural to get into a kind of role or script about it as a way to keep feeling safe: as the clothes come off, a subtle mask often comes on. But to be really open while all the intensities of sex—sensation, emotion, desire—tremble inside, bare nerve endings exposed to the eyes and touch of your lover, is incredibly exciting. It makes sex fresh again, every time.

Because love is the most tender of the intensities of sex, it is both the most thrilling and the most tempting to veil. For many of us, it is easy to be sexual, easy to be loving—but hard to be both at the same time. Nonetheless, in daily life, the seeming domain of love alone, can you sometimes open the gates of sexuality inside, letting the tingle of eros be present between you and your husband as you make a meal together, hand off a child, or say good-bye on your way to work? Or, when being sexual, can you and your mate open wide the gates of love? Then you touch with a cherishing in lips and fingertips, the giving of your bodies opening your hearts. Now raising children together adds to your love life instead of subtracting from it: you feel warmed by appreciation for each other, your sexuality an inherent part of the circle of love that is your family.

PART FIVE
Managing the Marathon of Motherhood

Motherhood is a long journey, a marathon, not a sprint. It begins before your first child is born: that incredible moment when you know you've conceived a new being, the long pregnancy, fixing up the baby's room, finally the birth itself, and then the little breathing bundle, the life delivered into your arms. The details differ a bit if you've adopted a child, but the essentials are the same: anticipation, nervousness, and an extraordinary love.

Some parts are a blur and others a long slow grind. Feeding, diapers, long nights with the baby, the first steps, the first words, the first everything. Tantrums, story time, bouncing a ball, wiping a chin, high chairs, tiny chairs, wiping crayons off chairs. Day care, nursery school, the first day of first grade, watching that sturdy back trudge down the hall to class. Camps, Cub Scouts, Girl Scouts, bullies, buddies, soccer games, Little League, balls caught, dropped, kicked, and lost. Chores, bedtimes, discipline, angry words and loving forgiveness. The grades tick by, good teachers and bad, science fairs and spelling lists, too much homework or not enough, that great moment when your child knows the answer to a question and you don't. Somewhere in there your youngest turns eight or ten and you think, *It's half over, where has the time gone?* Middle school, high school, pimples and makeup and dating and fingernails chewed after midnight until you hear a step at the door. Strange music and stranger friends, coltish and gawky, solemn and wise. All the while, the birthdays have ticked by, some with numbers that echo: one, two, six, ten, thirteen, sixteen. Then the eighteenth: what now?

The marathon doesn't end there, though it becomes more meandering and less consuming. Loans that are really gifts, advice that is rejected loudly and followed quietly, graduations, postcards from Mexico or Maui, the bittersweet joy of watching your child walk down a wedding aisle, a downpayment with your name on it. If your children have kids, your journey takes on a second sort of mothering. You age and your children don't seem to. There comes that time when the trajectory of your life is clearly falling back to earth as your children's ascends. You drift into old age and there is a subtle shift of care and power. And then the final moments come, your veined and aged hands in the strong ones of your children, squeezing, a kiss, a final blessing, a farewell, an ending to the path you walked as a mother, and the beginning of a mysterious new one.

It's a long, long road. That's why it's so important to have a few good tools for the practical problems that make your journey harder than it really needs to be. We've seen one bunch of problems, in particular, wear on women year after year: those involved in juggling home and work. In the next chapter, we'll look at how you can solve them while still being a highly giving mother.

Juggling Motherhood and Work

MANY WOMEN THESE DAYS ARE STRUGGLING to find ways to balance motherhood and work.* Whether you took a short leave and are now back at work full-time, have gone to a part-time schedule (perhaps switching careers to do so), or work at home, the juggle is never easy. If you don't currently work at a job, the decision to be a stay-at-home mom was likely a complicated one—as will be any return to work down the road. Consider these mothers we've known:

Donna had two daughters, seven and four, and a full-time job as a checker in a supermarket; she and her husband had separated a year after their second child was born. She came to see Jan about a cold that wouldn't go away. Jan asked what her days were like, and Donna replied matter-of-factly: *They're insane. There's no other word for it. Mario has the girls a couple days a week, but one's on the weekend, so your basic day has me up early to get things ready, drop them off at two different day cares, and get to work I hope on time. They're cranky because I have to hustle them along just to make the schedules work. And God help us if one is sick: Is she well enough for day care? Am I a bad person for infecting the other kids? Can I afford to stay home again this month? What if they call me and I have to leave work? There's no one else, I've got no family here. We get home and we're all fried, I can't be the kind of mom I want to be since I'm so tired, I put them to bed and half the time fall asleep with them and wake up groggy in the middle of the night with my neck scrunched into a corner of the bed. The whole thing's like a Swiss watch: if every little part works perfectly with every other part, then the day's OK. But how often does that happen?*

---

*Obviously, mothers "work" at home as well as "work" for pay in their occupation, but for simplicity, we'll use the word *work* in this chapter to refer collectively to one's job, career, or business. Many of the points made would also apply to an avocation that has a central place in a mother's life, such as art or a spiritual practice.

Astrid, a lawyer, had planned to return to work a few months after her first child, Sean, was born. But, as she put it to Rick when Sean was about six months old: *I just can't. I'm totally surprised I feel this way, but he's so little and I love him so much that I don't want to be away from him. I thought I'd nurse him for a month or so and then wean, but we're still going and it's so important I don't want to stop that either. But all this is creating a problem in my marriage. My husband wants me to go back to work because it's beyond tight without my income. But every day, Sean does something different and amazing, and I don't want to miss that or have some nanny be the one who gets to see it all.*

Cora was staying home with her two-year-old daughter, Tatiana, but, as she said at a talk Rick gave to a mothers' club: *It's getting old, and I'm starting to feel very restless at home. Put clothes on, take them off. Make a meal, clean up, and make it again. We go out for a walk, but no one's around, just us and the birds. I want to go back to work as a dental hygienist, but my husband thinks Tatiana is too young and his family agrees.*

Mandy had received an unexpected surprise at age forty-two: she was pregnant. Now, several years later, she was the full-time mother of a bouncy four-year-old boy, Isaac, having left her career as an art director for a major ad agency. She said to Rick: *I feel guilty about it—because being a mom is supposed to be wonderful and all, but I really miss my old job, the bustle of the office, the travel, the intensity, even the deadlines. It was like the world of an exciting color, you know, red. I totally love my son and I'm happy I'm here with him, but I get pretty bored being home all day, like my world has become beige. And me, as well: for example, my husband and I recently had dinner with people from his office. We introduced ourselves, everybody had interesting jobs, and then it got to me. I said I was mother and homemaker, they said, "Oh, how nice," and the conversation moved on. During dinner, people asked each other about their work, but no one asked me about raising Isaac. I felt dismissed and like I had nothing to offer. It made me mad.*

Claire worked at home as a freelance writer while raising Tim, just turned six, and Tammy, "age three, going on thirteen." Claire told Ricki: *People say I've got the best of both worlds, but it's more like the worst of both. I get calls at all hours, but especially in the morning since many of my clients are on the East Coast and everybody needs last-minute changes, so I have to take the calls. I heard Tammy once tell a little boy, "My mom's job is she's on the phone." Tim's in first grade, that's finally working, but child care for Tammy is one problem after another. She's in a great preschool, but the day care is expensive (and I miss her, I admit it). So I get her early, but then it's hard to do more than bits and pieces of work, and definitely no calls: try talking to an editor while your child keeps calling "Mommy"!*

Problems like these are so commonplace that it's natural to take them as a given. But until the last hundred years or so, motherhood and career were woven together into one seamless tapestry in which most women worked with their young children mainly nearby. While we couldn't endorse more strongly the principle that women should have the right to leave home for a job—or emphasize the fact that fathers could just as readily stay home with children—it remains that the modern division between home and work is completely unnatural. Yes, the industrialization that's driven these changes has brought many benefits, like safer childbirth, but one of its costs has been an unprecedented tension in the lives of many women between two callings. If a mother works, she misses her children. Yet if she stays home, she misses the income, camaraderie, and fulfillment of work.

So if you're feeling pulled in two directions, the first step is to let go of any guilt or self-blame: the tug-of-war between family and work is a modern invention, and none of it is your fault. Nor should it all be on your shoulders to fix or solve or bear—as it's construed so often, both in the media and across the dinner table—since it's a father's job just as much as it is a mother's to balance the need to have bread on that table with the need for vulnerable young children to have the attentive and loving care of someone who adores them.

In the swirl and press of raising a family, in the middle of a society that is breaking new ground each day, you can feel pressured to make quick decisions, go along with the views of a persuasive person or group, or simplify complicated matters by fastening upon one compelling "reason" for one choice or another. But that's not what would be most nurturing for you, plus it often leads to a less than ideal arrangement. Every mother has *options*: for example, even if you're a single mom or your family can't live without two incomes, there are almost always ways to work a little more or less, or manage your child care differently. In the next few pages we'll analyze the pros and cons of the options today and see how they fit with your deepest purposes in life and the needs of your family. And once you've made your choices—about a job, schedule, or child care—we'll explore the steps you can take to have them work for you. (If you are already clear about the choices you've made about staying home or working, you could skip ahead to the next section on making it work to stay home, p. 322, or to the section after that on making it work to work, p. 325.)

The work world has evolved as if employees had no families.

—*Marcia Killien, R.N., Ph.D.*

Making Choices About Working

A good deal of research has been done on the options for working and child care (see the boxes, pp. 314 and 317), which can help you make an informed decision, but even with all the knowledge in the world, you still have to thread your way through a messy bunch of tradeoffs.

For instance, studies have found that mothers who work are healthier than mothers who do not.* Sounds simple, right? But behind that headline, there's a more complex truth. Research findings are almost always about the *averages* of groups.† Yet you are a person, not an average! If you read a statement like "mothers who work are healthier than those who do not," you might conclude, reasonably enough, that you will be healthier if you return to work. But the statement really means only that "the average mother who works is healthier than the average mother who does not." In fact, many mothers who do not work are healthier than many mothers who do. The crux is always individual: What's right for *you* and *your family* in *your particular situation?* Let's look at the details that have to be considered to come up with the answer.

The Benefits of Working

The many rewards of working start with the enjoyment and fulfillment you experience from the work itself. There could be the feeling that you are using an important capacity within yourself, like a technical or managerial talent. Working offers the satisfaction of accomplishing a specific ambition (e.g., to be a teacher), and some lines of work give you the sense that you are making a contribution to society beyond your family. Certain jobs or careers also have prestige or social status. Last and usually not least, there's the additional money a job brings. As Ann Crittenden has shown in her book *The Price of Motherhood,* our nation's laws and policies place economic burdens and risks on all mothers, but they weigh most heavily on those who stay home with their children.

There are also pluses for the children of a working mother. Some of the physical or psychological health benefits she enjoys from working will spill over onto them—like her feeling more fulfilled, or less cranky from being cooped up with a child all day. A second paycheck means more money to buy them things, like better food and health care, or enriching experiences. Child care carries the benefit of

---

*Though this apparent benefit is inflated by other factors; for example, women who work are likely to be better educated, which is associated with better health practices and less illness. They also tend to have been healthier in the first place, since ill people are less likely to seek work.

†We're using the word *average* as a shorthand term for the various statistical measures of the central tendencies of groups.

time with other kids and caregivers, and some breathing room from mom.* Then there are future benefits to a child if his mom works when he's little: by not stepping off the career track—especially the fastest ones—she will probably have a larger salary when he's older.

There are other things about working that are good for a mother, but it's possible to enjoy each of them without going off to a job, depending on the all-important details of your own situation. Knowing this gives you the choice of seeking that benefit through work or through other arrangements.

- *Access to health resources.* A good job (usually) offers health insurance and money for doctors, but your husband's occupation may already provide those without you needing to work.

- *Sense of equality and clout with your husband.* Bringing home a paycheck can help you to feel that you are on an equal footing with him and give you more say in how money is spent and the family is run, but some relationships operate that way when the mother doesn't work.

- *General sense of accomplishment and recognition.* This need may already be fully satisfied by being a full-time mother.

- *Camaraderie and support with other people.* You may already be fortunate to have a strong sense of community with friends, neighbors, and other mothers.

- *Respite from children.* Definitely a benefit, but it's usually possible to get a break by taking steps such as swapping child care with a friend or enrolling your child in one more morning at the preschool.

The Costs of Working for You

Now comes the other side of the balance sheet: the benefits of working need to be netted against its costs. Physically demanding work—involving heavy lifting or exertion, or standing on your feet all day—has been associated with poorer health in mothers, especially during the first year after giving birth. Jobs that offer the employee little say in when and how specific tasks are done, especially low-level clerical positions, are a risk factor for cardiovascular problems in mothers. Moving from physical to mental health, you could feel uneasy, worried, or even upset at be-

---

*Though, in all fairness, this can be accomplished without child care, through spending informal time with other children and parents. Nor does one need to work to get a baby-sitter or put a child in preschool.

The Options for Working

The main options include:

- **No work at all.** Your partner, others (such as relatives), or savings support the family financially. Maybe you deliberately take on some debt, knowing you can return to work in a few years, and that a person's income normally rises as she gets older and more experienced. *Benefits:* Provides maximum time with your child, and easiest way to keep breast feeding. *Drawbacks:* You may feel isolated, unstimulated, or stressed with no relief.

- **Be a student.** More flexible scheduling than most jobs, often with more child care. Class load can be increased or decreased depending on the needs of you and your family. Much schoolwork can be done at home, or all of it through distance learning. Classes could be related to current career, or you could go in a new direction; check with your accountant, but the costs may be tax deductible. *Benefits:* A very direct way to satisfy the hunger for intellectual stimulation. *Drawbacks:* No income from you, additional costs for tuition and books, and a potential disruption of nursing.

- **Part-time.** You could cut back your hours, job share, or work as a temp. Perhaps the most common job choice for mothers of young children. *Benefits:* You get to keep one leg planted in the world of work and bring in some money. *Drawbacks:* Usually means stepping off the fast track of career advancement, a fairly rapid weaning (if your baby is still breast feeding), and additional income is offset by extra child care costs.

- **Full-time.** *Benefits:* Maximum income and career opportunities. *Drawbacks:* Maximum dependence on child care, time away from children, and potential tension between home and office. Even greater impact on breast-feeding than part-time work.

- **Telecommuting.** *Benefits:* Eliminates the commute and allows you to shift gears more smoothly between mother mode and work mode. *Drawbacks:* Can be hard to fend off a young child who knows you're in the house, and hard to get much work done. Often goes well if you have in-home child care, or if child is being cared for elsewhere some of the time you're home.

- **Self-employed.** Could be full- or part-time, at home or at your own office. *Benefits:* You're the boss, so it's not necessary to persuade anyone that you need some time off. Offers the satisfaction and potential financial rewards of building your own business. *Drawbacks:* Burden of responsibility and financial risks.

ing separated from your child. Or guilty, perhaps, at not being the sort of mother you want to be.

If nothing else, working means spending less time with your child, and sometimes missing special moments or milestones, like the first steps; to have as much time as possible with her children, an employed mother typically sleeps about five or six hours a week less than a stay-at-home mom. Working also means spending more time in traffic (unless you work at home), with the aggravations and expenses of commuting.

Meanwhile, the hassles of investigating, managing, or changing child care usually land on you; as the difficulty of arranging for child care rises, a mother's health tends to decline. Once everything is set up and work looks like clear sailing, your job still gets disrupted when a child is sick or needs to be taken to a doctor, and your partner can't or won't handle it. And if you are already heavily burdened, such as by a colicky baby who keeps you up at night or personal health problems, a job could be the proverbial straw that breaks your back. Adding it all up, it's not surprising that full-time employed mothers of infants report greater stress than do full-time homemakers with infants, and they often neglect their own health to cope with their total workload.

The Costs of Working for Both You and Your Family

Stresses from work can wear you down so you have less to give at home. Business travel causes separations that could be upsetting to you and your children. Going to work also means needing to find places and occasions to pump breast milk if you have continued nursing. These hassles are a major reason why returning to work (especially full-time) usually leads a mother to wean earlier than she otherwise would, which means losing the benefits of breast-feeding. In addition to the ways that nursing can be emotionally fulfilling for a mother and her child, continuing to breast-feed seems to help shield a woman from the effects of stress. The other benefits for children include a boost in IQ and fewer illnesses—some of the reasons why the American Academy of Pediatrics recommends that mothers nurse for at least one year, and the World Health Organization recommends at least two years.

For the family as a whole, mornings and evenings get especially frenzied when both parents work. At the beginning of the day, everybody zooms around getting dressed, packing lunches, and schlepping kids to child care. At the other end of the day, you've got to shove *so* much into a small sliver of time: hugs and kisses for children, questions like *How did it go at preschool?* or *Was Rory nice to you today?* and housework tasks that get pushed into the evening or weekend. When—finally—you get the kids to bed and the last dishes done or the laundry folded, it's hard to have much energy left for yourself or your relationship.

Adding to your stress, kids are often cranky from long hours in child care and more frequently ill from exposure to other children who are sick—and this brings us to the complex, sometimes touchy subject of the impact on kids of child care. Some research has found that moderate, high-quality child care, especially past the first birthday, has, on average, some benefits for language and social development without disrupting the attachment relationship between a typical parent and child, though it does seem to make some kids more aggressive. But the actual child care the majority of kids experience is completely different: it lasts for many hours each day, sometimes 7 a.m. to 7 p.m.; it is performed—often by one adult for four to six children—by poorly trained, poorly educated, and poorly paid staff with high rates of turnover; and it starts when children are just a few months old. Plus, the research instruments used to assess potential psychological injury to children cannot fully measure many subtle issues, such as a person's lifelong capacity for a deep, trusting intimacy. Then, even if one assumes there is no injury to a child, no lasting impact, there is still the matter of suffering: most young children do *not* like being separated from both of their parents. Finally, research on child care may not apply to your own child, who may be more sensitive or vulnerable than some other kids.

Our point here is not to make anyone feel guilty about using child care. Your child may do very well in child care or preschool, especially if it's a well-run program. And if your options are not so great but you still need child care, you pick the best setting possible and compensate for any less-than-perfect care in other ways. It's simply that child care needs to be used with a sensitivity to the possible impacts on your own unique child, for her sake as well as yours.

Resources for Child Care

The Anxious Parents' Guide to Quality Childcare by Michelle Ehrich
The Unofficial Guide to Childcare by Ann Douglas
The Nanny Book by Susan Carlton and Coco Myers
Child-Care Research in the 1990's by Deborah Vandell
National Network for Childcare: www.nncc.org
National Childcare Information Center: nccic.org
Single Parent Central: www.singleparentcentral.com/childcare.htm
www.home-childcare.com

Your Options for Child Care

The main options include:

- **Mr. Mom:** Dad stays home and watches the kids, either full- or part-time. Besides being the ultimate way for the father to fully engage the parenting role, this option sometimes makes economic sense, since a growing number of women make more money than their husbands.*

- **Relatives:** Could be the child's grandparents, older stepsister, aunt or uncle, or other kin. Care by people who consider the child "family."

- **Nanny, baby-sitter:** Possibilities range from a live-in, professional nanny to an older, good-hearted child who plays with a preschooler while Mom does work at home. The caregiver is not distracted by other children, but is often more expensive than a child care center. Also lacks the safeguards against potential abuse that exist in child care centers with other people present. Generally zero state regulation. You are legally responsible for paying employer taxes.

- **Home child care:** Frequently in the neighborhood close by. Convenient, informal, inexpensive. Often run by a kindly woman who is a mother herself. Typical ratios of one adult to two to six young children; caregivers may be spread thin. If solo caregiver, no checks and balances provided by other caregivers. Depending on the state, zero to moderate regulation.

- **Child care centers:** Sometimes conveniently located at job sites or preschools. More formal and usually more expensive than home child care. Usually moderate state regulation.

- **Preschools:** Same pluses and minuses of child care centers, plus a more explicit educational component (e.g., Montessori, Waldorf), and sometimes a religious one. Moderate state regulation.

---

*This option and the two that follow naturally need to include appropriate time for your child with other children.

Summing Up the Pros and Cons

The sensible way to think about work and motherhood is to consider different options—work or not? full- or part-time? this job or that one?—in terms of *this* mother with *this* child and *this* partner in *this* family with *this* child care possibility at *this* time. Let's suppose a mother, Jane, is debating whether to return to work or to continue staying home with her toddler, Tommy, and his big sister, Grace. If Jane is bored out of her skull staying home + Tommy is easygoing and would adapt quickly to child care + her husband is up for doing more housework + Grace is doing fine in preschool + there's a good home day care site just down the street + Jane already weaned Tommy months ago = Returning to work probably makes more sense than staying home. But what if the opposite were true? If Jane feels deeply satisfied with being a full-time mom + Tommy is anxious and clingy + her husband works very long hours + Grace is jealous of her brother and wants a lot of time with Mom + and Tommy is still nursing = staying home probably makes more sense.

Of course, in real life, the case for one option or another is usually a closer call: suppose Jane is climbing the walls at home and her husband is fine with doing more housework, but Tommy is anxious about separation and the child care options don't look very good. The needs of children must be balanced against the needs of their parents, who have rights, feelings, and wants that count, too. Even when you consider only the child, there are still tradeoffs: sometimes a "cost" to a child (such as adequate but less than optimal care) in one area is balanced by an even greater gain to the child in another area (such as a mother's greater patience because she is less stressed). Complicating things, there are the tradeoffs between present costs and benefits, and future ones: perhaps Tommy will be quite stressed at this time by Jane working, but he'll benefit in a few years from the additional income and seniority she'll have from continuing to work.

Overall, it's a tough decision, and either way Jane goes there will be problems. But the right decision for any mother, whatever it is, will be the one that considers all aspects of her situation—and then evaluates them *in light of her purposes and priorities in life.*

Using Purpose and Priorities to Inform Your Choices

When you are clear about your purposes and priorities, it is enormously easier to make fundamental decisions about working or not, and to inform daily choices. Say your boss offers you a plumb assignment, but it entails a day or two of business travel each month. If you know that your priority right now is maxing time with your family and you're deliberately treading water in your career, then you'll feel more peace of mind about turning down the opportunity. On the other hand, if you've decided to put more energy into your career, you'll feel easier inside about telling your child every few weeks that you have to go on a trip overnight, but you'll be back really, really soon.

When you have a clear direction in life, you don't have to continually reevaluate your choices, or agonize over the ones you've made. It helps you deal with people who are questioning, sniping at, or resisting the choices you've made; you know what you feel in your heart, and you're more able to explain your actions (if you need to). Even if you can't fulfill an important purpose right now or be entirely true to your priorities, clarity about what's awry helps you let go of self-blame, feel entitled to mourn what's missing, and be motivated to work on creating a life structure that's a better fit with your values.

So how do you come up with your essential purposes and priorities? Just like one sort of job might suit you but not another person, some ways of clarifying life purposes will speak to you while others will not. Therefore, here's a sampler of different methods (please see the resources on the next page for additional ideas):

- Imagine that you're nearing the end of your life. What do you want to make sure you are glad about, in terms of the choices you have made? What do you want to make sure you don't regret?

- Consider what you love doing: *What are my passions? What situations or activities make me very happy?*

- Reflect on your moral commitments: *What do I care about deeply? What larger cause(s) do I want to serve? How do I want to make a difference?*

- Consider how improving your functioning in some regard, such as remedying physical depletion, or cultivating psychological growth and wisdom, could be the catalyst or foundation for many positive things. Perhaps that form of personal healing or development should be a priority for the next few years.

- Think about the people you admire, your role models and your heroes and heroines. What are the characteristics or actions that inspire you? What might you like to emulate, in your own way, in one or more of these people?

- If this is meaningful to you, ask God for guidance as to what you're meant to do with your life in general, or with regard to work at this time.

- Make a collage from pictures and words cut or torn from magazines. You can do this on poster board or on individual sheets of paper in a notebook. The theme could be very broad, such as your purpose in life, or quite specific, such as how you want your transition back to working half-time to go.

- Ask your mate what he thinks your priorities should be at this time. He may have a fresh angle, but don't be overly swayed; the heart of the matter is what's in *your* heart.

- In one sentence (present tense), try to state your overall purpose in life.* It's not set in stone, and you can have a different purpose later on. Some examples: *My family is healthy and happy, and so am I. I live a life of health, happiness, and contribution. My life is an expression of Radiant Being. I am love, communication, and aliveness. I leave the world a better place. I live with integrity, humor, love, and grace.* Also, try to state your purpose as a *mother.*

- Consider how the priorities of family and career may not be in conflict, but could serve each other. For example, being successful at your job could be an important model for your children. Similarly, creating a solid, loving foundation at home could help you feel secure in venturing forward in your career.

Resources for Life Purpose and Priorities

A Year to Live by Stephen Levine
The 7 Habits of Highly Effective People by Stephen Covey
Do What You Love, the Money Will Follow by Marsha Sinetar
Creative Visualization by Shakti Gawain
The Road Less Traveled by M. Scott Peck
Gift from the Sea by Anne Morrow Lindbergh
East of Eden by John Steinbeck

Once you've clarified your purposes, it's worth taking some time to acknowledge the losses that are inherent in any choices you've made or will make. You can't have more of one thing without less of another, and we've never known a perfect arrangement of home and work for any mother.

---

*A variation on this method is found in Stephen Covey's discussion of a personal mission statement in *The 7 Habits of Highly Effective People.*

Next, we suggest you step back and take a long, honest look at your life. Start by asking yourself where you are living true to your purposes. Let yourself feel really good about that. Then—big breath—ask yourself where you are not. When you reflect on any gaps between your ideals and your actions, consider first whether it is possible, in fact, to close them. Maybe it just isn't right now: perhaps your family simply can't manage without your paycheck, or no matter how much you want to get back to your career, a chronically ill child needs you at home. If you can't pursue some important purpose at this time, the best you can do is to be compassionate with yourself about that, reach out for support, and keep trying to figure out how to fulfill your dreams.

On the other hand, maybe you *could* actually accomplish your purposes. Then it's really important for your well-being to try. If the problem is external, like no transportation to get to work, you could look into ride sharing or other jobs that are closer to bus lines. If it's internal, like feeling too shy to call people you once worked with to ask if they know about any jobs, you could use the techniques in chapters 2 and 3 to work on it. Usually there's some action, internal or external, that will give you a jump start and get the snowball rolling. For instance, a shy person could invite her former colleagues out for a casual lunch, and then, once the ice is broken, she could steer the conversation to her going back to work and see if they have any ideas.

Above all, seek the balance of family and work that will be truest to your nature, rather than conforming to what other people think. Perhaps you've run into one-size-fits-all thinking in the form of social pressure to work, or to stay at home. Advocates for either side can talk as if there's just one natural way to be, and selectively use scientific studies to make their case. But in truth, there is wide variation among women in their natural interest in mothering and working. One of Rick's clients had to muster up her courage to tell him: *I feel really bad about saying it, but a lot of the time, taking care of my daughters is really tiresome and irritating, and I just want to get away. There's no doubt I love them. But when I hear other moms go on about the bliss of motherhood, that's just not me. I have to work, or I'd go crazy—and that wouldn't be good for them, either.*

On the other hand, a different mom (who used to be a stockbroker) was laughing gently at herself one day in his office: *About a month before I was due with my first child, I sent out a letter to my clients saying I'd be back full-time after six weeks, not to worry. But I just fell in love with the little guy and something completely changed inside me. What had I been thinking?! There was no way I could be away from him all day and leave him with people who could never love him the way I did. Forget it! So we cut back, I stayed home, and I can hardly believe it, but now, several years later, I've become fulfilled by being a mother in a way I never imagined was possible. I can see a time ahead, maybe when he's in grade school, when I'll want to work again, but that's a ways off, and when it comes, it'll be natural.* The shape of your nature—as individual in its contours as a baby's footprint—may not fit neatly into the hole defined by one cultural model or another, and trying to jam it in or act like there's no friction puts needless stress on you and your family.

Making It Work to Stay Home

If you've decided to stay home full- or part-time, let's assume you're using the skills of inner competence discussed in chapters 2 and 3 to manage your stress, stay as relaxed as possible, and take in all the delicious rewards of this time. Additionally, your husband needs to understand that your role is not a piece of cake, and to be helpful when he's home. Perhaps most important of all, you need community (see p. 54), especially with mothers. That's what will break up the monotony of your day, give you emotional support and a helping hand, and satisfy the tug in your heart for the company of other moms.

With these as a foundation, let's look at practical steps you can take to have staying home work for you:

- *Leave your work mind behind.* This point is obvious, but it's so important we have to say it anyway: mothering is not like working. Just like your job calls for a specific set of skills and attitudes, so does staying home with children, which has totally different activities and priorities. You just can't do motherhood like a day at work. The same pace will frazzle your nerves. Nor should you demand the same kind of concentration or memory from yourself. A lack of mental clarity is natural when you're fatigued, depleted, or surfing big hormonal waves. But a deeper intelligence will replace that businesslike acuity, a maternal wisdom that naturally knows what to do most of the time.

- *Use your work skills.* On the other hand, there's no sense in forgetting the work skills you've got that could be useful at home, including creating policies, putting things on a calendar, and so on. As one mother said: *When I have to deal with the outside world, even just talking with the pediatrician, I kind of put on my business mind and let it do the talking. I'll even imagine that I'm wearing my business clothes. It helps me be more organized and confident.*

- *Take it easy and let yourself enjoy this time.* No doubt, there are the hard parts of staying home with children. Yet there are all the wonderful parts, too. Some mothers feel guilty about savoring these, as if they ought to be suffering the whole time, like everybody else is (supposedly) at work. But each day, you handle situations that are harder than anything most people deal with in a day of work, so when you get a chance to put up your feet and relax, grab it and linger. You don't have to keep the house spotless or prepare a fabulous meal every night in order to justify your (supposed) "vacation" as a homemaker: it's not a vacation, as anyone well knows who has taken care of young kids all day. You earned this time with your children, and it won't last forever. Finally, you *need* to rest and even laze about during the few times each day when you actually get the chance, in order to settle down the stress chemistry in your body and nurture your health and well-being.

- *Feed your mind.* There are lots of ways to keep your mind alive while tending to children or doing housework. Many women pursue a natural subject: child development, health, and family relationships. With the Internet, this knowledge is just a click away. Alternately, you could return to an interest or hobby you had before children, such as playing a musical instrument, writing letters to help free political prisoners, reading about history, or gourmet cooking. Or take up a new interest, even if it's only to the extent that you subscribe to a new magazine or spend more time in the local library. You could also take steps to stay current in your field so that any future reentry to work goes as well as possible, by maintaining subscriptions to trade journals, looking at Web sites, or going out to lunch with a friendly colleague every few months to catch up on the latest news.

  To be sure, some of these activities are hard to do with children nearby—unless you really like duets on the piano with a two-year-old!—but you can always find slivers of time for them, perhaps by enlisting your partner or others. And some things that feed your mind can be enjoyed with kids close at hand, such as listening to public radio or new kinds of music, or doing certain crafts. Reading books to preschoolers (especially older ones) can capture your imagination as well as theirs, especially with the intellectual challenge of simplifying vocabulary and dropping in necessary background explanations as you go along; we've enjoyed doing this with our own kids, and favorite books included *Peter Pan, The Hobbit* and *The Lord of the Rings,* and *Watership Down.*

- *Manage the boredom.* For us, the most unpleasant part of taking care of children all day is that it is often amazingly BORING. You do the same laundry, work the same puzzle, clean the same counter, jiggle the same mobile, read the same book, play the same game, over and over. That's when the desire to do *anything else* gets especially shrill. But what worked for us and other parents we know is to pay *closer* attention, noticing tiny details you'd normally overlook. This makes the activity suddenly more interesting and draws you into a more peaceful, contemplative awareness. Similarly, by putting your awareness into your body and releasing any tension or discomfort you find, you'll feel more comfortable and less eager to be somewhere else.

  It also helps to look for the nice parts in an activity, or nudge it in a more playful and stimulating direction. For example, you could goof around by putting puzzle pieces in upside down, and see what your toddler does. Or make up a song while she puts them in the right way.

- *Find respites.* Make sure to get some relief from interacting with your child every day. The possibilities include your partner giving him a bath while you read a good book or watch TV, another mom coming over with a child that will play with your own, or formal child care. In particular, study the conditions that drag the needle on your internal stress meter into the Red Zone, like more than four hours alone in your house with an oppositional three-year-old, and do everything in your power to change them so you never "redline" with stress.

- *Nurture your sense of worth.* To the extent that your job gave you a sense of accomplishment, status, or worth, staying home means finding other sources of self-esteem. The first place to look, of course, is your role as a mother: it's the plain truth that you are making an extraordinary contribution to your children, with results that are visible every time you see them, and the honor due you for that is magnified by any personal sacrifices you've made to be a mother.

  Widening the circle, you could get involved in your children's activities, such as by becoming a room-parent in preschool, soccer coach, or teacher in Sunday school. Besides being an excellent way to meet other mothers and families, it would give you a greater sense of making a difference in the world. These benefits also apply to other forms of community service, whether it's ladeling soup once a month at a homeless shelter or sitting on the board of a worthy nonprofit.

Finally, it's often possible to use some important capacity within yourself—some way that work stretched you—at home as well. For example, if you enjoyed applying your analytical intelligence to solve problems at work—perhaps you were a CPA, scientist, or computer programmer—you could read fascinating but mentally challenging books such as *Gödel, Escher, Bach* or *A Brief History of Time.* If you worked in TV, try volunteering with community access television. If you liked public speaking, consider arranging to spend an evening each week with a local chapter of Toastmasters.

For other suggestions on maintaining your sense of worth, see chapter 3, pages 76 to 85.

- *Check in with yourself.* Keep paying attention to how it's actually going for you. Are you feeling isolated? Is there a frustrated sense of the world passing you by? If you try some of the suggestions above and you still feel that something important is missing, it could be a sign that you need to shift gears, perhaps by returning to work.

Making It Work to Work

The foundation of staying sane while working is the same as if you were at home full-time: solid stress relief skills, support from your partner, and community with other mothers and families. On top of that, here are some practical actions you can take to have working work for you:

- *Finding a family-friendly workplace.* Sometimes you're stuck with a job, but usually, you've got some options. Before a planned pregnancy, you could look around for an employer that's more family-friendly than your current one, or start a business of your own; the same applies if you've taken significant time off your old job before returning to work. If you've come back to work some time ago, but the current situation is far from ideal, look around, using the want ads, headhunters, or resources on the Internet. You may also want to make a longer term plan and get specific training or experiences that will improve your skills and give you more options in the labor market.

When you evaluate different opportunities, consider the family-related aspects of each job (in addition to the standard ones): Paid pregnancy leave? On-site child care? Flextime? Telecommuting? Would your boss be sympathetic to your commitment to your children? Chance to avoid frequent business travel? Timesaving conveniences on the corporate campus, like ATMs, gyms, laundry services, or stores? The way you're likely to feel when you get home at the end of a day? Bottom line—what's the wear and tear going to be on your body and mind?

- *Managing maternity leave.* The Family Medical Leave Act (FMLA) requires businesses with fifty or more employees to give women twelve weeks of unpaid leave, but many companies are not affected by the FMLA, and those that are vary in their individual policies. Make sure you are crystal clear on the details that apply to you, keep a copy of the employee manual or any other applicable records, and take written notes of relevant conversations with a benefits manager or your boss. Once you know what you're working with, try to make a plan that's as flexible as possible, because there's a lot of inherent uncertainty about how you will feel and how it will go with your baby, especially if you're a first-time mom. You don't have to give in to pleas or pressure from people at work to return sooner than you'd like: just keep listening to that wise voice inside you that knows what's best for you and your family.

- *Continuing to breast-feed.* As we've seen, there are many benefits to you and your child of continuing to nurse while going off to a job. In some cases, you could nurse her at your work site (through on-site child care or a nanny bringing her to you), zip over to see her if you live (or she's in child care) nearby, or just go down the hall if you work at home. But more commonly, breast-feeding while working means pumping at work. Unfortunately, most workplaces are at best unhelpful when it comes to pumping, without any place more private than the ladies' rest room, and some are downright hostile.* Happily, many resources can help you continue with breast-feeding while you work, including articles in *Mothering* magazine (look to their Web site, www.mothering.com, for a listing), or the LaLeche League. A lactation consultant (your OB/GYN or midwife can refer you to one) can advise you about pumping or storing breast milk. Finally, for most mothers, feeling encouraged to continue breast-feeding—by a partner, other mothers, and hopefully coworkers—is vital, and it's appropriate to ask openly for the support you and your baby need.

---

*Besides stressing mothers, this attitude is shortsighted from a strictly business perspective. For example, one study found that working mothers who pumped breast milk had lower absentee rates than comparable mothers who weaned their babies (due to fewer colds and other illnesses in their children that required Mom to come home).

- *Dealing with coworkers who grumble that you're getting special treatment.* There's no need to skulk around or pretend that you're childless, but you could also take reasonable steps to stay off their radar screens, like scheduling doctor appointments after work or during your lunch hour (if possible), and not using work time to chat about children. Do what's reasonable to make up any missed work. If you can't attend a meeting or go on a business trip, tell your manager in advance so you and she can make other arrangements, and talk with any coworkers that may be affected.

- *Standing up for your rights.* If you feel that you are being discriminated against at work due to being a mother—such as unreasonable exclusion from certain meetings, career opportunities denied, or outright demotion or firing—contact the National Partnership for Women and Families (202-986-2600; www.nationalpartnership.org) and they can help you understand your rights.

- *Stopping work from spilling over onto home.* The occasional call from the office is one thing, but it's another to have already limited time with your children and husband routinely interrupted and consumed by work. You may need to create a polite but firm boundary at your job, delegate more, or insist on increasing staffing so that the tasks that somehow can't wait at 5:30 p.m. get done earlier in the day, when they should have been. Even without the phone ringing, if you're preoccupied by a problem at work, it could help to talk about it briefly with your mate, perhaps blowing off some steam, so you can set it aside for the next day.

- *Working at home.* But what do you do if you work *at* home? Four million or more corporate employees work from home at least part-time—lots of them mothers—and many other moms run home-based businesses. To stay both relaxed and productive, try to minimize interruptions that are not work-related, like letting the phone machine pick up a call from a friend that you'll return later. Make it clear to your children, friends, and husband that even though you're home you're still in worker mode and need to have your time and focus of attention respected. If you feel isolated, call or e-mail people at the office, get out of your home—even if it's only to do some business reading over lunch—or perhaps arrange for a coworker or assistant to come see you. It's especially important to keep your manager posted on your output if you're not in the office. Finally, don't let work fill your home like a bad case of bermuda grass: schedule specific times to be on the job, and keep work materials in specific places, like inside a home office or on a particular desk.

- *Stopping home from spilling over onto work.* Fathers seem generally able to drop any concerns about children on their way out the door, but many mothers have a harder time doing that because of their visceral connection to their kids. If there's something you really need to pay attention to during the day, like the status of a child who may be too sick to stay in child care, then so be it: make discreet phone calls and give your manager a heads-up that you might have to take a long lunch or go home early.

  But if it's one of those common but more diffuse problems—like wondering why your four-year-old still has a case of the terrible twos—you could make a mental appointment with yourself to think or worry or plan about it at a specific time that day, like during lunch, or at your desk for fifteen minutes (no one has to know what you're pondering). And do what you can to have your husband handle a big piece of the problem himself: maybe it makes more sense for him to set up an appointment with a doctor, or make a few calls to start the ball rolling on getting a different baby-sitter.

  Some work sites are friendly places where people feel quite open about their personal situations, whether it's grousing about a balky car or comparing notes to see whose child is the pickiest eater. But some aren't so chatty, and it's prudent to err on the side of caution because—unfair as it is—it's not hard to stir up doubts about a woman's capacity to focus on her job if there are any issues with her children. You can always choose to explain something in the future, but once you've spilled your guts about a problem at home, it's all out on the table and there's no way to unsay it. Besides, it's your private life. You don't need to apologize, or preempt anticipated criticism from others by doing it first to yourself: *I'm so sorry, my baby got sick again.* Babies get sick, toddlers freak out because they just can't stand it any longer not seeing their mommy, and preschoolers fall off of jungle gyms—and not one bit of it is because of you, and a fair-minded and neutral person would say that it's always more important in the larger scheme of things to take care of your child that day than it is to take care of some task at work. If you've got to leave to handle something, make your apologies with dignity, and then take care of any unfinished work as soon as you're able. That's all anyone can do.

- *Shifting gears from work to home.* During the transition from work to home, use the commute to send your mind in a more relaxing direction by listening to books on tape, inspirational talks, or soothing music. Think about your children, how nice it will be to see them, and how you'd like the evening to go. When you get home or to the child care center, perhaps wait a few minutes to clear your mind, go for a short walk, or simply relax in your car with a magazine. Walking up to your front door, imagine that you are placing any job worries into a basket outside your home, where you can retrieve them on your way to work in the morning—if you really want to. When you first see your children, whether at child care or in your living room, try to let them have your full attention for a while; once they've had a recharge of mommy juice, it's usually easier to slip away for a bit to change clothes, flip through the mail, or make a quick call.

- *Getting help from your husband.* When you're going off to work, you *really* need a partner who does his share at home. While fathers whose wives work tend to do more than fathers whose wives are full-time mothers, working mothers still typically do more total work than their husbands. If you feel your partner should pitch in more, try the techniques in chapters 6 and 7. You could also tell him that researchers have found that dads who help more with children have greater well-being than dads who do not.

- *Handling business travel.* The biggest transition from work to home occurs when you walk through the door after a business trip. This scenario is more common than ever, since millions of women—many of them mothers—take one each year. To ensure that going out of town doesn't mean going out of your mind, try to arrange the details in advance with your husband, like a written note listing the kids' vitamins. Many dads step up without a quibble, but if your husband grumbles, remind him that your business trip is a both-of-us-problem, not a me-problem, and it's more than fair for him to do his part without dropping any guilt bombs on you.

  For the kids, you could show them on a calendar when the trip is coming up, the day(s) you'll be gone, and when you'll be back. Try to be understanding with any distress; on the other hand, while you may regret that you need to travel, you don't need to be guilty or apologetic. For your time away, try to leave daily notes and treats from Mom, and maybe a present to open each night. Most children old enough to talk will appreciate a daily phone call, perhaps both morning and night; some out-of-town moms also like to send e-mails. Or—wild idea—take the kids with you. Maybe your spouse could come along, or a friend with children, who'd be happy to take your child along on day trips while you're in meetings. If it's just you and your child, look into child care in the city you're traveling to or neat activities for kids; perhaps your employer will pick up some or all of the bill.

For yourself, really enjoy the nice parts of business travel, like room service, peace and quiet, and someone else doing the laundry. This is a chance to catch up on some long-overdue self-nurturing. And you might like to bring stuff from home to feel connected: photos, kids' drawings, a mug decorated by a child, and so on. Stop your imagination from running away into catastrophic thinking—*Ohmigod, the house has burned down*—but feel free to call home, even at odd hours, to reassure yourself. If any guilty or anxious feelings persist, use the techniques in chapter 3.

Nonetheless, even with all the clever strategies in the world, sometimes it's just not right to go out of town: maybe there's a performance in the Christmas play at preschool, or the third trip in four months is simply too much. You're not alone in saying no; two in three parents have turned down a business trip that conflicted with some activity of their children's. Talk with your manager as soon as possible, and see if anyone else can go or if there are any alternatives, like videoconferencing. Over the long term, you may want to join other parents at work to push for policies on business travel that take families into account, like not having to spend an extra night in order to save on airfare.

- *Helping kids feel connected to you at work.* When you drop a baby or toddler off at child care, tell him how much he's in your thoughts and your heart while you're at work, and how he can feel your love inside him all day long; in a mysterious way, he may get the gist of what you are saying, and he will certainly sense your care and love.

   With a preschooler, make sure he has a photo of you at school (maybe of you working). You could also tuck a picture or note into his lunchbox each day, and perhaps call to check in, as long as that doesn't make him upset. If possible, arrange for him to visit your office, maybe on a Saturday when things are less hectic. He could meet your colleagues at company events, or you could have one or two over for dinner. Explain what you do, tell stories about coworkers, or describe the physical setting of your job; you could even bring a disposable camera to work and take a series of photos, starting with the outside of your workplace, then moving through doors or down hallways to where you work, maybe with pictures of some of your coworkers. At night, have him imagine a glowing, golden rope connecting him to you throughout the day; in the morning, remind him that whenever he wants, he can feel that cord joining you together.

- *Picking up signals.* Keep your radar out for signs that two parents working is taking a toll at home, like a toddler who's getting increasingly clingy or a five-year-old becoming quiet and withdrawn. Some changes may simply be necessary, like Dad coming home sooner or you starting work later. Both of you might have to give the kids more one-to-one attention every day, no matter how tired you are. For a reality check, estimate how much time daily *each* kid receives from *each* parent that's *child-centered* (following the child's interests, and not task-focused, correcting, or scolding); if it's less than fifteen minutes (the minimum a child needs—and many could really use more), you and your mate should make some adjustments if it's at all humanly possible: besides being good for your child, it will prevent problems that will take even more of your time in the future.

- *Learning from others.* Over the years, many women have blazed trails for working mothers. At your job, there are probably other moms—perhaps even your supervisor—who can mentor you about the ins and outs of juggling home and work at your company. Some corporations have support groups for mothers who work there. Part-time professionals can link up with each other, like attorney mothers who work part-time having a brown-bag lunch each month at a different law firm.

- *Using your time well.* At the most practical level, having a job means finding ways to get more done in less time, from shopping later at night when the supermarket's empty to hiring a responsible teenager with a car to run errands for you a few hours each week. This is such a universal problem that just about every issue of a magazine for women is loaded with tips, and you can learn more from some of the books listed on the next page under Resources for Working Mothers.

- *Saying goodbye to "Supermom."* It's hard for a working mother to avoid the traps of feeling that she has to go overboard at home to make up for having a job, or to be a superstar at work to make up for having a family. Sometimes the prick of guilt feels more like a knife in the ribs. For instance, one mother said: ***I'd been buried under a pile of work for a couple of weeks, but finally I had a chance to catch up on things. Then I found an invitation to a birthday party in all the stuff my son brings home from kindergarten—that had happened three days ago. He really liked the boy and I felt horrible about him not going. I started to cry, I was so mad at myself.*** Sure, it's important to do what you can to stay on top of the details at work or home. But it's almost impossible to avoid some stuff slipping through the cracks. Most of us need to accept the fact that we cannot be outstanding in each of two separate areas, in both our career and our parenthood. Still, a person can be outstanding at the *package* of the two, *outstanding at being a parent who works.* When you redefine your overall job description that way, it's a challenge you can actually succeed at. Sometimes an excellent performance in the *total* job requires doing less at work or at home. Or saying *No,* even if that means disappointing a coworker, spouse, or child. Or making a special effort to nurture yourself in one setting—such as by slowing down, connecting with others, or focusing on activities you particularly enjoy—so that you can excel in the other one, year after year, throughout the marathon of motherhood.

Resources for Working Mothers

Mothering magazine (www.mothering.com)
Working Mother magazine
LaLeche League International, (800) 525-3243
www.bluesuitmom.com
The Womanly Art of Breastfeeding by Gwen Gotsch and Judy Torgus
Nursing Mother, Working Mother by Gale Pryor
Working Mothers 101 by Katherine Wyse Goldman
Time Management from the Inside Out by Julie Morgenstern
Be Your Best: The Family Manager's Guide to Personal Success by Kathy Peel
Organizing from the Inside Out by Julie Morgenstern
Chore Wars: How Households Can Share the Work and Keep the Peace by
       James Thornton
Home Comforts : The Art and Science of Keeping House by Cheryl Mendelson

AFTERWORD

The most immediately effective ways to nurture yourself are personal, like getting enough sleep, and that's why we've focused on those. But no one raises her children in a vacuum, and we need to acknowledge the impersonal forces that stress and deplete mothers.

For example, poverty, injustice, and war strain and frighten families worldwide. The persistent devaluing of women and their work, notably raising children, burdens mothers emotionally and financially. Sweeping changes in the social environment in which humans evolved to raise families have eroded the community support that once lightened the loads and lifted the spirits of mothers.

Therefore, Mother Nurture is, fundamentally, a *societal* issue. A nation that truly nurtured mothers, families, and marriages would value childrearing in its deeds, not just its words. It would have policies like those found in many modern, industrialized countries, such as paid parental leave, subsidized child care, and community property laws in the case of divorce. It would strongly encourage fathers to have a major role in the care of young children and to pull their weight at home. In the broadest sense, it would protect the world its children will inherit through preserving peace, justice, and the environment.

This vision of a nation that nurtures its mothers is not idealistic, but hardheaded pragmatism. Yes, the work of mothers is moral: tending to vulnerable children whose beings are entrusted to our care. But it is also highly practical, raising young people to be productive citizens, creating the "human capital" that is the basis of progress and prosperity. A society fulfills its ethical obligations to its children, as well as makes a shrewd investment in its future, when it spends the time, the money, and the caring to nurture its mothers.

Whenever you nurture yourself or your family, are kind to children and mothers and fathers, support organizations that help families, or otherwise contribute to a safe and peaceful world, you take a stand for such a society, and ripples spread out from your actions. If enough of us take those stands, our country and this earth will become a better place to raise children, and to be a parent.

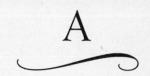

Defining Depleted Mother Syndrome

W HEN A MOTHER'S DEPLETION is long-standing, severe, and harmful to her health, we propose that she has the Depleted Mother Syndrome (DMS).

What Is a Syndrome?

A syndrome is a group of signs and symptoms that occur together and can help predict a person's prognosis and guide her treatment. Examples of syndromes include premenstrual syndrome (PMS) and acquired immune deficiency syndrome (AIDS).

A syndrome is typically not as well defined as a "disease" or a "disorder." It can be caused by more than one thing, present a variety of symptoms, take a varying course, and respond to more than one treatment. And it can incorporate several individual disorders within its overarching umbrella. For example, a person with chronic fatigue syndrome may have arthritic conditions and insomnia as well as fatigue itself. Similarly, a woman with DMS may have nutritional deficiencies, sleep disturbance, infection in her digestive tract, and depression, each of which is a health problem in its own right. The various elements of a syndrome appear together because they have underlying causes in common, or they lead to each other.

In sum, we suggest that the elements of maternal depletion form a coherent whole, organized in self-perpetuating ways, that is a diagnostically distinct and meaningful condition.

Diagnosis of Depleted Mother Syndrome

Depleted Mother Syndrome is defined as *a biopsychosocial condition in which the combination of a mother's outpouring, stresses, vulnerabilities, and (low) resources drain and dysregulate her body.* Specifically, we propose the following criteria for a diagnosis of DMS:

1. ***History of outpouring, stress, vulnerabilities, or low resources related to raising children.*** Indicated by the combination of:
   - *Outpouring:* Such as two or more pregnancies, or extended nursing
   - *Stress:* Such as raising young children, caring for a child with a challenging temperament or a health problem, or serious conflicts with her partner.
   - *Vulnerabilities:* Such as a history of trauma, preexisting physical or mental health problems, or a reactive or sensitive temperament
   - *Low resources:* Such as poor nutrition, little chance for rest, minimal help from her partner, little care of children by others, or lack of community.

2. ***Drained nutrients.*** Indicated by laboratory findings of low levels of important nutrients, such as vitamins, minerals, amino acids, or essential fatty acids.

3. ***Dysregulated systems.*** Indicated by signs and symptoms that one or more of the following systems are significantly dysregulated: gastrointestinal, nervous, endocrine, or immune.

4. ***Rule out other medical conditions.*** The drained nutrients or dysregulated systems are not caused by another medical condition (although other medical conditions may coexist with DMS).

Individual Variations

DMS can vary from woman to woman in terms of its severity, duration, and course.

Differential Diagnosis

Postpartum depression (PPD). The current (somewhat controversial) definition of PPD is that it is a major depressive episode that begins within four weeks of delivery and is resolved within six to twelve months after the baby's birth.* DMS differs from postpartum depression in several ways:

- DMS is based on physical depletion (which is not part of the definition of PPD).
- The symptoms of DMS do not necessarily include depression.
- DMS often appears a year or more after the baby has been born, because of the gradual accumulation of depletion.
- DMS can linger long after the first year postpartum.

The "maternal depletion syndrome." Several years after Rick coined the term "depleted mother syndrome," we found references to a "maternal depletion syndrome" suffered by malnourished women in Third World countries who commonly bear and breast-feed multiple children with short birth intervals. DMS differs from the maternal depletion syndrome (MDS) in two regards. First, we use the term *depletion* to refer to specific, moderate to severe nutritional deficiencies in an otherwise reasonably well fed person, while in the context of MDS, depletion generally refers to an overall condition of (sometimes extreme) malnutrition. Second, our definition of depletion includes disturbed bodily systems; MDS focuses on nutritional shortages. In essence, DMS is a broader and milder condition than MDS, and it is rooted in the social context of industrialized nations. Clearly, we were not the first people, by any means, to be concerned about the depletion of mothers. Whether the construct of DMS can be applied in Third World settings far removed from our professional experience remains to be seen, and we offer it respectfully for consideration by scholars and professionals working in that area.

---

*Shoshana Bennett, Ph.D., and other professionals argue that postpartum-related mood disorders might well have an onset later than four weeks after childbirth, symptoms that are more volatile and complex than those of a major depressive episode, and a course that continues past the baby's first birthday.

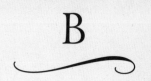

Resources for Your Health and Well-Being

*T*REMENDOUS RESOURCES ARE AVAILABLE these days for anyone who wants to take an active role in her own health and well-being, from laugh-out-loud memoirs of motherhood to consumer-oriented Web sites, medical reference books, or disease prevention handouts from your doctor. We think the ones mentioned below are the cream of the crop.

Reflecting on Motherhood

The foundation of caring for your health as a mother is understanding the whys and wherefores of everything that's happened to you since you became a mom. There are many excellent books out there, and here are some that we've gotten a lot out of ourselves.

Personal Experiences

Operating Instructions, Anne Lamott. Fawcett Books, 1994. Intimate, hilarious, inspiring description of life as a new mother.

Mothers Who Think, Camille Peri and Kate Moses, eds. Villard, 1999. Excellent collection of first-person stories of motherhood by gifted writers.

A Slant of Sun, Beth Kephart. William Morrow, 1998. Beautifully written account of raising a child with special needs.

Mother's Nature, Andrea Alban Gosline, Lisa Burnett Bossie, and Ame Mahler Beanland, eds. Conari Press, 1999. Wonderful gathering of heart-warming passages from many authors.

Scholarly Perspectives

The Birth of a Mother, Daniel N. Stern, M.D., Nadia Bruschweiler-Stern, M.D., and Alison Freeland. Basic Books, 1998. Sensitive description of the inner transition to motherhood.

Of Woman Born, Adrienne Rich, Ph.D. W. W. Norton, 1976. Ground-breaking discussion of "motherhood as experience and institution."

The Mask of Motherhood, Susan Maushart, Ph.D. The New Press, 1999. Passionate, funny, erudite tour of the hard parts of being a mother and the social prohibitions aganst acknowledging them.

The Transition to Parenthood, Jay Belsky, Ph.D., and John Kelly. Follows three couples as they become parents; excellent integration of personal details and research findings.

The Chalice and the Blade, Riane Eisler. Harper & Row, 1987. Fascinating, eye-opening exploration of the hunter-gatherer cultures in which humans evolved—and in which women and mothers, arguably, played a much more central role than they do today.

The Postpartum Period

What to Expect the First Year, Arlene Eisenberg, Heidi E. Murkoff, and Sandee Hathaway, B.S.N. Workman Publishing, 1989. Thorough, sensible suggestions from the authors of *What to Expect While You're Expecting.*

Postpartum Survival Guide, Ann Dunnewold, Ph.D. and Diane G. Sanford, Ph.D. New Harbinger Publications, 1994. Practical guide, particularly focused on coping with postpartum emotional issues.

After the Baby's Birth—A Woman's Way to Wellness, Robin Lim. Celestial Arts, 1991. Thoughtful, holistic suggestions for well-being during the challenging first year with a baby.

For help with postpartum depression (PPD), contact these organizations:

POSTPARTUM SUPPORT INTERNATIONAL
(805) 967-7636
927 North Kellogg Avenue
Santa Barbara, CA 93111
www.postpartum.net
   Offers referrals to support groups, advocates for mothers, and presents conferences.

THE MARCÉ SOCIETY
P.O. Box 30853
London, W12 OXG
United Kingdom
www.marcesociety.com
> *For professionals who research or treat postpartum mental health problems; holds biennial conference.*

Raising a Family

The cliché that children don't come with a manual carries a profound truth: every parent is thrust into the most difficult and the most important job in the world as a complete beginner who has to figure out how to do it all on the fly. These books have helped guide our learning—and prevented a few disasters.

The Continuum Concept, Jean Liedloff. Addison-Wesley Publishing Company, 1977. Classic exposition of the natural child rearing environment that fosters secure attachment and child well-being.

Natural Family Living, Peggy O'Mara. Pocket Books, 2000. Excellent resource by the publisher of *Mothering* magazine, who is a staunch advocate for mothers and a gifted writer.

Your Baby and Child, Penelope Leach, Ph.D. Knopf, 1997. Thorough, sensible guide to raising children, from newborns to five-year-olds.

The Interpersonal World of the Infant, Daniel N. Stern, M.D. Basic Books, 2000. Scholarly but highly readable integration of research and psychoanalysis that offers useful insights into the experience of an infant with his or her mother.

Raising Your Spirited Child, Mary Sheedy Kurcinka. HarperPerennial Library, 1992. Encouraging, practical suggestions for children with a high-energy temperament.

Positive Discipline, a series of books by Jane Nelsen and others. Depending on the ages of your children, you'll find loving and effective ways to cultivate good values and good behavior.

Skills for Your Mind and Your Relationships

Though written for anyone, these books contain helpful perspectives and tools that can be applied to the specific issues of a mother and her partner.

Kitchen Table Wisdom: Stories That Heal, Rachel Naomi Remen, M.D. - Riverhead Books, 1997. Collection of brief (most are one to three pages) stories of personal challenge and healing, told in the author's warm, comforting, and wise voice.

The Road Less Traveled, M. Scott Peck, M.D. Simon and Schuster, 1997. A soul-searching blend of psychology and spirituality.

The HeartMath Solution, Doc Childre and Howard Martin, with Donna Beech. HarperSanFrancisco, 1999. Presents practical techniques for lowering stress, releasing negative emotions, and tapping the native intelligence of the human heart.

The 7 Habits of Highly Effective People, Stephen R. Covey. Fireside, 1990. A classic for good reason. Penetrating consideration of core principles of mental health and interpersonal effectiveness.

Wherever You Go, There You Are: Mindfulness Meditation in Everyday Life, Jon Kabat-Zinn. Hyperion, 1995. An accessible, commonsense, and warmly written introduction to meditation and mindfulness.

Emotional Intelligence, Daniel Goleman, Ph.D. Bantam Books, 1997. Fascinating survey of how the brain processes emotion, with plenty of practical applications.

Focusing, Eugene T. Gendlin, Ph.D. Bantam Books, 1982. Describes a fundamental method for becoming highly aware of one's experience and helping it shift into a more positive direction.

The Dance of Anger: A Woman's Guide to Changing the Patterns of Intimate Relationships, Harriet Lerner, Ph.D. HarperCollins, 1997. A calm, clear guide to managing anger in relationships.

You Just Don't Understand, Deborah Tannen, Ph.D. Ballantine Books, 1990. Fascinating guidebook to the different ways that men and women tend to communicate; full of practical suggestions.

Why Marriages Succeed or Fail: And How You Can Make Yours Last, John Gottman, Ph.D., and Nan Silver. Fireside, 1995. Excellent combination of research information and practical advice, from a leading researcher on marriages.

Health Care Information

The Internet has hundreds of Web sites offering research information and suggestions about how to improve your health. Here's a sampling of our favorites:

- National Institutes of Health; www.nih.gov
- Centers for Disease Control and Prevention; www.cdc.gov
- National Women's Health Information Center; www.4woman.gov
- National Women's Health Network; www.womenshealthnetwork.org
- Yale Library: Selected Internet resources; info.med.yale.edu/library
- National Center for Complementary and Alternative Medicine, a division of the National Institutes of Health. Has fact sheets for consumers, results of clinical trials, and a wealth of other information; www.nccam.nih.gov Also see www.noah-health.org for information about complementary treatments for numerous health conditions.
- The Richard and Hinda Rosenthal Center at Columbia University; cpmcnet.columbia.edu/dept/rosenthal
- The Research Council for Complementary Medicine; www.rccm.org.uk
- American Botanical Council; for information about herbs, see www.herbalgram.org
- Transitions for Health Women's Institute. Knowledgeable about hormone imbalance, and a good source of referrals to professionals who are experienced with the spectrum of care; www.tfhwomensinstitute.com
- www.medscape.com—Extensive information on health care subjects for physicians and other professionals; some handouts on selected topics for consumers; search engine
- www.medmd.com—Consumer oriented website loaded with health care information

You can also read about your health in these books:

Women's Bodies, Women's Wisdom (2nd Ed.), Christiane Northrup, M.D. Bantam Books, 1998. Thorough, friendly handbook on women's health.

Encyclopedia of Natural Medicine (2nd Ed.), Michael Murray, N.D., and Joseph Pizzorno, N.D. Prima Publishing, 1997. Excellent coverage of nutritional medicine (with hundreds of research citations), including in-depth summaries of how to treat seventy conditions.

Staying Healthy with Nutrition, Elson Haas, M.D. Celestial Arts, 1992. Great detailed reference book on nutrition.

Nutrition Made Simple, Robert Crayhon, M.S. M. Evans & Co., 1996. Excellent introduction to nutrition; easy reading and filled with useful information.

Fats that Heal and Fats that Kill, Udo Erasmus. Alive Books, 1999. Everything you ever wanted to know (and more) about fats. Quite technical.

Smart Fats: How Dietary Fats and Oils Affect Mental, Physical and Emotional Health, Michael Schmidt, D.C. Frog Ltd., 1997. Lots of information about fats and oils. Readable for a beginner, but still full of important material.

The Web That Has No Weaver (2nd Ed.), Ted Kaptchuk. Contemporary Books, 2000. Beautiful introduction to Chinese medicine.

Everybody's Guide to Homeopathic Medicines (3rd Ed.), Stephen Cummings and Dana Ullman. J. P. Tarcher, 1997. Easy-to-use guide for homeopathic remedies.

The Family Guide to Homeopathy, Andrew Lockie and William Shevin. Fireside, 1993. Another well-done introduction to homeopathy, with attention to children's health.

Health Care Professionals

The Insider's Guide (appendix E) discusses the spectrum of licensed health care providers. For referrals to physicians in general, see:

- American Medical Women's Association. Focus on women's health; www.amwa-doc.org
- American Medical Association. The largest association of physicians in America; www.ama-assn.org

For referrals to licensed professionals oriented toward complementary and alternative medicine, see:

- American Association of Naturopathic Physicians. Graduates of accredited naturopathic medical schools and licensed in a limited number of states. Usually very knowledgeable in nutrition and the alternative methods in the spectrum of care; www.naturopathic.org
- American College for the Advancement of Medicine. Association of physicians practicing complementary medicine; www.acam.org

- American Association of Colleges of Osteopathic Medicine. National association of colleges that train osteopaths, with information about osteopathy; www.aacom.org

- American Holistic Medical Association. Physicians and other licensed health care providers; www.holisticmedicine.org

For other professional groups, see:

- National Certification Commission for Acupuncture and Oriental Medicine. Certifies acupuncturists for licensure in most states; www.nccaom.org

- American Association of Oriental Medicince. Professional association of acupuncturists; www.aaom.org. You could also try state associations for referrals.

- American Academy of Medical Acupuncture. Association of physicians who perform acupuncture; www.medicalacupuncture.org

- American Chiropractic Association. National association of chiropractors; www.amerchiro.org. Or try state associations for referrals.

- National Center for Homeopathy. Directory of licensed practitioners who use homeopathy; www.healthy.net/nch

- American Psychological Association. National association of psychologists, plus great information about mental health; www.apa.org

- American Psychiatric Association. National association of psychiatrists; with some information for consumers; www.psych.org

Specialized Medical Tests

These are the specialized tests mentioned in chapter 5:

- **Food sensitivities, other allergies:** Blood testing of IgG antibodies for food sensitivities. Blood can also be tested for allergies to potential airborne allergens, such as pollen or mold.

- **Stool:** Assesses beneficial and pathogenic microbes, including yeast, parasites, and bacteria, and other markers of digestion, absorption, and intestinal health.

- **Amino acids:** Measures amino acid levels, and also produces nutritional and metabolic information.

- **Organic acids:** Analyzes urine for by-products of pathogenic intestinal microbes, as well as some markers for vitamins, neurotransmitter metabolites, and energy metabolism.

- **Essential fatty acids:** Evaluates your levels of omega-3 and omega-6 fatty acids, and the metabolic pathways associated with them.

- **Minerals:** Various tests assess mineral levels in blood, urine, or hair, both those that are too high (toxic) and those that are too low (nutritionally deficient).

- **Salivary hormones:** Analyzes saliva for cortisol, DHEA, estrogen, progesterone, and melatonin; especially useful for evaluating levels of "free" (available and active) hormones. Some labs do an extended test of ovarian hormones across the menstrual cycle.

- **Estrogen metabolites:** Assesses markers of estrogen metabolism that may be associated with disease.

- **Thyroid:** Twenty-four-hour urine test for thyroid that measures the levels of this hormone that are "free."

- **Immune markers:** Detailed assessment of cells in your immune system.

Labs use test kits that can be sent back to them overnight from anywhere in the United States, so the location of a lab should not be a concern. But in most cases, you'll need a licensed health professional to order and interpret these tests. Your doctor could order a test, but if he or she is unfamiliar with it or otherwise disinclined to order it, please see appendix E for how to locate an appropriate, licensed practitioner; you could also contact the labs below and ask them for a referral to a professional in your area who uses their tests.

Medical Laboratories

There are hundreds of medical laboratories around the country. We list here those that do the specialized tests described above. We are familiar with these labs, but there are others that also do specialized testing, and your practitioner may prefer to use a lab other than the ones in the following list.

GREAT SMOKIES DIAGNOSTIC LABORATORY
(800) 542-3526
63 Zillicoa Street
Ashville, NC 28801
www.gsdl.com

> *Excellent full-spectrum, "functional medicine" laboratory; very good interpreta-tion and clinical support for providers. This may make it easier for your practi-tioner to use tests with which he or she is not that familiar.*

THE GREAT PLAINS LABORATORY
(888) 347-2781
The Great Plains Laboratory
11813 West 77th
Lenexa, KS 66214
www.greatplainslaboratory.com

> *Great Plains developed the organic acid test in its present form. This test was ini-tially used with autistic children, but it can be quite informative for adults with compromised health.*

AERON LIFE CYCLES
(800) 631-7900
933 Davis Street, Suite 310
San Leandro, CA 94577
www.aeron.com

> *Excellent hormonal assessment; highly experienced with saliva testing.*

ZRT LABORATORY
(530) 466-2445
1815 NW 169th Place, Suite 5050
Beaverton, OR 97006
www.salivatest.com

> *Salivary hormone assessment.*

DOCTOR'S DATA
(800) 323-2784
3755 Illinois Avenue
St. Charles, IL 60174-2420
www.doctorsdata.com

> *Focuses on mineral assessment, but also does stool and other metabolic tests.*

MERIDIAN VALLEY LABORATORY
(253) 859-8700
515 West Harrison Street, Suite 9
Kent, WA 98032
www.meridianvalleylab.com
> *Offers a wide spectrum of testing.*

METAMETRIX
(800) 221-4640
5000 Peachtree Ind. Blvd.
Norcross, GA 30071
www.metametrix.com
> *Full range of tests with good support.*

AAL REFERENCE LABORATORIES
(800) 522-2611
1715 Wilshire, Suite 715
Santa Ana, CA 92705
www.antibodyassay.com
> *Innovative testing of the immune and endocrine system. Will not give referrals to local professionals who use their tests.*

PARASITOLOGY CENTER
(480) 777-1078
903 South Rural Road
Tempe, AZ 85281
www.parasitetesting.com
> *Specializes in detection of parasites.*

Sources for Supplements and Herbs

Supplements and herbal products are available at our Web site, www.nurturemom.com, which also offers new information about nurturing mothers and families, and links to other, high-quality Web sites.

Additionally, most of the supplements we've discussed are available at good health food stores, which may carry Chinese herbal formulas as well. Chinese formulas will also be available from an acupuncturist and at stores specializing in

Chinese herbs (which can be found in most large cities), or they may be purchased from:

SHEN NONG HERBS
(510) 849-0290
1600 Shattuck Avenue, Suite 125
Berkeley, CA 94709
E-mail: shennong@pacbell.net

Natural hormone products are available at:

TRANSITIONS FOR HEALTH, INC.
(800) 888-6814
621 SW Alder, Suite 900
Portland, OR 97205

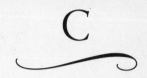

A Safe Room in Your Mind

*T*HIS EXERCISE SHOULD TAKE about ten to thirty minutes, depending on how deeply you get into it, so try to do it when you won't be interrupted. You can use it for expressing your feelings, thoughts, and desires. If you are getting more upset, not less, please immediately stop the exercise and do something calming and soothing.

The Exercise

Find a comfortable place to sit or lie down, and close your eyes. Take a minute or more to relax your body.

Visualize a completely safe room, either one that is familiar or one from your imagination. Make it as real as possible by visualizing the details, such as thick walls, a strong door, or a force field around the entire room. Keep deepening your sense of the utter safety of this room. You are completely in charge of it. Only you can decide what can come in. You have total control over what happens in the room, and you can decide at any time to send something back out.

Experiment with bringing a safe, supportive person into the room, perhaps someone you know or an imagined being such as an angel of light. See if that helps you feel even safer and stronger. But do not yet bring in anyone that you feel uncomfortable with, including the person your feelings may be directed at.

When you feel ready, let yourself experience some of the feelings you want to release. Keep remembering that you are utterly safe and secure, that you have complete control over everything that happens in your safe room, and that you can turn the feelings up or down as you choose.

Then express your feelings in whatever way works for you. You could imagine saying them softly, firmly, or loudly, or in a hurt, anxious, sad, or angry tone. You can scream your head off if you like within the safe room in your mind. You can also imagine expressing emotion symbolically through pounding on the floor, tearing things apart, breathing fire, and so on.

Perhaps that alone will feel complete. If not, you could bring the person(s) that your feelings may be related to into your safe room. Remind yourself that you have complete control within this space, and then imagine the person in the room with you. Make him or her as real in your mind as you are comfortable with. Either ask the person for a willingness to hear your feelings and imagine receiving it, or skip that step and just start communicating. You can imagine the other person acting in a loving way, or being very small, immobilized, or mute. You can vent your feelings through physical contact, such as by hugging the person tightly, hitting, or kicking; but stay focused on your purpose of releasing feelings rather than taking pleasure in hurting another person. When you feel a sense of completion or that you need to move on, wrap up your communications to the person. See if there is anything left to express, especially deeper, more vulnerable feelings or wants.

You can repeat this process with other people or communicate with several people at once. You can vary the format and immediately bring individuals into your safe room without first venting on your own. And you can have the supportive beings in your room say things to you or to the other person. See if you can find an intuitive wisdom inside that knows what will be most valuable for you to do, and also what your limits are.

You can completely let yourself go in your safe room. But there is a fine line between releasing an emotion and intensifying it. If you find that your feelings are getting stronger rather than dissipating, shift to a different mode within the exercise. Try expressing them more gently, sincerely, vulnerably. Or reach for the softer feelings under the harsher ones. Be gentle with yourself, especially if you have had any seriously distressing or traumatizing experiences. You can do this exercise again and again, if necessary, emptying the bucket of painful feelings one ladle full at a time.

When you are done, you could imagine that the other person has really heard, really received what you had to say. You can ask the person questions, and listen to what he or she says. Or you can have the person say things that you need to hear. If you like, acknowledge the person for being with you. Then send him or her out of your safe room.

Complete the exercise by seeing if there is anything else you would like to communicate, either into your safe room or to any supportive beings that are with you. Thank the supportive beings for their presence, and see if there is anything they have to say to you. Acknowledge yourself for making an effort and being brave. Notice how you feel. Relax even more deeply and let any uncomfortable feelings drain out of you. Focus on positive feelings and let them grow and fill you. End the exercise by saying a kind thought for yourself or brief prayer. Then recall the actual room you are in, rub your hands on your thighs and your feet on the floor, and open your eyes.

After the Exercise

Take a few minutes to let the experience settle before getting up and going about your day. You might like to do something relaxing at first, such as taking a shower.

Mother's Suggested Daily Values (MSDVs)

Nutrient	Daily Values (DV's)			MSDV's	Intensive Daily Dose (IDD)	Comments
	Standard	*Pregnant*	*Lactating*			
Vitamin A*	2300 IU	2500 IU	4290 IU	5000 IU	50,000 IU only for a few days	Do not exceed 5000 IU of Vitamin A if you are nursing, pregnant, or for several months before pregnancy
Vitamin B1 (Thiamine)	1.1 mg	1.4 mg	1.4 mg	30–50 mg	50–500 mg	
Vitamine B2 (Riboflavin)	1.1 mg	1.4 mg	1.6 mg	30–50 mg	50–500 mg	
Vitamin B3 (Niacin)	14 mg	18 mg	17 mg	30–100 mg		At higher dosages, use niacin-amide to avoid flushing.
Vitamin B5 (Pantothenic acid)	5 mg	6 mg	7 mg	50–100 mg	500–1000 mg	
Vitamin B6	1.3 mg	1.9 mg	2.0 mg	50 mg	100 mg of pyridoxine or 50 mg of P-5-P	P-5-P = pyridoxal-5-phosphate
Vitamin B12 (Cobalamine)	2.4 mcg	2.6 mcg	2.8 mcg	200 mcg	2000 mcg; take sublingually	
Folic Acid	400 mcg	600 mcg	500 mcg	800 mcg; 1200 mcg P		
Vitamin C	75 mg	85 mg	120 mg	1000–3000 mg	5000 mg up to bowel tolerance	Divide into 2–3 doses taken over the course of the day.
Vitamin D*	200 IU	200 IU	200 IU	400–600 IU		
Vitamin E*	22 IU	22 IU	28 IU	200–400 IU	800 IU	Try to get a supplement that has a variety of (e.g. "mixed") tocopherols and tocotrienois.
Vitamin K	90 mcg	90 mcg	90 mcg	75–150 mcg		
PABA				50 mg		
Biotin	30 mcg	30 mcg	35 mcg	500 mcg		
Choline	425 mg	450 mg	550 mg	500 mg		
Inositol				500 mg; 250 mg P/L		

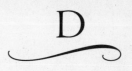

Nutrient	Daily Values (DV's)**			MSDV's	Intensive Daily Dose (IDD)	Comments
	Standard	Pregnant	Lactating			
Betacarotene				20,000 IU	100,000 IU	Consume as mixed carotenes in your foods,
Bioflavinoids				500 mg		Or as high quality supplements.
Coenzyme Q				60–100 mg		
Calcium	1000 mg	1000 mg	1000 mg	1200 mg; 1600 mg P/L		Try to get calcium citrate, malate, or hydroxyapatite.
Chromium	25 mcg	30 mcg	45 mg	400 mcg		Try to get chromium picolinate.
Copper	0.9 mg	1.0 mg	1.3 mg	2–3 mg	1 mg per 15 mg of zinc	
Iodine	150 mcg	220 mcg	290 mcg	300–400 mcg		
Iron	18 mg	27 mg	9 mg	18–30 mg; 60 mg P/L	Up to 60 mg if iron deficient on lab test	Best from organic liver; or take supplements of ferrous glycinate, succinate, or fumerate.
Manganese	1.8 mg	2.0 mg	2.6 mg	15 mg		
Magnesium	320 mg	360 mg	320 mg	500 mg	800–1000 mg (decrease if diarrhhea occurs)	Try to get magnesium citrate, malate, or glycinate; magnesium glycinate helps avoid diarrhea.
Molybdenum	45 mcg	50 mcg	50 mcg	500 mcg		
Potassium				2–5 grams from food		This amount from supplements would be dangerous.
Selenium	55 mcg	60 mcg	70 mcg	200 mcg	400 mcg	
Zinc	8 mg	11 mg	12 mg	30 mg	50 mg	
Omega 3 oils:						
As fish oil containing approximately 25% DHA				1000 mg	2000–4000 mg	
As flax oil				1 tablespoon	2 tablespoons	

NOTES: P = pregnant, L = lactating, P/L = both pregnant and lactating; IU = International Unit, mg = milligram, mcg = microgram
Blank DV's indicate no established level. Some minerals have their best forms suggested.

*For convenience, these daily values have been converted to International Units (IU's).

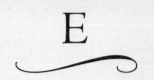

The Insider's Guide: Finding the Right Practitioners and Procedures for Your Unique Health Care Needs

THE PROSPECT OF GOING OUT and finding good care for your health problems can seem pretty overwhelming, especially if you are in the throes of DMS. It can be so tempting to listen to one person who gives you hope, close your eyes, and jump. But the days of the all-knowing doctor who had the time to get to know you thoroughly, while staying current in the latest research on every single modality within the spectrum of care, are long gone, if they ever existed at all. Your health will do best over the long run if you keep your own counsel while working with several good professionals, check out different approaches and weigh their evidence carefully, try cautious experiments, and set your course based on your own experience.

So, how should you go about choosing practitioners and approaches that are right for you? Let's begin with four key points that will help ensure that you're getting the most nurturing and effective care.

Four Guidelines for Navigating Within the Spectrum of Care

1. Do no harm. The more sensitive your body has become, the more you ought to start treatments at low levels, intensify them slowly (if at all), and consider modalities that have the least likelihood of side effects (such as Energetic or Dietary). On the other hand, you need to avoid the harm of using a weak or worthless intervention; this is the principle risk of alternative approaches, and one of the reasons why a physician should *always* be a member of your health care team. For example, Jan pursued an herbal treatment for her digestive parasites for six months that allowed the pathogens to become more entrenched; in retrospect, she should have immediately bombed them with antibiotics. We think you should routinely get a good assessment within the framework of Western medicine to make sure you aren't overlooking a health condition that's more serious than depletion.

You should also avoid the harm of treating symptoms while overlooking root causes. For example, many women have recurrent vaginal yeast infections that they treat topically—time after time—without ever addressing the underlying conditions that predispose them to these infections, such as a weakness in their immune system. The root causes of an illness commonly include stress and lifestyle factors (such as not exercising, or abusing alcohol), and you can improve these with the methods discussed in parts 2 and 3 of this book. A general imbalance or weakness in one or more systems of the body is frequently another fundamental source of illness—especially subclinical, chronic conditions—and these are often particularly helped by alternative approaches.

2. Use methods with good evidence. You'll often hear about some new treatment that's being trumpeted loudly—or seemingly debunked. It *might* benefit you (or not, if it's been dunked in debunking), but how do you know what's really true? With the Internet, you can look up the research on health topics by going to Pub Med (www4.ncbi.nlm.nih.gov/PubMed/), or to other sources given in appendix B for more specialized studies on nutrition or complementary medicine.

The chance that something will work for you increases as the evidence for it comes from sources higher up on this list:

- Careful meta-analyses of dozens or hundreds of studies
- Multiple, high-quality studies that converge in their findings
- One double-blind, randomized study with a control group
- One so-so study
- A professional's clinical experience with many patients
- Preliminary indications an intervention might help based on an understanding of the workings of the body
- Anecdotes about one person's response to an intervention

Nonetheless, much medical information today—particularly about innovative or alternative interventions—comes from sources below the top two above.* For ex-

> In God we trust.
> All others must
> have data.
>
> —*Dr. Yank Coble*

---

*Unless otherwise stated (e.g., "we've seen . . ."), the interventions we suggest are usually based on at least one study.

ample, the majority of the practices used day to day in Western medicine have not yet been evaluated in multiple, high-quality studies. And alternative treatments have generally received even less research (though European studies are often quite sophisticated), since most of them cannot be patented and thus pay back the costs of careful studies; this means that their benefit to you is more uncertain, but it does not mean there is certainly no benefit: as the saying goes, absence of evidence is not evidence of absence.

Sometimes the evidence for or against some intervention will be very solid. But often it will be more uncertain, especially when you consider more innovative or less-studied methods.* There's really no way around it: we all have to make decisions about our health care in which we weigh the odds of the potential benefits and costs. If the risks of an intervention are low—such as with most of the alternative modalities in the spectrum of care—then it may well be worth trying even when the evidence for its benefit is mixed, but if the risks are relatively high, then you should have stronger indications that it's likely to help.

3. *Work with the right people.* It's important to look for people who stay within their own area of knowledge while respecting the work of other professionals within the spectrum of care.† For example, few holistic practitioners have a deep understanding of the pharmacology of Western medicine, yet some might tell you not to take a prescription drug. Similarly, few physicians are trained in nutritional work, yet some might tell you to throw away your supplements. Whether it's an alternative practitioner or an M.D., watch out for arrogance, close-mindedness, or zealotry. In particular, a warning sign is when someone tries to talk you out of doing a certain test; it's one thing to recommend against an *intervention*, but we see little sense in recommending against *gathering information* that has a good chance of making your health care more focused and effective.

Fundamentally, you have options in your health care providers, and if you do not get the support and rational open-mindedness you need, look for other pro-

---

*For example, a methodological problem often occurs in those studies on nutrients that do not find a significant benefit, because many of these do not screen their subjects to see if there is a nutritional deficiency in the first place. If numerous participants already have high levels of the nutrient, they will usually get little advantage from consuming more—watering down the *average* benefit and thus perhaps making it appear that the nutrient has little to offer, when in fact it may have considerably helped those subjects who began the study with low levels. It would be like doing a study on Prozac in which a substantial fraction of the participants already were receiving moderate doses: the average impact of the drug would appear reduced.

†Unfortunately, many people have little choice about their health care professionals, usually for financial reasons. On the other hand, some managed care organizations are starting to include alternative methods, and many alternative care providers are relatively inexpensive. You can also educate yourself free of charge about the new options in health care using books or Internet access from your local library.

fessionals. Many people, including us, use several practitioners for different things. Perhaps an HMO doctor handles your annual physical exam or any urgent care, while other licensed individuals have primary responsibility for helping you with chronic, subclinical conditions such as DMS.

So who can help you to replenish your body and balance its systems? Many professionals trained in Western medicine can, including physicians (M.D.s), osteopaths* (D.O.s), nurse practitioners (N.P.s), and physician's assistants (P.A.s)—the last two work under a doctor's supervision. But ask about their experience with nutritional or functional medicine, since these subjects were probably not studied in depth in their formal training.

More often than not, though, you'll have to look to other licensed professionals for many of the methods you can use to reverse depletion. Acupuncturists (L.Ac.s) are sometimes knowledgeable about biochemistry and nutrition from the perspective of Western science, in addition to their expertise in a very different model. Many chiropractors (D.C.s) have a strong background in nutrition. Finally, some states have a license for Naturopathic Doctors (N.D.s), who receive training in both Western medicine (including pharmacology) and alternative methods (especially nutrition and herbs); if your state has such a license, an N.D. may be most able to offer the integrated approach we generally suggest.

If you are looking for a practitioner, you could start by asking your friends for referrals; the key words that flag licensed professionals who use an integrated approach include *complementary, nutritional, functional,* or *holistic* medicine. Your doctor or your child's pediatrician may be able to give you a referral even if he or she doesn't practice that sort of medicine. Or you could call the referral line for the national or county association of the profession you'd like to work with; that phone number will usually be shown prominently in the section of the Yellow Pages devoted to that profession (e.g., physician, naturopath, acupuncturist, chiropractor). Some alternative health care practitioners advertise in local newspapers or directories, particularly those that lean toward the holistic or progressive end of the spectrum.

4. Revise the approach based on your own results. A method with good research support could be useless for you or have overwhelming side effects; alternately, studies might be unable to find a statistically significant benefit for some intervention, but it works wonders for *you*.† Methods that were once helpful may stop

---

*These are doctors who have completed medical school as well as received specialized training in the musculoskeletal system.

†Occasionally this could be due to the "placebo effect," but that actually appears quite small in research studies, and it seems rare in clinical practice; you can usually tell if some intervention has helped you.

working, and others that used to do nothing for you could suddenly start making a real difference. Or you may get no benefit at first from a supplement or herb (these often take up to eight weeks to reveal their full effects), which over time becomes clearly helpful. In all these cases, your personal experience should be your ultimate guide as you tailor your care to your own individual needs.

Getting a Good Assessment

The foundation of effective health care is good assessment. There are many good tests available that can help your health care provider target specific imbalances in your body. It's like casting a net into the sea; if the mesh is too coarse or dropped in just one place, you may not catch the important fish you are looking for. Similarly, you need an assessment that is both *fine-grained* and *comprehensive*.

Who Does the Assessment

An assessment is only as good as the professionals who do it. There is something about being a mother that inclines some practitioners to offer reassurances instead of information, and then send you on your way. In addition to this "motherism," we know many women who have encountered a health professional who:

- Did not want to order tests that took time to interpret or cost money
- Held the patronizing belief that "all that information will just confuse you"
- Dismissed findings that did not fit his or her assumptions
- Did not try to figure out complex results
- Thought low results were just fine as long as they were within the broad, "normal range"

It's best to work with people who respect your intelligence, consider health in a comprehensive and holistic framework, actually try to figure out puzzling results, and explain their thinking. Persist in getting your questions answered and the help you need, or find another professional. Standing up to the health care system can feel daunting on a good day. It may help to have your partner or a friend come along for support.

Various health care providers might manage different aspects of your assessment. If several people are involved, one person, typically a physician, should integrate the findings into a coherent picture. A family doctor or gynecologist may be the right person to do this, or a specialist in women's health, but we suggest that

If you drag a net with a two-inch mesh through the sea, you will conclude there is no such thing as a fish that is shorter than two inches.

—*Arthur Eddington, Ph.D.*

you try to work with someone who is knowledgeable about good nutrition and optimizing gastrointestinal function, which are key to reversing depletion.

Medical labs vary in their quality, particularly if you are running a specialized test. Well-regarded labs are listed in appendix B, and your practitioners may know of others. You could ask them to use a particular lab, if you like. (Or you can work in the other direction by asking the lab you want for referrals to professionals nearby.)

Making Sense of the Findings

Here's a quick guide to assessment interpretation that you can use for your child's health as well as your own.

Avoiding mistakes. An assessment can miss the boat in two ways. *A false-positive* error occurs when it looks like there's a problem but there actually is not, which can lead to unnecessary treatments with potentially harmful side effects. A *false-negative* error happens when no problem is found but there actually is one, so undiagnosed conditions then go untreated. Depending on the test or medical laboratory, these errors can be surprisingly common. It is wise to ask practitioners about their estimates of the false-positive and false-negative rates in the tests they use. If they resent your question, do not understand it, or do not know how to get some kind of answer, that is a yellow flag about their support for you or their expertise.

Keeping tests in perspective. Laboratory tests are only part of a total assessment. You have a right to speak up if a professional dismisses your concerns and palpable symptoms because of test results that do not definitively indicate a problem. You also have a right to probe the thinking of your practitioner—who, frankly, has probably not had much time to analyze your testing—or ask questions about what the findings mean, like:

- What do these low numbers mean? How about these high numbers?

- Why should I worry about how much magnesium I have?

- What could be the relationship between X and Y (e.g., low tryptophan and depressed mood, low thyroid and achy joints)?

- Why are my minerals so low if I've been taking supplements?

Link current tests to your health history. Health professionals today usually have little time to put current findings in context. Keep a copy of your previous lab reports and bring them to your appointments. Then you can compare current test results to past ones and ask the professional to explain what is getting better, or worse, and *why.*

Compared to what? Many test results are interpreted in terms of where you stand within the *range* of a comparison group. For example, a five-year-old who can read five hundred words would be high within the range of other children her age, but a sixteen-year-old who can read only five hundred words would have a low score among others her age. The group your results are compared to is crucial to a correct understanding of your health status. If the range is skewed incorrectly in one direction or another, then a truly problematic test result may be erroneously considered "normal," which would be a false-negative finding. Therefore, try to ask about the sources of the "reference range" your lab uses. If your health professional or lab does not understand your question, dismisses it, or cannot track down an answer, that's a yellow flag.

In particular, we strongly suggest that you scrutinize so-called low-normal* results, especially of nutrients. The "normal range" is typically set between the 2.5 to 97.5 percentiles—based on the (questionable) assumption that 95 percent of the population is perfectly healthy. If your test results fall close to the high or low end of the "normal range," they will be ignored more often than not. We think that's misguided for several reasons. First, the population used for the reference range may not be especially healthy in the first place! For example, if your iron levels were at the twentieth percentile of women your age, that might seem acceptable until you consider that the majority of women are thought to be at least a little anemic. Second, low-normal conditions matter in their own right. For example, if your child's academic test scores were in the lower fifth of his or her class but above the 3rd percentile, how would you feel if a teacher told you everything was fine? Finally, mothers need good reserves in their bodies to cope with future stresses, so they should aim for the high-normal end of the range.

⌐

With these tools, you should be ready to go out in search of the care that you— that all of us—truly deserve. Because it probably took many months for your body to become depleted, it may also take some time to start feeling the effects of treatment. But with patience and a willingness to change course when something is obviously not working, over time you *will* begin to feel better. Please don't give up and decide to accept depletion as normal. You ought to feel good in your body and full of the energy you'll need for this long and lovely journey of motherhood.

---

*Occasionally, high—rather than low—is "bad"; for example, high-normal thyroid stimulating hormone (TSH) may indicate that you have low thyroid. The points in this paragraph would still apply, but with the percentiles reversed.

Page numbers in *italics* refer to tables and figures.

(The authors have identified sources of quotations as completely as possible. Additional information will be added to future printings.)   *Introduction* "Thy Lord" Koran 17:13.   *Chapter 1* "A baby" Mark Twain, letter to Annie Webster (September 1, 1876); "Improvements" Gladys Block and Barbara Adams, "Vitamin and mineral status of women of childbearing potential," *Annals of the New York Academy of Sciences* 678 (March 15, 1993): 251; "Compared to 1969" President's Council of Economic Advisors, quoted in U.S. Department of Labor, *Futurework* (1999): 36; "Evidence" Rosalind C. Barnett and Grace K. Baruch, "Women's involvement in multiple roles and psychological distress," *Journal of Personality and Social Psychology* 49 (July 1985): 137; "For many couples" Alison Fearnley Shapiro, John M. Gottman, and Sybil Carrere, "The baby and the marriage: identifying factors that buffer against decline in marital satisfaction after the first baby arrives," *Journal of Family Psychology* 14(1) (March 2000): 59.   *Chapter 2* "Helmer: First and foremost" Henrik Ibsen, *A Doll's House* (1879), act III; "When you are a mother" Sophia Loren, quoted in *For a Mother with Love* (Bloomington, MN: Garborg's Heart 'n Home, n.d.); "The quickest way" Lane Olinghouse, quoted in *A Mother's Journal: A Keepsake for Thoughts and Dreams* (Philadelphia: Running Press, 1985); "I see most women's spirits" Shoshana Bennett, founder, Postpartum Assistance for Mothers, personal communication, 2000; "There is no pleasure" Mary Little, quoted in *For a Mother with Love;* "I don't think" Christina Feldman, in *Spirit Rock Meditation Center Newsletter* (February–August 1998).   *Chapter 3* "Insanity" Sam Levenson, quoted in Harris, *The Pregnancy Journal;* "Parents are often so busy" Marceline Cox, quoted in Harris, *The Pregnancy Journal;* "It will be gone" Dorothy Evslin, quoted in *A Mother's Journal;* "We are, perhaps, uniquely" Lewis Thomas, "The Youngest and Brightest Thing Around," in *The Medusa and the Snail: More Notes of a Biology Watcher* (1979); "Motherhood brings" Marguerite Kelly and Ella Parsons, quoted in *A Mother's Journal.*   *Chapter 4* "Health is a state" Platform for Action of the Fourth World Conference on Women, Beijing, September 1995, quoted in C. S. Weisman, "Changing definitions of women's health: implications for health care and policy," *Maternal and Child Health Journal* 1,3 (1997): 183; "There never was a child" Ralph Waldo Emerson, quoted in *A Mother's Journal;* "I often feel" Simone Bloom, quoted in *A Mother's Journal;* "I can resist" Oscar Wilde, *Lady Windemere's Fan* (1892), act I; "Tobacco use" Centers for Disease Control and Prevention, quoted in R. Weissman, "Women and tobacco," *The Network News* of the Women's Health Network (March–April 2001): 1; "Alcoholism" Barry Zuckerman, "Women's health: key to a two-generational approach to child health and development, *Zero to Three* 18,5 (April–May 1998): 5–9; "At the end of a meal" Traditional.   *Chapter 5* "A Brief History" Internet posting, quoted in *The Family Therapy Networker* (May–June 2000): 19; "The road to health" Chip Watkins, personal communication, 2001.   *Chapter 6* "It is an amazing . . . thing" Source not found; "The test" George Bernard Shaw, *The Philanderer* (1893), act II; "Kind words" Mother Teresa, quoted in *For a Mother with Love.*   *Chapter 7* "Before I got married" Robert Carr, Lord Rochester (c.1590–1645), quoted in *A Mother's Journal;* "If evolution works" Ed Dussault, quoted in *A Mother's Journal;* "The real test" Margaret Mead, author's paraphrase (source not found); "A rich child" Danish proverb, quoted in *A Mother's Journal.*   *Chapter 8* "We are too busy" Anonymous mother, personal communication, 2000; "Men fall in love" Oscar Wilde (attributed; source not found); "Helpful husbands" Anonymous mother, personal communication, 2000.   *Chapter 9* "The work world" Marcia Killien, "Childbearing choices of professional women," in *Health Care for Women International* 8(2–3) (1987): 121–31.   *Appendices* "If you drag a net" Rupert Sheldrake, Ph.D., paraphrasing physicist Sir Arthur Eddington (1882–1944), in *Discover* magazine (August 200): 65; "In God we trust" Yank Coble, quoted in *Time* magazine, n.d.